Pancreatic Cancer

Shubham Pant

Editor

Pancreatic Cancer

Current Therapeutics and Future Directions

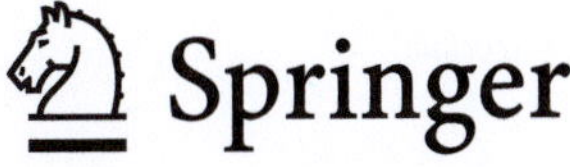

Editor
Shubham Pant
GI Medical Oncology
The University of Texas MD Anderson Canc
Houston, TX, USA

ISBN 978-3-031-38625-1   ISBN 978-3-031-38623-7   (eBook)
https://doi.org/10.1007/978-3-031-38623-7

This Springer imprint is published by the registered company Springer Nature Switzerland AG
The registered company address is: Gewerbestrasse 11, 6330 Cham, Switzerland

Paper in this product is recyclable

Introduction

Pancreatic cancer is the third most common cause of cancer mortality in the United States and is projected to become the second leading cause of cancer-related death in the coming years. Over the past decade, therapy for pancreatic cancer has undergone various advances with the advent of multiagent chemotherapy. In patients with resectable disease, adjuvant chemotherapy with 5-fluorouracil, leucovorin, irinotecan, and oxaliplatin (FOLFIRINOX) demonstrated median overall survival of 54 months. Patients who present with borderline resectable and locally advanced disease are candidates for chemotherapy, radiation therapy, and/or surgery. However, the optimal therapy regimen, length of treatment, and type of radiation (short or long course) are still to be determined.

For patients with advanced disease though, combination chemotherapies only provide modest improvement in overall survival of a few months. This contrasts with many other tumor types, such as breast and lung cancer in which novel therapies have enabled major improvements in survival durations.

Pancreatic cancer is challenging in that it is a complex disease characterized by a dense fibrotic stroma and an immunosuppressive tumor microenvironment, along with low neoantigen burden, which inhibit infiltration and recognition by effector T cells. Development and progression of tumor is further promoted by an abundance of tumor-associated macrophages and myeloid-derived suppressor cells. This overall regulatory immune population of cells creates a "cold," non-immunogenic tumor that is resistant to immunotherapies including checkpoint inhibitors.

Until recently, there were no predictive biomarkers to personalize selection of targeted or biologic therapies as a part of standard of care treatment. However, in the last few years, there has been substantial progress in our understanding of the role of mutations in the pathogenesis of diseases, leading to an increased adoption of germline and next-generation sequencing to identify mutations and fusions to optimize selection of therapies and select patients for clinical trials of targeted agents.

On account of these significant challenges, there lies a need to review existing therapeutics and shed light on future directions to improve outcomes in this devastating disease. This book will provide a comprehensive, global overview on current therapies for pancreatic cancer and focus on the "Next" in drug development including molecularly targeted therapy and efforts at "Drugging the Undruggable": the KRAS mutation. It will also address efforts at targeting the inhospitable stroma to improve drug delivery to the tumor cells and challenges and opportunities in incorporating ct DNA (liquid biopsies) in the care of patients and updates on immunotherapy in pancreatic cancer. Importantly we will also discuss updates in supportive care, management of pain, nutrition, and the importance of physical exercise in patients undergoing therapy for this disease.

Shubham Pant

Contents

Resectable Pancreatic Cancer: Neoadjuvant and Adjuvant Therapy

Jacob L. van Dam and Bas Groot Koerkamp

Introduction

Pancreatic ductal adenocarcinoma (PDAC) is a highly lethal malignancy with rising incidence. In Europe and the United States, the 5-year overall survival (OS) after diagnosis is 7–10% [1, 2]. PDAC is projected to become the second leading cause of cancer death in 2030 [3]. Contrary to other cancer types, survival outcomes for PDAC have improved little in the past decades [4].

Non-metastatic, localized PDAC is generally classified according to the extent of vascular involvement on cross-sectional imaging. Categories include resectable, borderline resectable, and locally advanced disease. In the 10–20% of patients that present with resectable disease, upfront surgery is the standard of care [5, 6]. Despite optimal surgery, recurrence rates are high. Apparently, most patients with resectable PDAC have systemic disease at diagnosis [7].

In an effort to improve outcomes, adjuvant therapy has been developed, and its use is supported by level 1 evidence from multiple randomized controlled trials (RCTs). The main problem with adjuvant therapy is that up to half of patients are unable to receive it as result of complications from surgery with clinical deterioration and early recurrence. Therefore, there is a high interest in in the use of neoadjuvant therapy (i.e., before surgery) and perioperative therapy (i.e., both neoadjuvant and adjuvant) to improve outcomes.

J. L. van Dam · B. Groot Koerkamp (✉)
Department of Surgery, Erasmus MC Cancer Institute, Rotterdam, The Netherlands
e-mail: j.l.vandam@erasmusmc.nl; b.grootkoerkamp@erasmusmc.nl

S. Pant (ed.), *Pancreatic Cancer*, https://doi.org/10.1007/978-3-031-38623-7_1

Staging Resectable Pancreatic Cancer

Staging of localized PDAC is historically based on the extent of arterial and venous tumor contact as visible on cross-sectional imaging. In most staging systems, resectable PDAC is defined as the absence of any arterial contact and no or limited venous contact (Table 1.1) [5, 8–10]. The National Comprehensive Cancer Network (NCCN) definition is most permissible as it allows up to 180° of venous contact.

In recent years, there is increasing interest in expanding the anatomy-based staging of localized PDAC with inclusion of biological and conditional factors [11]. For example, several studies have demonstrated that patients with elevated carbohydrate antigen (CA) 19-9 above 500 or 1000 have decreased survival that is similar to patients with borderline resectable disease [12–14]. Similarly, patients with a low performance status have worse survival [12, 14].

The NCCN and American Society of Clinical Oncology (ASCO) guidelines both advice to include CA 19-9 in the decision making between upfront surgery or neoadjuvant therapy in patients with resectable disease [5, 6]. The NCCN guideline states to consider neoadjuvant therapy particularly in patients with high-risk features, including a "markedly elevated CA 19-9." The ASCO guideline recommends upfront surgery only if patients have a CA 19-9 level "suggestive of potentially curable disease." Both guidelines do not provide a precise cut-off level for CA 19-9 above which neoadjuvant therapy is recommended.

Table 1.1 Definitions of resectable PDAC at diagnosis

	NCCN	AHPBA/SSAT/SSO	MD Anderson	DPCG
Arterial	No arterial contact	No arterial contact	No arterial contact	No arterial contact
Venous	No tumor contact with the SMV or PV or ≤180° contact without vein contour irregularity	No SMV or PV abutment, distortion, tumor thrombus, or venous encasement	Patent SMV/PV	No tumor contact with the SMV or PV or ≤90° contact

NCCN National Comprehensive Cancer Network, *AHPBA/SSAT/SSO* Americas Hepato-Pancreato-Biliary Association/Society of Surgical Oncology/Society for Surgery of the Alimentary Tract, *DPCG* Dutch Pancreatic Cancer Group, *SMV* superior mesenteric vein, *PV* portal vein

Adjuvant Therapy for Resected Pancreatic Cancer

Although earlier trials were performed [15–18], the first RCTs that definitively demonstrated chemotherapy after resection could improve survival were the ESPAC-1 and CONKO-001 trials [19, 20]. Key clinical trials of adjuvant therapy are discussed below and summarized in Table 1.2.

Trials of Adjuvant Chemotherapy

The **ESPAC-1** trial was a multicenter trial in 11 European countries that investigated 5-fluorouracil (5-FU) with folinic acid (FA) chemotherapy and chemoradiotherapy (20 Gray with 5-FU). Between 1994 and 2000, patients were randomized to four arms: 69 to observation, 73 patients to chemoradiotherapy alone, 75 to chemotherapy alone, and 72 patients to both chemoradiotherapy and chemotherapy [19]. After a median follow-up of 47 months, the median OS was 16.9 months with observation, 13.9 months with chemoradiotherapy alone, 21.6 months with chemotherapy alone, and 19.9 months with chemoradiotherapy and chemotherapy. When the 142 patients who received chemotherapy (with or without chemoradiotherapy) were compared with the 147 patient who did not (with or without chemoradiotherapy), adjuvant 5-FU/FA chemotherapy was associated with a superior median OS of 20.1 versus 15.5 months (hazard ratio [HR] 0.71, 95% CI 0.55–0.92, $p = 0.009$).

The **CONKO-001** trial randomized 368 patients to 6 cycles of adjuvant gemcitabine or to observation in 88 centers in Germany and Austria [20]. After a median follow-up of 53 months, the trial did show an improvement in median disease free survival (13.4 vs. 6.9 months, $p < 0.001$), but did not demonstrate a statistically significant OS benefit (22.1 vs. 20.2 months, $p < 0.06$) [21]. After a longer follow-up of 136 months, however, adjuvant gemcitabine was associated with superior OS (HR 0.76, 95% CI 0.61–0.95, $p = 0.01$). The 5-year OS was 20.7% in the gemcitabine group and 10.4% in the observation group.

The Japanese **JSAP-02** trial had a similar design as the CONKO-001 as it compared adjuvant gemcitabine with observation, but the adjuvant treatment duration was three rather than six cycles. Between 2002 and 2005, 118 patients were randomized in 10 centers. The primary outcome of disease-free survival was significantly improved (11.4 vs. 5.0 months, HR 0.60, 95% CI 0.40–0.89, $p = 0.01$), but a difference in OS could not be demonstrated (22.3 vs. 18.4 months, HR 0.77, 95% CI 0.51–1.14, $p = 0.19$). The 5-year OS rate was 23.9% with gemcitabine and 10.6% with observation.

Table 1.2 Key randomized controlled trials of adjuvant therapy for resected pancreatic cancer

Trial	Inclusion period	No. of patients	Intervention	Comparator	Median OS (months)		5-year OS (%)		HR (95% CI), p value
					I	C	I	C	
Chemotherapy									
ESPAC-1	1994–2000	289	5-FU/FA	No chemotherapy	20.1	15.5	21.1	8.4	0.71 (0.55–0.92), p = 0.009
CONKO-001	1998–2004	354	GEM	Observation	22.8	20.2	20.7	10.4	0.76 (0.61–0.95), p = 0.01
JSAP-02	2002–2005	118	GEM	Observation	22.3	18.4	23.9	10.6	0.77 (0.51–1.14), p = 0.19
ESPAC-3	2000–2007	1088	5-FU/FA	GEM	23.0	23.6	15.9	17.5	0.94 (0.81–1.08), p = 0.39
JASPAC-01	2007–2010	377	S-1	GEM	46.5	25.5	44.4	24.4	0.57 (0.44–0.72), p < 0.001
CONKO-005	2008–2013	436	GEM/erlotinib	GEM	24.5	26.5	25	20	p = 0.61[a]
CONKO-006	2008–2013	122	GEM/sorafenib	GEM	17.6	17.5	–	–	p = 0.48[a]
ESPAC-4	2008–2014	730	GEM/CAP	GEM	27.7	26.0	28	20	0.84 (0.70–0.99), p = 0.049
PRODIGE-24/ CCTG PA.6	2012–2016	793	mFOLFIRINOX	GEM	53.5	35.5	43.2	31.4	0.64 (0.48–0.86), p < 0.001
APACT	2014–2016	866	GEM/nab-P	GEM	41.8	37.7	38	31	0.80 (0.68–0.95), p = 0.009
Chemoradiotherapy									
GITSG	1974–1982	43	CRT followed by maintenance 5-FU	Observation	21.0	10.9	19	5	p = 0.03[a]
EORTC 40891	1987–1995	120	CRT	Observation	17.1	12.6	20	10	0.76 (0.52–1.12), p = 0.099
ESPAC-1	1994–2000	289	CRT	No chemoradiotherapy	15.9	17.9	10.8	19.6	1.28 (0.99–1.66), p = 0.05
RTOG 9704	1998–2002		GEM followed by 5-FU CRT (50.4 Gy) followed by GEM	5-FU followed by 5-FU CRT (50.4 Gy) followed by 5-FU	20.5	17.1	22	18	0.82 (0.65–1.03), p = 0.09

5-FU/FA 5-fluorouracil with leucovorin, *CAP* capecitabine, *CI* confidence interval, *CRT* chemoradiotherapy, *GEM* gemcitabine, *HR* hazard ratio, *mFOLFIRI-NOX* modified 5-fluorouracil with leucovorin, irinotecan and oxaliplatin, *nab-P* nab-paclitaxel

[a] HR not reported

As both gemcitabine and 5-FU/FA were proven effective as adjuvant therapy, the **ESPAC-3** trial compared both treatments in 1088 patients from 159 centers in 17 countries [22]. After a median follow-up of 34.2 months, the median OS was not different with 23.6 months in the gemcitabine group and 23.0 in the 5-FU/FA group (HR 0.94, 0.81–1.08, $p = 0.39$). Due to the higher rate of adverse events in the 5-FU/FA group, gemcitabine became the preferred adjuvant regimen.

The **JASPAC-01** trial compared adjuvant S-1 with adjuvant gemcitabine in 385 patients in 33 centers in Japan. The median OS was 46.5 months with S-1 and 25.5 months with gemcitabine (HR 0.57, 95% CI 0.44–0.72, $p < 0.0001$) [23]. The 5-year OS rate was 44.1% in the S-1 group and 24.4% in the gemcitabine group. These results made S-1 the preferred adjuvant regimen for Japanese patients. A difference in pharmacokinetics of S-1 in Asian and Western populations and a lack of registration limit the use of S-1 in Western countries.

The **CONKO-005** and **CONKO-006** trials studied whether the addition of erlotinib or sorafinib to adjuvant gemcitabine could improve survival in patients who underwent R0 and R1 resection, respectively [24, 25]. Both trials failed to show an OS benefit of adding erlotinib or sorafinib to gemcitabine as adjuvant therapy.

The **ESPAC-4** trial randomized 730 patients in 92 centers to the combination of gemcitabine with capecitabine or gemcitabine monotherapy as adjuvant therapy [26]. After a median follow-up of 60 months, the median OS showed a modest improvement with 27.7 months in the gemcitabine/capecitabine group as compared with 26.0 months in the gemcitabine monotherapy group (HR 0.84, 95% CI 0.70–0.99, $p = 0.049$) [27]. The 5-year OS rate was 28% in the gemcitabine/capecitabine group and 20% in the gemcitabine group.

In 2011, the PRODIGE 4 ACCORD 11 trial showed an improvement in OS with FOLFIRINOX compared with gemcitabine in patients with metastatic PDAC [28]. On the basis of these results, the French-Canadian **PRODIGE-24/CCTG PA.6** trial was initiated to compare 12 cycles of adjuvant modified FOLFIRINOX with 6 cycles of adjuvant gemcitabine in 493 patients in 77 centers [29]. After a median follow-up of 33.6 months, median OS was an unprecedented 54.4 months with mFOLFIRINOX and 35.0 months with gemcitabine (HR 0.64, 95% CI 0.48–0.86, $p = 0.003$) [29]. In the long-term analysis with a median follow-up of 69.7 months, these results were confirmed with a 5-year OS of 43.2% with mFOLFIRINOX and 31.4% with gemcitabine [30].

In 2013, the MPACT trial demonstrated improved survival with the addition of nanoparticle albumin-bound paclitaxel (nab-paclitaxel) to gemcitabine in metastatic PDAC [31]. Following these results, the **APACT** trial investigated the addition of nab-paclitaxel to adjuvant gemcitabine [32]. Between 2014 and 2016, 866 patients were randomized to 6 cycles of adjuvant gemcitabine with nab-paclitaxel or to 6 cycles of gemcitabine alone in North America, Europe, Asia, and Australia. The trial did not meet its primary endpoint of improving independently assessed disease free survival (HR 0.88, 95% CI 0.73–1.06, $p = 0.18$) [33]. After a median follow-up of 63.2 months, however, the median OS was 41.8 months with gemcitabine/nab-paclitaxel compared with 37.7 months with gemcitabine alone (HR 0.80, 95% CI 0.68–0.95, $p = 0.009$) [32]. The 5-year OS was 38% with gemcitabine/nab-paclitaxel and 31% with gemcitabine monotherapy.

Trials of Adjuvant Chemoradiotherapy

The **GITSG** trial compared adjuvant 5-FU chemoradiotherapy (total 40 Gray) followed by maintenance 5-FU during a maximum of 2 years with observation in 43 patients with margin-negative resected PDAC [34]. Median OS was 21 months with adjuvant chemoradiation and 10.9 months with observation ($p = 0.03$). At 5-year follow-up, 19% of patients were alive in the chemoradiotherapy group and 5% in the observation group [34].

The **EORTC 40891** trial compared adjuvant 5-FU chemoradiotherapy with observation in 218 patients with pancreatic and periampullary cancer [17]. In the long-term analysis, no improvement in OS was observed in the 120 patients with PDAC (median OS 17.1 vs. 12.6 months, HR 0.76, 95% CI 0.52–1.12) [35].

The **ESPAC-1** trial investigated both chemotherapy and chemoradiotherapy, as described in the previous section on chemotherapy. The chemoradiotherapy group included 145 patients and the no chemoradiotherapy group 144 patients. Chemoradiotherapy was associated with worse survival with a median OS of 15.9 months in the chemoradiotherapy group as compared with 17.9 months in the no chemoradiotherapy group (HR 1.28, 95% CI 0.99–1.66, $p = 0.05$) [19]. On the basis of these results, adjuvant chemoradiotherapy became controversial and its use declined.

The **RTOG 9704** trial investigated whether the addition of adjuvant gemcitabine to adjuvant 5-FU chemoradiation could improve survival. Between 1998 and 2002, 451 patients were randomized in 164 centers in the United States and Canada [36]. In the long-term analysis, the median OS was 20.5 months in the gemcitabine group as compared with 17.1 months without gemcitabine (HR 0.82, 95% CI 0.65–1.03, $p = 0.09$) [37].

Neoadjuvant Therapy for Resectable Pancreatic Cancer

Until recently, the best available evidence for neoadjuvant therapy consisted of meta-analyses of mostly non-randomized studies [38, 39]. These meta-analyses consistently demonstrated similar or improved OS with neoadjuvant therapy even though resection rates were lower. The first phase three trials that completed accrual and reported results are the PREOPANC and Prep 02/JSAP-05 trials [40, 41]. More recently, results of the SWOG S1505, NEONAX, and PANACH01-PRODIGE48 trials have been reported [42–44]. Key RCTs of neoadjuvant therapy for resectable PDAC are discussed below and presented in Table 1.3.

Table 1.3 Key studies of neoadjuvant therapy for resectable pancreatic cancer

Trial/study	Inclusion period	No. of patients	Intervention (no. of cycles)	Comparator (no. of cycles)	Median OS (months)		HR (95% CI), p value	Resection rate (%)	
					I	C		I	C
RCTs									
Prep 02/ JSAP-05[a]	2013–2016	362	Neoadj. GEM/S-1 + adj. S-1 (6 mo.)	Adj. S-1 (6 mo.)	36.7	26.6	0.72 (0.55–0.94), $p = 0.015$	86	87
PREOPANC[a]	2013–2017	246	Neoadj. GEM-based CRT + adj. GEM (4)	Adj. GEM (6)	15.7	14.3	0.73 (0.56–0.96), $p = 0.025$	61	72
SWOG S1505	2015–2018	102	Periop. mFOLFIRINOX (6+6)	Periop. GEM/ nab-P (3+3)	22.4	23.6	NR	73	70
NEONAX	2015–2019	118	Periop. GEM/nab-P (2+4)	Adj. GEM/nab-P (6)	25.2	16.7	NR	70	78
PANACHE01-PRODIGE48	2017–2020	146	Neoadj. mFOLFIRINOX (4) Neoadj. FOLFOX (4)	Adj. mFOLFIRINOX (12)	1-yr OS: mFOLFIRINOX, 84.1 FOLFOX, 71.8	1-yr OS: 80.8%	NR	mFOLFIRINOX, 71 FOLFOX, 68	81
Retrospective cohort study									
TAPS cohort	2012–2019	346	mFOLFIRINOX	–	31.2	–	–	71	–

Adj adjuvant, *CI* confidence interval, *CRT* chemoradiotherapy, *FOLFOX* 5-fluorouracil, leucovorin, and oxaliplatin, *GEM* gemcitabine, *HR* hazard ratio, *mFOLFIRINOX* modified 5-fluorouracil with leucovorin, irinotecan, and oxaliplatin, *nab-P* nab-paclitaxel, *NR* not reported, *OS* overall survival
[a] Includes patients with both resectable and borderline resectable pancreatic cancer

Trials of Neoadjuvant Chemotherapy

In the Japanese phase 3 **Prep 02/JSAP-05** trial, 362 patients with resectable or borderline resectable PDAC were randomized to neoadjuvant chemotherapy or to upfront surgery [41]. Patients in the neoadjuvant chemotherapy arm received two cycles of neoadjuvant gemcitabine with S-1. In both arms, 6 months of adjuvant S-1 was administered after resection. In an abstract publication from 2019, the median OS was 36.7 months for the neoadjuvant arm compared with 26.6 months with upfront surgery (HR 0.72, 95% CI 0.55–0.94, $p = 0.015$). The resection rates were similar (86% vs. 87%).

The first published RCT that compared two neoadjuvant multi-agent regimens in resectable PDAC was the phase 2 **SWOG S1505** trial. The trial compared neoadjuvant mFOLFIRINOX with neoadjuvant gemcitabine/nab-paclitaxel in 147 patients. After central review, 44 patients were excluded, and 1 patient withdrew informed consent leaving 102 patients for analysis. No difference in OS was observed with a median OS of 23.2 with mFOLFIRINOX and 23.6 months with gemcitabine/nab-paclitaxel. The resection rate was 73% in the mFOLFIRINOX group and 70% in the gemcitabine/nab-paclitaxel group. Compliance with adjuvant therapy was low as 56% started adjuvant therapy in the mFOLFIRINOX group and 55% in the gemcitabine/nab-paclitaxel group.

The first RCT to compare perioperative with adjuvant administration of multi-agent chemotherapy is the phase 2 **NEONAX** trial. The trial compared 6 cycles of perioperative gemcitabine/nab-paclitaxel (2 neoadjuvant, 4 adjuvant) with 6 cycles of adjuvant gemcitabine/nab-paclitaxel in 127 patients with resectable PDAC from 22 German centers [45]. According to an abstract published in 2022, median OS was 25.2 months with perioperative treatment compared with 16.7 with adjuvant treatment [43]. The resection rate in the perioperative arm was 70% compared with 78% in the adjuvant arm. In the perioperative arm, 54 (91.5%) started neoadjuvant therapy, while in the adjuvant arm, only 25 patients (42.4%) started adjuvant therapy.

The three-arm phase 2 **PANACHE01-PRODIGE48** trial randomized (2:2:1) 153 patients to 4 cycles of neoadjuvant mFOLFIRINOX, 4 cycles of neoadjuvant FOLFOX, or 12 cycles of adjuvant mFOLFIRINOX for resectable PDAC [46]. Additional adjuvant chemotherapy (8 cycles) was scheduled in the neoadjuvant therapy arms. Following the interim analysis, the FOLFOX arm was closed early for lack of efficiency. In an abstract publication in 2022, the 1-year OS rates were 84.1%, 71.8%, and 80.8%, and the resection rates were 74%, 68%, and 81%, respectively [44].

Trials of Neoadjuvant Chemoradiotherapy

The Dutch phase 3 **PREOPANC** trial compared neoadjuvant gemcitabine-based chemoradiotherapy with upfront surgery in 246 patients with resectable and borderline resectable PDAC. Neoadjuvant chemoradiotherapy consisted of three cycles of neoadjuvant gemcitabine combined with 36 Gy radiotherapy in 15 fraction during the second cycle. Following surgery, patients received four cycles of adjuvant gemcitabine. In the upfront surgery group, patients received six cycles of adjuvant gemcitabine. After a median follow-up of 27 months, median OS was 16.0 months with neoadjuvant chemoradiotherapy and 14.3 months with adjuvant gemcitabine (HR 0.78; 95% CI 0.58–1.05, $p = 0.096$) [47]. However, after a median follow-up of 59 months, 5-year OS was 20.5% with neoadjuvant chemoradiotherapy compared with 6.5% with adjuvant gemcitabine (HR 0.73; 95% CI 0.56–0.96, $p = 0.025$) [40]. Only 51% started adjuvant therapy in the adjuvant gemcitabine group.

A recent meta-analysis including 6 RCTs including 938 patients with resectable or borderline resectable PDAC found improved OS with neoadjuvant therapy (HR 0.66, 95% CI 0.52–0.85, $p = 0.001$) [48]. In the subgroup of patients with resectable PDAC, however, no significant treatment effect was found (HR 0.77, 95% CI 0.53–1.12, $p = 0.18$). A limitation of the meta-analysis was that none of the trials included adjuvant mFOLFIRINOX as the trials were started before the publication of the PRODIGE 24/CCTG PA. 6 trial.

Few non-randomized studies reported on neoadjuvant FOLFIRINOX for resectable PDAC [14, 49]. The largest study is a retrospective study by the Trans-Atlantic Pancreatic Surgery consortium from five centers in the United States and the Netherlands [14]. The study included 346 patients with resectable PDAC who received neoadjuvant (m)FOLFIRINOX. The median OS was 31 months and the resection rate was 71%.

Comparing Neoadjuvant and Adjuvant Therapy

Advantages of Neoadjuvant Therapy

The most important advantage of neoadjuvant therapy is that patients are guaranteed to receive systemic chemotherapy. Nationwide studies show that a considerable proportion of patients who underwent successful resection for PDAC do not receive adjuvant therapy. In a National Cancer Data Base study from the United States including 7967 patients who underwent resection between 2010 and 2012, 47% did not receive adjuvant chemotherapy. In a more recent nationwide analysis from the Netherlands, 433 of 1306 (33%) patients who underwent resection between 2014–2017 did not receive adjuvant therapy. Compliance remains the main concern with adjuvant therapy.

Second, the time period of neoadjuvant therapy allows for the tumor biology to declare itself. Patients with tumors that progress during neoadjuvant therapy are unlikely to have benefitted from a pancreatic resection. Consequently, neoadjuvant therapy allows for a better selection of those patients who may benefit from a potentially morbid operation.

Third, neoadjuvant therapy improves the R0 resection rate. In the PREOPANC trial, the R0 resection rate was 72% in the neoadjuvant CRT arm vs. 43% in the upfront surgery arm ($p < 0.001$).

Fourth, neoadjuvant therapy may reduce postoperative complications. An analysis of the PREOPANC trial found 0% postoperative pancreatic fistula after neoadjuvant chemoradiotherapy and no increase in overall major complications [50]. Several other non-randomized studies had similar results [51, 52].

Disadvantages of Neoadjuvant Therapy

Upfront surgery with adjuvant therapy has some small advantages over neoadjuvant therapy.

First, neoadjuvant chemotherapy requires a tissue diagnosis of PDAC, while most patients with a hypo-intense pancreatic mass on CT undergo a resection without tissue diagnosis. Diagnostic procedures to obtain tumor tissue are endoscopic ultrasound-guided fine needle aspiration (EUS-FNA) or bile duct brushing. These procedures are associated with complications including acute pancreatitis, hemorrhage, and perforation of the gastrointestinal tract [53].

Second, both cross-sectional imaging and a biopsy cannot distinguish periampullary cancer from PDAC with 100% accuracy. In a nationwide analysis from the Netherlands, the misdiagnosis rate was 13% in patients who were preoperatively thought to have PDAC. With upfront surgery, the full histopathology specimen is available for the correct diagnosis and appropriate adjuvant treatment.

Third, the majority of patients with resectable PDAC present with obstructive jaundice. These patients need a stent for biliary decompression to tolerate neoadjuvant therapy. Placement of a biliary stent with endoscopic retrograde cholangiopancreatography is associated with a non-negligible risk of complications and even death. Biliary drainage can be omitted in patients treated with upfront surgery. An RCT showed an increased rate of complications in patients with tumors in the pancreatic head who underwent preoperative biliary drainage as compared with patients who proceeded to surgery without drainage [54].

Comparing Neoadjuvant and Adjuvant Trials

Survival is lower in RCTs investigating neoadjuvant and perioperative treatment as compared with RCTs that compare only adjuvant therapy (Tables 1.2 and 1.3). Some have misinterpreted this as evidence of inferior survival after neoadjuvant therapy [55]. For example, the median survival in the PREOPANC trial (comparing a neoadjuvant with adjuvant treatment) of patients in the adjuvant gemcitabine arm was 14 months, while the median survival in the PRODIGE 24/CCTG PA.6 trial (comparing two adjuvant regimens) of patients in the same adjuvant gemcitabine arm was 36 months (Tables 1.1 and 1.2) [29, 40]. This large difference is explained by an entirely different selection of patients for an RCT comparing one or more neoadjuvant regimens with an RCT with only adjuvant regimens. Adjuvant RCTs include only a subgroup of all patients who would have been eligible for a neoadjuvant trial. In order for a patient presenting with resectable PDAC to become eligible for inclusion in an adjuvant RCT, the patient has to overcome many hurdles: (1) no occult metastases at staging laparoscopy (about 5–10% drops out), (2) a resection without postoperative mortality (about 2–5% drops out), (3) recover sufficiently from surgery to receive adjuvant chemotherapy (about 30% drops out), (4) no early recurrence on postoperative CT scan (about 5% drops out), and (5) no elevated postoperative CA 19-9 levels (about 5% drops out). In summary, up to 50% of all patients randomized in an RCT with one or more neoadjuvant treatment arms would have never become eligible for an RCT comparing only adjuvant therapy.

Most trials of neoadjuvant therapy have demonstrated a lower resection rate as compared with upfront surgery. This is explained by patients that progress during neoadjuvant therapy. Some argue that this is a disadvantage of a neoadjuvant approach. However, it is unlikely that patients who progress during neoadjuvant therapy would have benefitted from a pancreatic resection. These patients would likely have developed disease recurrence within 3–6 months after upfront resection.

Future Directions

Ongoing Clinical Trials

Several ongoing studies investigate neoadjuvant and adjuvant therapy for resectable PDAC (Table 1.4).

The **NorPACT-1** trial investigates perioperative mFOLFIRINOX for resectable PDAC. In the intervention arm, patients receive four cycles of neoadjuvant mFOL-FIRINOX followed by surgery. After surgery, eight cycles of mFOLFIRINOX are planned. In the comparator arm, patients receive 12 cycles of adjuvant mFOLFIRI-NOX. In the original design, the adjuvant therapy was gemcitabine/capecitabine, but this was changed after the publication of the PRODIGE-24/CCTG PA.6 trial results. Between 2016 and 2020, 140 patients were randomized in Norway, Sweden, Finland, and Denmark, and results are expected at the end of 2022.

The Dutch **PREOPANC-2** compared neoadjuvant FOLFIRINOX with neoad-juvant gemcitabine-based chemoradiotherapy. In the intervention arm, patients receive neoadjuvant FOLFIRINOX without adjuvant therapy. The comparator arm is based on the superior arm of the PREOPANC-1 trial, consisting of 3 cycles of neoadjuvant gemcitabine whereby the second cycle is combined with 36 Gray radiotherapy in 15 fractions. After surgery, four cycles of adjuvant gemcitabine are planned. The trial included patients with both resectable and borderline resect-able PDAC. Between 2018 and 2021, 368 patients were randomized and results are expected in 2023.

The **ALLIANCE A021806** trial from the United States compares perioperative mFOLFIRINOX with adjuvant mFOLFIRINOX. In the intervention arm, patients receive eight cycles of neoadjuvant mFOLFIRINOX, and after surgery, four cycles of adjuvant mFOLFIRINOX are planned. In the comparator arm, 12 cycles of adju-vant mFOLFIRINOX are planned. The trial opened for accrual in July 2020, and as of 1 August 2023, 193 patients have been randomized.

Table 1.4 Ongoing or pending randomized controlled trials of (neo)adjuvant therapy for resectable pancreatic cancer

Trial name and registration	Inclusion period	Target sample size	Primary outcome	Intervention (no. of cycles)	Comparator (no. of cycles)
Adjuvant trials					
RTOG 0848 NCT01013649	2009–2014	545	DFS	Adjuvant CRT after adjuvant GEM	Adjuvant GEM without CRT
ESPAC-6 NCT05314998	Not yet recruiting	394	DFS	Adj. GEM/CAP (6) or adj. mFOLFIRINOX (12) based on transcriptomic signature	Adj. mFOLFIRINOX (12)
Neoadjuvant trials					
NorPACT-1 NCT02919787	2016–2020	140	OS at 18 months	Periop. mFOLFIRINOX (4+8)	Adj. mFOLFIRINOX (12)
PREOPANC-2[a] EudraCT 2017-002036-17	2018–2021	368	OS	Neoadj. FOLFIRINOX (8)	Neoadj. GEM-based CRT + adj. GEM (4)
ALLIANCE A021806 NCT04340141	2020–	352	OS	Periop. mFOLFIRINOX (8+4)	Adj. mFOLFIRINOX (12)
PREOPANC-3 NCT04927780	2021–	378	OS	Periop. mFOLFIRINOX (8+4)	Adj. mFOLFIRINOX (12)

Adj adjuvant, *CRT* chemoradiotherapy, *DFS* disease free survival, *GEM* gemcitabine, *OS* overall survival, *mFOLFIRINOX* neoadj, neoadjuvant, modified 5-fluorouracil with leucovorin, irinotecan, and oxaliplatin, *periop* perioperative

[a] Includes patients with both resectable and borderline resectable pancreatic cancer

The **PREOPANC-3** trial from the Netherlands investigates perioperative mFOL-FIRINOX and has a similar design as the ALLIANCE A021806 trial with 378 patients needed. The trial opened for accrual in August 2021, and as of 1 August 2023, 171 patients have been randomized.

The **RTOG 0848** trial investigates whether the addition of adjuvant chemoradiotherapy after adjuvant gemcitabine improves OS in patients with resected PDAC. In the two-step design, patients were first randomized to adjuvant gemcitabine or to adjuvant gemcitabine with erlotinib. Patients were restaged after five cycles of gemcitabine and, if without progression, randomized again to one cycle of gemcitabine followed by adjuvant capecitabine or 5-FU-based chemoradiotherapy (50.4 Gray) or to one cycle of gemcitabine. The results of step 1 were reported in 2020 and did not show a benefit of adding erlotinib to gemcitabine [56]. The step 2 result on the use of adjuvant chemoradiotherapy is pending.

The **ESPAC-6** trial from Germany investigates whether selecting an adjuvant regimen based on tumor characteristics can improve survival. In the intervention arm, patients will either receive adjuvant mFOLFIRINOX or adjuvant gemcitabine with capecitabine based on the transcriptomic signature of the tumor. In the comparator arm, patients receive adjuvant mFOLFIRINOX. The trial plans to accrue 394 patients.

Neoadjuvant Therapy Based on Treatment Response

Neoadjuvant therapy allows for evaluating treatment response. This provides the opportunity to adapt or "switch" the neoadjuvant regimen in the absence of treatment response. As radiologic indicators of treatment response are generally unreliable in localized PDAC [57], serum CA 19-9 is often used to assess response.

Several studies have reported on the effect of a treatment "switch" of the neoadjuvant regimen. A single-institution study included 25 patients with borderline resectable and locally advanced PDAC who were switched from FOLFIRINOX to gemcitabine nab-paclitaxel [58]. Of the 25 patients, 21 showed radiographic or CA 19-9 response after switching and 11 patients underwent resection. Another study described the outcomes of 468 patients with borderline resectable and locally advanced PDAC of whom 139 (30%) had chemotherapy switch [59]. The majority (89%) switched from 5-FU-based therapy (FOLFIRINOX or FOLFOX) to gemcitabine with nab-paclitaxel. Of the 139 patients with chemotherapy switch, 100 underwent resection, and their survival was not different from the patients without chemotherapy switch (36.4 vs. 41.4 months; $p = 0.94$).

Several ongoing studies are investigating whether adaptive neoadjuvant therapy can improve survival. A study from the University of Wisconsin (NCT03322995) investigates whether switching based on treatment response can improve outcomes in patients with resectable or borderline resectable PDAC. Treatment response is assessed using CT imaging, serum CA 19-9, and performance status. All patients start with FOLFIRINOX. In case of response, patients continue with FOLFIRINOX. In case of stable disease, patients switch to gemcitabine-based therapy. In case of local progression, patients receive chemoradiation. The primary outcome of the study is completion of all neoadjuvant therapy and resection. Another study, from the Oregon Health and Science University (NeoOPTIMIZE; NCT04539808), follows the same principle. Patients with localized PDAC start with four cycles of FOLFIRINOX, and in case of progression at evaluation (by CT imaging or increase of CA 19-9 >30%), they switch to gemcitabine with nab-paclitaxel. The primary endpoint is the proportion of patients that undergo R0 resection. Finally, a study from the University of Cincinnati (NCT04594772) investigates whether a neoadjuvant chemotherapy switch improves the resection rate in 32 patients with resectable and borderline resectable PDAC.

Adjuvant Therapy After Neoadjuvant therapy

Current guidelines recommend a total duration of systemic therapy (combining neoadjuvant and adjuvant therapy) of 6 months [5, 6]. This recommendation is based on extrapolation of treatment duration in the metastatic and adjuvant setting. No RCTs are available that investigate the duration of chemotherapy for PDAC or the use of adjuvant therapy after neoadjuvant therapy and resection.

An international, multi-institutional, retrospective analysis investigated adjuvant therapy after neoadjuvant FOLFIRINOX and resection in 520 patients of all stages of localized PDAC [60]. Adjuvant therapy was gemcitabine-based in 59% and 20% received FOLFIRINOX. Improved survival with adjuvant chemotherapy was observed only in patients with node-positive disease (median OS, 26 vs. 13 months, $p = 0.004$). Another study, based on the National Cancer Database, included patients who underwent a resection between 2004–2016 and used propensity score matching to account for selection bias [61]. A total of 2016 patients who received adjuvant therapy after neoadjuvant therapy and resection were successfully matched to 2016 patients who did not. Median OS was 29.4 months in patients who received adjuvant therapy compared with 24.9 months in patients who did not ($p < 0.001$). These results were irrespective of nodal or margin status. A total neoadjuvant therapy approach is increasingly used, because it avoids the challenge of administering adjuvant chemotherapy to all patients.

Conclusions

Progress has been made over the last decades in the treatment of resectable PDAC. Systemic therapy in the form of neoadjuvant or adjuvant therapy is an integral part of multimodality treatment and improves OS. The main concern with adjuvant therapy is compliance, and neoadjuvant therapy has the potential to improve outcomes in this regard. Two phase 3 RCTs have shown improved survival with neoadjuvant therapy, but both trials used single-agent systemic therapy. In patients with resectable PDAC, high-quality evidence for a survival benefit of neoadjuvant therapy over upfront surgery with multi-agent adjuvant therapy is therefore lacking. Current RCTs, including the ALLIANCE A021806 and PREOPANC-3 trials, will answer the question whether perioperative mFOLFIRINOX improves OS compared with upfront surgery with adjuvant mFOLFIRINOX.

References

1. Siegel RL, Miller KD, Fuchs HE, Jemal A. Cancer statistics, 2021. CA Cancer J Clin. 2021;71(1):7–33.
2. Lepage C, Capocaccia R, Hackl M, Lemmens V, Molina E, Pierannunzio D, et al. Survival in patients with primary liver cancer, gallbladder and extrahepatic biliary tract cancer and pancreatic cancer in Europe 1999-2007: results of EUROCARE-5. Eur J Cancer. 2015;51(15):2169–78.
3. Rahib L, Smith BD, Aizenberg R, Rosenzweig AB, Fleshman JM, Matrisian LM. Projecting cancer incidence and deaths to 2030: the unexpected burden of thyroid, liver, and pancreas cancers in the United States. Cancer Res. 2014;74(11):2913–21.
4. Latenstein AEJ, van der Geest LGM, Bonsing BA, Groot Koerkamp B, Haj Mohammad N, de Hingh I, et al. Nationwide trends in incidence, treatment and survival of pancreatic ductal adenocarcinoma. Eur J Cancer. 2020;125:83–93.

5. National Comprehensive Cancer Network. NCCN clinical practice guidelines in oncology: pancreatic adenocarcinoma (version 1.2022) 2022. Available from https://www.nccn.org/professionals/physician_gls/pdf/pancreatic.pdf.

6. Khorana AA, McKernin SE, Berlin J, Hong TS, Maitra A, Moravek C, et al. Potentially curable pancreatic adenocarcinoma: ASCO clinical practice guideline update. J Clin Oncol. 2019;37(23):2082–8.

7. Sohal DP, Walsh RM, Ramanathan RK, Khorana AA. Pancreatic adenocarcinoma: treating a systemic disease with systemic therapy. J Natl Cancer Inst. 2014;106(3):11.

8. Varadhachary GR, Tamm EP, Abbruzzese JL, Xiong HQ, Crane CH, Wang H, et al. Borderline resectable pancreatic cancer: definitions, management, and role of preoperative therapy. Ann Surg Oncol. 2006;13(8):1035–46.

9. Callery MP, Chang KJ, Fishman EK, Talamonti MS, William Traverso L, Linehan DC. Pretreatment assessment of resectable and borderline resectable pancreatic cancer: expert consensus statement. Ann Surg Oncol. 2009;16(7):1727–33.

10. Versteijne E, van Eijck CH, Punt CJ, Suker M, Zwinderman AH, Dohmen MA, et al. Preoperative radiochemotherapy versus immediate surgery for resectable and borderline resectable pancreatic cancer (PREOPANC trial): study protocol for a multicentre randomized controlled trial. Trials. 2016;17(1):127.

11. Seo YD, Katz MHG. Preoperative therapy for pancreatic adenocarcinoma-precision beyond anatomy. Cancer. 2022;128(16):3041–56.

12. Tzeng CW, Fleming JB, Lee JE, Xiao L, Pisters PW, Vauthey JN, et al. Defined clinical classifications are associated with outcome of patients with anatomically resectable pancreatic adenocarcinoma treated with neoadjuvant therapy. Ann Surg Oncol. 2012;19(6):2045–53.

13. Anger F, Doring A, van Dam J, Lock JF, Klein I, Bittrich M, et al. Impact of borderline resectability in pancreatic head cancer on patient survival: biology matters according to the new international consensus criteria. Ann Surg Oncol. 2020;28(4):2325–36. https://doi.org/10.1245/s10434-020-09100-6.

14. Janssen QP, van Dam JL, Doppenberg D, Prakash LR, van Eijck CHJ, Jarnagin WR, et al. FOLFIRINOX as initial treatment for localized pancreatic adenocarcinoma: a retrospective analysis by the Trans-Atlantic pancreatic surgery consortium. J Natl Cancer Inst. 2022;114(5):695–703.

15. Gastrointestinal Tumor Study Group. Further evidence of effective adjuvant combined radiation and chemotherapy following curative resection of pancreatic cancer. Cancer. 1987;59(12):2006–10.

16. Bakkevold KE, Arnesjo B, Dahl O, Kambestad B. Adjuvant combination chemotherapy (AMF) following radical resection of carcinoma of the pancreas and papilla of Vater–results of a controlled, prospective, randomised multicentre study. Eur J Cancer. 1993;29(5):698–703.

17. Klinkenbijl JH, Jeekel J, Sahmoud T, van Pel R, Couvreur ML, Veenhof CH, et al. Adjuvant radiotherapy and 5-fluorouracil after curative resection of cancer of the pancreas and periampullary region: phase III trial of the EORTC gastrointestinal tract cancer cooperative group. Ann Surg. 1999;230(6):776–82. discussion 82-4.

18. Takada T, Amano H, Yasuda H, Nimura Y, Matsushiro T, Kato H, et al. Is postoperative adjuvant chemotherapy useful for gallbladder carcinoma? A phase III multicenter prospective randomized controlled trial in patients with resected pancreaticobiliary carcinoma. Cancer. 2002;95(8):1685–95.

19. Neoptolemos JP, Stocken DD, Friess H, Bassi C, Dunn JA, Hickey H, et al. A randomized trial of chemoradiotherapy and chemotherapy after resection of pancreatic cancer. N Engl J Med. 2004;350(12):1200–10.

20. Oettle H, Neuhaus P, Hochhaus A, Hartmann JT, Gellert K, Ridwelski K, et al. Adjuvant chemotherapy with gemcitabine and long-term outcomes among patients with resected pancreatic cancer: the CONKO-001 randomized trial. JAMA. 2013;310(14):1473–81.

21. Oettle H, Post S, Neuhaus P, Gellert K, Langrehr J, Ridwelski K, et al. Adjuvant chemotherapy with gemcitabine vs observation in patients undergoing curative-intent resection of pancreatic cancer: a randomized controlled trial. JAMA. 2007;297(3):267–77.

22. Neoptolemos JP, Stocken DD, Bassi C, Ghaneh P, Cunningham D, Goldstein D, et al. Adjuvant chemotherapy with fluorouracil plus folinic acid vs gemcitabine following pancreatic cancer resection: a randomized controlled trial. JAMA. 2010;304(10):1073–81.
23. Uesaka K, Boku N, Fukutomi A, Okamura Y, Konishi M, Matsumoto I, et al. Adjuvant chemotherapy of S-1 versus gemcitabine for resected pancreatic cancer: a phase 3, open-label, randomised, non-inferiority trial (JASPAC 01). Lancet. 2016;388(10041):248–57.
24. Sinn M, Bahra M, Liersch T, Gellert K, Messmann H, Bechstein W, et al. CONKO-005: adjuvant chemotherapy with gemcitabine plus erlotinib versus gemcitabine alone in patients after R0 resection of pancreatic cancer: a multicenter randomized phase III trial. J Clin Oncol. 2017;35(29):3330–7.
25. Sinn M, Liersch T, Riess H, Gellert K, Stubs P, Waldschmidt D, et al. CONKO-006: a randomised double-blinded phase IIb-study of additive therapy with gemcitabine + sorafenib/placebo in patients with R1 resection of pancreatic cancer - final results. Eur J Cancer. 2020;138:172–81.
26. Neoptolemos JP, Palmer DH, Ghaneh P, Psarelli EE, Valle JW, Halloran CM, et al. Comparison of adjuvant gemcitabine and capecitabine with gemcitabine monotherapy in patients with resected pancreatic cancer (ESPAC-4): a multicentre, open-label, randomised, phase 3 trial. Lancet. 2017;389(10073):1011–24.
27. Neoptolemos JP, Palmer DH, Ghaneh P, Valle JW, Cunningham D, Wadsley J, et al. ESPAC-4: a multicenter, international, open-label randomized controlled phase III trial of adjuvant combination chemotherapy of gemcitabine (GEM) and capecitabine (CAP) versus monotherapy gemcitabine in patients with resected pancreatic ductal adenocarcinoma: five year follow-up. J Clin Oncol. 2020;38(15):4516.
28. Conroy T, Desseigne F, Ychou M, Bouche O, Guimbaud R, Becouarn Y, et al. FOLFIRINOX versus gemcitabine for metastatic pancreatic cancer. N Engl J Med. 2011;364(19):1817–25.
29. Conroy T, Hammel P, Hebbar M, Ben Abdelghani M, Wei AC, Raoul JL, et al. FOLFIRINOX or gemcitabine as adjuvant therapy for pancreatic cancer. N Engl J Med. 2018;379(25):2395–406.
30. Conroy T, Hammel P, Turpin A, Belletier C, Wei A, Mitry E, et al. LBA57 Unicancer PRODIGE 24/CCTG PA6 trial: updated results of a multicenter international randomized phase III trial of adjuvant mFOLFIRINOX (mFFX) versus gemcitabine (gem) in patients (pts) with resected pancreatic ductal adenocarcinomas (PDAC). Ann Oncol. 2021;32:S1334.
31. Von Hoff DD, Ervin T, Arena FP, Chiorean EG, Infante J, Moore M, et al. Increased survival in pancreatic cancer with nab-paclitaxel plus gemcitabine. N Engl J Med. 2013;369(18):1691–703.
32. Tempero M, O'Reilly E, Van Cutsem E, Berlin J, Philip P, Goldstein D, et al. LBA-1 phase 3 APACT trial of adjuvant nab-paclitaxel plus gemcitabine (nab-P + Gem) vs gemcitabine (Gem) alone in patients with resected pancreatic cancer (PC): updated 5-year overall survival. Ann Oncol. 2021;32:S226.
33. Tempero MA, Reni M, Riess H, Pelzer U, O'Reilly EM, Winter JM, et al. APACT: phase III, multicenter, international, open-label, randomized trial of adjuvant nab-paclitaxel plus gemcitabine (nab-P/G) vs gemcitabine (G) for surgically resected pancreatic adenocarcinoma. J Clin Oncol. 2019;37(15):4000.
34. Kalser MH, Ellenberg SS, Pancreatic cancer. Adjuvant combined radiation and chemotherapy following curative resection. Arch Surg. 1985;120(8):899–903.
35. Smeenk HG, van Eijck CH, Hop WC, Erdmann J, Tran KC, Debois M, et al. Long-term survival and metastatic pattern of pancreatic and periampullary cancer after adjuvant chemoradiation or observation: long-term results of EORTC trial 40891. Ann Surg. 2007;246(5):734–40.
36. Regine WF, Winter KA, Abrams RA, Safran H, Hoffman JP, Konski A, et al. Fluorouracil vs gemcitabine chemotherapy before and after fluorouracil-based chemoradiation following resection of pancreatic adenocarcinoma: a randomized controlled trial. JAMA. 2008;299(9):1019–26.
37. Regine WF, Winter KA, Abrams R, Safran H, Hoffman JP, Konski A, et al. Fluorouracil-based chemoradiation with either gemcitabine or fluorouracil chemotherapy after resection of pancreatic adenocarcinoma: 5-year analysis of the U.S. Intergroup/RTOG 9704 phase III trial. Ann Surg Oncol. 2011;18(5):1319–26.

38. Gillen S, Schuster T, Meyer Zum Buschenfelde C, Friess H, Kleeff J. Preoperative/neoadjuvant therapy in pancreatic cancer: a systematic review and meta-analysis of response and resection percentages. PLoS Med. 2010;7(4):e1000267.
39. Versteijne E, Vogel JA, Besselink MG, Busch ORC, Wilmink JW, Daams JG, et al. Meta-analysis comparing upfront surgery with neoadjuvant treatment in patients with resectable or borderline resectable pancreatic cancer. Br J Surg. 2018;105(8):946–58.
40. Versteijne E, van Dam JL, Suker M, Janssen QP, Groothuis K, Akkermans-Vogelaar JM, et al. Neoadjuvant chemoradiotherapy versus upfront surgery for resectable and borderline resectable pancreatic cancer: long-term results of the Dutch randomized PREOPANC trial. J Clin Oncol. 2022;40(11):1220–30.
41. Unno M, Motoi F, Matsuyama Y, Satoi S, Matsumoto I, Aosasa S, et al. Randomized phase II/III trial of neoadjuvant chemotherapy with gemcitabine and S-1 versus upfront surgery for resectable pancreatic cancer (Prep-02/JSAP-05). J Clin Oncol. 2019;37(4):189.
42. Sohal DPS, Duong M, Ahmad SA, Gandhi NS, Beg MS, Wang-Gillam A, et al. Efficacy of perioperative chemotherapy for resectable pancreatic adenocarcinoma: a phase 2 randomized clinical trial. JAMA Oncol. 2021;7(3):421–7.
43. Ettrich TJ, Uhl W, Kornmann M, Algül H, Friess H, Koenig A, et al. Perioperative or adjuvant nab-paclitaxel plus gemcitabine for resectable pancreatic cancer: updated final results of the randomized phase II AIO-NEONAX trial. J Clin Oncol. 2022;40(16):4133.
44. Schwarz L, Bachet J-B, Meurisse A, Bouché O, Assenat E, Piessen G, et al. Resectable pancreatic adenocarcinoma neo-adjuvant FOLF(IRIN)OX-based chemotherapy: a multicenter, non-comparative, randomized, phase II trial (PANACHE01-PRODIGE48 study). J Clin Oncol. 2022;40(16):4134.
45. Ettrich TJ, Berger AW, Perkhofer L, Daum S, Konig A, Dickhut A, et al. Neoadjuvant plus adjuvant or only adjuvant nab-paclitaxel plus gemcitabine for resectable pancreatic cancer - the NEONAX trial (AIO-PAK-0313), a prospective, randomized, controlled, phase II study of the AIO pancreatic cancer group. BMC Cancer. 2018;18(1):1298.
46. Schwarz L, Vernerey D, Bachet JB, Tuech JJ, Portales F, Michel P, et al. Resectable pancreatic adenocarcinoma neo-adjuvant FOLF(IRIN)OX-based chemotherapy - a multicenter, non-comparative, randomized, phase II trial (PANACHE01-PRODIGE48 study). BMC Cancer. 2018;18(1):762.
47. Versteijne E, Suker M, Groothuis K, Akkermans-Vogelaar JM, Besselink MG, Bonsing BA, et al. Preoperative chemoradiotherapy versus immediate surgery for resectable and borderline resectable pancreatic cancer: results of the Dutch randomized phase III PREOPANC trial. J Clin Oncol. 2020;38(16):1763–73.
48. van Dam JL, Janssen QP, Besselink MG, Homs MYV, van Santvoort HC, van Tienhoven G, et al. Neoadjuvant therapy or upfront surgery for resectable and borderline resectable pancreatic cancer: a meta-analysis of randomised controlled trials. Eur J Cancer. 2022;160:140–9.
49. Talamonti MS, Baker MS, Posner M, Roggin K, Matthews J, et al. Primary systemic therapy in resectable pancreatic ductal adenocarcinoma using mFOLFIRINOX: a pilot study. J Surg Oncol. 2018;117(3):354–62.
50. van Dongen JC, Suker M, Versteijne E, Bonsing BA, Mieog JSD, de Vos-Geelen J, et al. Surgical complications in a multicenter randomized trial comparing preoperative chemoradiotherapy and immediate surgery in patients with resectable and borderline resectable pancreatic cancer (PREOPANC Trial). Ann Surg. 2020;275(5):979–84. https://doi.org/10.1097/SLA.0000000000004313.
51. Hank T, Sandini M, Ferrone CR, Rodrigues C, Weniger M, Qadan M, et al. Association between pancreatic fistula and long-term survival in the era of neoadjuvant chemotherapy. JAMA Surg. 2019;154(10):943–51.
52. Marchegiani G, Andrianello S, Nessi C, Sandini M, Maggino L, Malleo G, et al. Neoadjuvant therapy versus upfront resection for pancreatic cancer: the actual spectrum and clinical burden of postoperative complications. Ann Surg Oncol. 2018;25(3):626–37.
53. Early DS, Acosta RD, Chandrasekhara V, Chathadi KV, Decker GA, et al. Adverse events associated with EUS and EUS with FNA. Gastrointest Endosc. 2013;77(6):839–43.

54. van der Gaag NA, Rauws EA, van Eijck CH, Bruno MJ, van der Harst E, Kubben FJ, et al. Preoperative biliary drainage for cancer of the head of the pancreas. N Engl J Med. 2010;362(2):129–37.

55. Schneider M, Neoptolemos JP, Buchler MW. Commentary: Neoadjuvant treatment of resectable pancreatic cancer: lack of level III evidence. Surgery. 2020;168(6):1015–6.

56. Abrams RA, Winter KA, Safran H, Goodman KA, Regine WF, Berger AC, et al. Results of the NRG Oncology/RTOG 0848 adjuvant chemotherapy Question-Erlotinib+Gemcitabine for resected cancer of the pancreatic head: a phase II randomized clinical trial. Am J Clin Oncol. 2020;43(3):173–9.

57. Katz MH, Fleming JB, Bhosale P, Varadhachary G, Lee JE, Wolff R, et al. Response of borderline resectable pancreatic cancer to neoadjuvant therapy is not reflected by radiographic indicators. Cancer. 2012;118(23):5749–56.

58. Vreeland TJ, McAllister F, Javadi S, Prakash LR, Fogelman DR, Ho L, et al. Benefit of gemcitabine/nab-paclitaxel rescue of patients with borderline resectable or locally advanced pancreatic adenocarcinoma after early failure of FOLFIRINOX. Pancreas. 2019;48(6):837–43.

59. Alva-Ruiz R, Yohanathan L, Yonkus JA, Abdelrahman AM, Gregory LA, Halfdanarson TR, et al. Neoadjuvant chemotherapy switch in borderline resectable/locally advanced pancreatic cancer. Ann Surg Oncol. 2022;29(3):1579–91.

60. van Roessel S, van Veldhuisen E, Klompmaker S, Janssen QP, Abu Hilal M, Alseidi A, et al. Evaluation of adjuvant chemotherapy in patients with resected pancreatic cancer after neoadjuvant FOLFIRINOX treatment. JAMA Oncol. 2020;6(11):1733–40.

61. Kamarajah SK, White SA, Naffouje SA, Salti GI, Dahdaleh F. Adjuvant chemotherapy associated with survival benefit following neoadjuvant chemotherapy and pancreatectomy for pancreatic ductal adenocarcinoma: a population-based cohort study. Ann Surg Oncol. 2021;28(11):6790–802.

Borderline Resectable and Locally Advanced Pancreatic Cancer

2

Ching-Wei D. Tzeng and Laura Prakash

Introduction

The 5-year overall survival of all patients with pancreatic adenocarcinoma (PDAC) remains 12% in 2023 [1]. Those with localized disease have however benefited from the combination of more effective chemotherapy regimens and continued advances in local therapies including aggressive surgical and radiation techniques with 5-year survival rate that can approach 44% in patients with good prognostic characteristics. Over 20 years ago, CONKO-001 showed that surgery alone is an inadequate treatment for localized PDAC, and thus chemotherapy is now a required component of multimodality therapy for all localized disease, regardless of radiographic "resectability" [2]. With recent advances, in well-selected contemporary patients, reported median overall survival (OS) has increased from 18–24 months historically to 43–54 months in duration [3, 4]. While multimodality therapy is the standard, resection when possible remains the most critical component of this multidisciplinary plan. Even for patients with localized disease, long-term survival without resection is nearly impossible. In this chapter, the workup, staging, and treatment options of borderline resectable (BR) and locally advanced (LA) disease will be reviewed.

Borderline Resectable Pancreatic Adenocarcinoma

Diagnosis and Clinical Staging

The term "borderline resectable" is an everyday part of our vocabulary in describing the clinical stage of PDAC patients, but the standardization of this terminology is

C.-W. D. Tzeng (✉) · L. Prakash
Department of Surgical Oncology, The University of Texas MD Anderson Cancer Center, Houston, TX, USA
e-mail: CDTzeng@mdanderson.org

© The Author(s), under exclusive license to Springer Nature Switzerland AG 2023
S. Pant (ed.), *Pancreatic Cancer*, https://doi.org/10.1007/978-3-031-38623-7_2

19

barely 15 years old. Introduced by Katz et al. at MD Anderson Cancer Center (MDACC), this clinical staging of PDAC combines three aspects of clinical classification into an "A-B-C" system, which stratifies anatomy, biology, and condition, for localized PDAC [5–9]. A patient may have features of one or more of these subtypes. While tumor anatomy at presentation is commonly the focus of surgeons, we argue that to assess the likelihood of a safe margin negative resection (R0) with maximum survival benefit, condition supersedes all and biology trumps anatomy.

As mentioned above, BR type C patients are those with preexisting comorbidities or depressed performance status who have the opportunity for optimization during the neoadjuvant therapy period [10]. BR type B patients present with clinical findings suspicious but not diagnostic of metastatic disease. These include enlarged regional nodes, indeterminate lesions in the liver or lungs, and/or an elevated carbohydrate antigen (CA)19-9 above 500U/ml in the setting of a normal total bilirubin level. Our experience is that less than half of BR type B patients get a resection with the majority manifesting disease progression during the neoadjuvant therapy period, thus saving them from the adverse effects of a futile pancreatectomy [7].

Finally, BR type A is characterized by involvement of the mesenteric vasculature to a limited degree that may require venous or arterial resection at pancreatectomy. MDACC definition differs slightly from NCCN (National Comprehensive Cancer Network) and AHPBA/SSAT/SSO (American Hepato-Pancreato-Biliary Association/Society for Surgery of the Alimentary Tract/Society of Surgical Oncology) and includes encasement of a short segment of the hepatic artery, without evidence of tumor extension to the celiac axis and/or tumor abutment of the SMA [6]. In isolation, BR type A is perhaps the most straightforward for a surgeon requiring a well-planned operation with negative margins, venous reconstruction patency, and leak-free pancreatic reconstruction. Patient selection for surgery is thus based on comprehensive assessment of radiologic, serological, and patient's condition determining improvements or stability in each of these A-B-C categories at each restaging visit [5, 10].

In most of the population, CA19-9 is a useful tumor marker; however, 10% are non-producers due to a genetic mutation in the Lewis antigen gene and another 10% have normal levels regardless of tumor burden. Once the bilirubin is normalized (<2.0 g/dL), CA 19-9 levels as baseline are routinely used to assess future response to chemotherapy and surveillance for recurrence post-resection. Normalization of CA 19-9 during neoadjuvant therapy has been associated with improved outcomes [11, 12]. Staging laparoscopy at a time preceding the planned pancreatectomy may be utilized to obtain clarity on tumor biology when CA 19-9 is rising, but radiological assessment is inconclusive for disease progression. However, in those with normalized CA19-9, the yield of laparoscopy is quite low, and thus laparoscopy performed at a separate time may not be cost-effective [13].

Locally Advanced (Unresectable) Pancreatic Adenocarcinoma

Diagnosis and Clinical Staging

Approximately 35% of patients with PDAC present with LA disease which is traditionally considered unresectable due to local but extensive involvement of adjacent vessels or organs [14]. While definitions vary slightly in the extent of tumor contact, there is consensus on extended tumor to artery interface and/or unreconstructable vein involvement resulting in a high probability of a gross positive margin with attempted upfront resection. This stage presents with a unique therapeutic challenge as the majority of patients do not undergo an attempted resection. The term unresectable however is less preferable to LA because while some tumors remain unamenable to resection even following administration of systemic therapy, 12–35% may successfully "downstage" by retraction of the tumor away from the vessels making a margin-negative resection possible when performed at specialized centers by experienced surgeons [15].

In addition to determining the tumor size, a multiphase contrast-enhanced computed tomography (CT) is the modality of choice for assessment of resectability. However, it may be inadequate in differentiating between residual tumor and fibrosis after induction chemotherapy [16]. Therefore, serum CA 19-9 levels and staging laparoscopy are often used in conjunction with CT scans in making decisions at resection attempts. A diagnostic laparoscopy can be useful since up to 20–30% of patients with LA PDAC are found to have occult peritoneal metastases at diagnosis [17]. LA as a stage includes patients with varying prognoses with survival heavily associated with the ability to undergo resection. In patients with tumors that remain unresectable, the focus is on management of tumor-related symptoms, quality of life, and palliative chemotherapy and/or local therapy to reduce tumor burden and/or offer a systemic therapy break [18].

Multimodality Therapy

Induction Systemic Chemotherapy

Multiagent systemic chemotherapy is considered the standard of care for first-line treatment of patients with BR and LA PDAC. The rationale for use of systemic chemotherapy includes early treatment of micro-metastatic disease, possible tumor shrinkage in size and away from blood vessels, and selection of patients with physiology and tumor biology who would be most likely to benefit from surgery [19]. In well-selected patients, no increased surgical morbidity has been associated with an induction chemotherapy approach [20].

Following favorable results in randomized phase III trials for metastatic disease such as PRODIGE for a combination of 5-fluorouracil, leucovorin calcium (folinic acid), irinotecan hydrochloride, and oxaliplatin (FFX) compared to gemcitabine monotherapy (11.1 vs 6.8 months; $P < 0.001$) [21] and MPACT for albumin-bound paclitaxel plus gemcitabine (GA) (8.7 vs 6.6 months; $P < 0.0001$) [22], these regimens are recommended by NCCN guidelines for patients with advanced localized disease by extrapolation [18, 23]. While the translation of these regimens to earlier stages was empirical, several case series have shown encouraging results suggesting that this more aggressive approach may be useful in patients with BR and LA PDAC resulting in longer median survival, higher resection rates, and significantly better objective response rates [24–26]. Radiographic response to therapy is evaluated using Response Evaluation Criteria in Solid Tumor (RECIST) version 1.1; these guidelines define complete response as the disappearance of the visible tumor, partial response as greater than 30% reduction in tumor load, progressive disease as an increase of greater than 20%, and any disease that does not meet the abovementioned criteria are deemed stable disease [27].

FFX appears to provide better objective response when compared to GA and in one study probable survival benefit in patients that are ultimately unresectable [28]. However, the outcomes are reportedly similar for patients who subsequently undergo surgical resection [24, 28]. In current practice at MDACC, the decision to initiate treatment with FFX or GA is based on multidisciplinary discussion and centered on patients' overall performance status, underlining comorbidity profile and patient preference. If the first-line treatment has been exhausted, not well tolerated, or no improvement/progression is seen in radiographic and/or biological disease, the subsequent treatment recommended is switching between FFX and GA. Current NCCN guidelines recommend all patients with PDAC be tested for germline mutations, alterations in germline BRCA and PALB2 (partner and localizer of BRCA2) are detected in up to 9% of patients with PDAC and platin-based therapy has been shown to be efficacious in these cases [29].

Role of Radiation

The role of radiotherapy (RT) in LA PDAC remains controversial but is recommended in the NCCN guidelines for BR [23]. The rationale for use of RT with neoadjuvant intent is potential treatment of occult disease in regional lymph nodes and sterilization of periphery tumor to increase the likelihood of an R0 resection [30]. In 2018, the results of the first prospective randomized controlled trial comparing upfront surgery and neoadjuvant RT were published and showed a significantly better median survival (21 vs 12 months; $P = 0.028$) in patients treated with chemoradiation [31]. While these findings were not replicated in subsequent randomized trials such as PREOPANC I [32], improved pathological metrics such as rates of R0 resection and decreased risk of locoregional recurrence were reported and collaborated by several retrospective studies [33–35].

Since PDAC is a systemic disease, a chemosensitizer is often administered concomitantly with RT, SCALOP (Selective Chemoradiation in Advanced Localized Pancreatic Cancer) trial showed capecitabine may be preferable to gemcitabine in the context of consolidation [36]. At our institution, we routinely administer sequential treatment with induction chemotherapy prior to radiation either with external

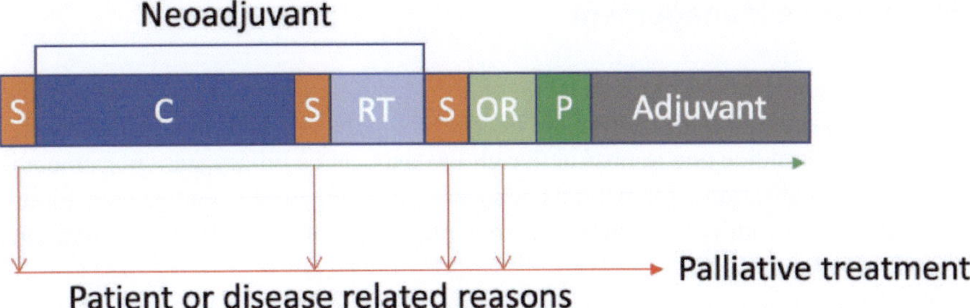

Fig. 2.1 Algorithm for multimodality therapy of borderline and locally advanced patients at MD Anderson Cancer Center. *S* staging or re-staging, *C* chemotherapy, *RT* radiation therapy, *OR* operation room, *P* pancreatectomy

beam RT (EBRT) and more recently stereotactic body RT (SBRT) (Fig. 2.1). While concerns of retroperitoneal fibrosis were induced by RT persist, we have previously shown that neoadjuvant RT is not associated with an increase in 90-day morbidity of mortality and may even reduce the rate of pancreatic fistula following distal pancreatectomy [20].

Pancreatoduodenectomy

While the pancreatoduodenectomy (PD), or "Whipple" procedure, was invented in 1935, it was Dr. John Cameron from Johns Hopkins University who made it a mainstream operation in the United States and internationally [37, 38]. The critical complication for PD's remains the same today—the risk of postoperative pancreatic fistula (POPF), which is the primary cause of subsequent cascade of complications that leads to significant morbidity and even mortality [39]. In the modern surgical setting, patients do not expect to die from elective operations. However, PD mortality remains 7–10% even in the United States and Europe [40, 41], especially in 30–90-day outcomes, not just inpatient mortality. The inability to centralize care for high-risk procedures is perhaps impossible to fix in the US healthcare system [42–44].

Our pancreatic surgery group has advocated a standardized approach to the PD with resection occurring in a clockwise fashion and the reconstruction in a counterclockwise direction [45]. With the six steps of extirpation and three steps of anastomoses, it is easy to reproduce the operation with trainees and OR staff. Reducing complications globally including POPF and death would improve OS for all surgical patients more than any new cytotoxic therapy.

Preoperative Management

Presenting symptoms of PDAC depend on the location of the tumor and the disease stage. Most of the tumors arise in the head of the pancreas with patients often presenting with jaundice due to obstructive cholestasis, and a biliary stent placement is required for palliation. For patients who present with plastic endoscopic biliary stents these are routinely exchanged from plastic to metal to prevent cholangitis episodes [46].

Pre-habilitation programs have been established for all patients regardless of age or performance status [47, 48]. For the elderly, geriatrics evaluations are added as needed to test cognitive function and ensure medical optimization for surgery. Nutrition counseling is required to monitor nutritional status of patients and aid in either building muscle mass in cachectic patients or losing excess fat in obese patients [49, 50]. All these services are available after the initial visit with the surgeon.

Operative Steps

Pancreatoduodenectomy

Step 1 starts with opening the lesser sac to identify the pancreas which can sometimes be buried underneath fat or fibrosis. The middle colic vein can be followed until its insertion into either the superior mesenteric vein (SMV) directly or into a gastrocolic trunk (combined with the gastroepiploic vein). The "tunnel" under the neck of the pancreas is nearby. Many surgeons will ligate the middle colic vein or gastrocolic trunk at this step to avoid avulsion later. Some surgeons will expose the SMV up to the tunnel or below a known area of SMV encasement to ensure a proper landing zone caudally. Step 1 continues with separation of the right colon from the duodenum (as if performing a right hemicolectomy). A formal Cattell-Brasch maneuver is not necessary, but mobilization of the entire right colon is ideal to show the duodenum.

Step 2 is the Kocher maneuver to mobilize the pancreatic head, to expose the inferior vena cava (IVC), and to find the superior mesenteric artery (SMA) coming off the aorta.

Step 3 is the portal dissection. Removing the station 8a lymph node, known as the common hepatic artery (CHA) node, exposes the CHA adventitia to then find the proper hepatic artery (PHA). The right gastric artery comes off superficially and can be ligated. At the CHA-PHA junction is where the gastroduodenal artery (GDA) comes off. Once an adequate length of GDA stump is safely exposed, it can be doubly ligated and/or sutured before dividing. Upon the division of the GDA, the PHA can be lifted to allow dissection of nodal issue between the CHA/PHA and portal vein (PV) below. On the right side of the hepatoduodenal ligament, the station 12p nodes (portocaval nodes) can be lowered toward the specimen. Then the common bile duct (CBD) is encircled. One must reconfirm that there is no aberrant right hepatic artery running posterolateral. The CBD can be divided at or near the cystic duct junction. The metal or plastic biliary stent can be removed and cultured. Some surgeons will do a bile and stent culture to direct antibiotics as needed.

Step 4 is the division of the distal stomach or proximal duodenum. There is no oncologic difference in these techniques. There is debate on their respective impact on postoperative delayed gastric emptying (DGE) [51]. We tend to create a 2-staple line Hofmeister shelf to sew the eventual gastrojejunostomy to the lower shelf at a natural angle that facilitates stomach emptying.

Step 5 is the mobilization of the ligament of Treitz and division of the proximal jejunum about 10–15 cm from the ligament.

Step 6 is the most important and longest step of the operation. At this time, the pancreatic neck tunnel is created carefully using instruments. Sometimes, if there is tumor at the portal vein (PV)–superior mesenteric vein (SMV)–splenic vein junction, the planned transection line will need to be a tunnel over the splenic vein under the true pancreatic body for an "extended" PD. Once the pancreas is divided with cautery, the pancreatic duct can be identified at this point. If too small to see, often looking on the specimen side will offer a clue. The SMV is then skeletonized on its anterior surface all the way to the turn of the duodenum. If not already, the gastro-colic trunk will be ligated and divided. The lower extent of the dissection starts at the 1st (posterior most often) jejunal vein. For tumors stuck to the SMV, this 1st jejunal vein will need to be ligated. However, for AR tumors, this can be saved, noting that there are usually several tiny veins draining the uncinate which should be carefully taken with energy device or ties. Once cleared, this is the most distal point of SMA dissection to start. For the SMA, there are two general philosophies of exposure. Once can go from the right side "under the SMV" while pulling the SMV to the left or from the left side (straight down) while pulling the SMV to the right. The latter requires division of all colic drainage into the SMV to allow the SMV to be pulled to the right with vessel loops.

A SMA-first technique is useful to learn for BR tumors that are abutting or attached to the PV-SMV. The author's personal preference is to do a right-sided approach with dissection of the SMA base off the aorta first to clear its lymphatic tissue and to show the "target area" for dissection from the distal SMA. Going back to the distal SMA, the peri-adventitial tissue (which wraps the artery like insulation) should be dissected until the bare white adventitia is seen. In obese patients or men with a lot of visceral fat, this dissection can be several mm. There are studies which show tumor cells penetrating past the uncinate to this tissue along the SMA [52]. That is why simple palpation and using an energy device or stapler along this peri-arterial tissue without seeing bare white adventitia is leaving a gross margin behind. The surgeon can march "up" cephalad along the bare SMA, clearing at least 180 degrees but never 360°, looking for at least 1–2 additional pancreatic arteries. This completes the SMA-first approach.

The remaining specimen is hanging on the SMV-PV. The lymphatics under the PV can be cleared with an energy device or ties. Then, there is the actual pancreas head (and tumor) on the SMV-PV. The question is whether the tumor can be dissected off sharply with scissors in a desmoplastic plane (with or without vein clamping) or if a true vein resection is needed. If a true vein resection is needed, will it be a side repair, side patch, end-to-end, or interposition graft. If there is going to be flow narrowing, we discourage side repairs. Side patches are rarely used as well. End-to-end repairs preserve laminar flow the best. Interposition grafts (preferentially using the internal jugular vein) are reserved for long distances of 5 cm or more. Table 2.1 outlines pearls and pitfalls of these six steps.

Table 2.1 Key maneuvers of MD Anderson's six-step pancreatoduodenectomy

Steps	Key maneuvers	Tips	Trouble
1	Lesser sac entry and right colon mobilization	• Follow middle colic vein to SMV • Expose pancreatic head and separate duodenum from mesocolon	• Middle colic vein avulsion leads to SMV bleed • SMV tear from aggressive traction before full exposure
2	Kocher maneuver	• Show the IVC, left renal vein, aortocaval groove • Undermine pancreatic head until you feel the SMA	• Not dissecting to the aorta-SMA takeoff and thus not ready for Step 6 later
3	Portal dissection	• Follow PHA and CHA to find GDA • Check right posterolateral to bile duct for aberrant right hepatic artery	• Ligating GDA before ensuring proper hepatic artery or dipping right hepatic artery protected • Dividing bile duct before ensuring aberrant RHA is protected
4	Distal gastrectomy	• Create "shelf" for reconstruction angle when stapling	• Bleeding from gastric staple line
5	Proximal jejunum transection	• Staple minimal length of jejunum	• Resecting too little or too much jejunum
6	Pancreatic division and SMA–SMV (retroperitoneal) dissection	• Not all SMV-PV tunnels are the same. Watch for tumor into neck thus requiring division at the proximal body • SMA dissection begins distally at the level of the posterior jejunal vein • Bare white SMA should be exposed for 180 degrees	• Finger dissection in the tunnel can rip the SMV-PV • Poor SMA visualization leading to pancreatic artery tears coming off SMA, which then requires sutures directly on SMA arteriotomies • Tumor venous congestion if all venous tributaries are ligated before SMA branches taken • Leaving tissue along SMA due to fear of SMA injury • Stapler or energy device along the uncinate while leaving visible tissue on SMA

Considerations for Vein Involvement

For a minimal vein involvement situation such as BR tumors with downsizing to abutment without invasion, there is sometimes a need to clamp the SMV–PV–splenic vein junction with a side-biting clamp for the final detachment of the pancreatic head from the SMV-PV. The side-biting clamp preserves partial venous flow to the liver for the anesthesiologist. This is not as physiologically stressful as a "Pringle" maneuver since the hepatic artery remains open the whole time you are working on the SMV–PV–splenic vein. If the clamp can be placed caudal to the splenic vein, then the PV gets at least that flow while only the SMV is restricted. We typically circulate 50 units of heparin per kg intravenously for 5 min before vein clamping and manipulation. Scissors will often be sufficient to take the specimen off the SMV-PV for abutment cases, and a bit of true wall can be taken for true invasion cases. This can be repaired while clamped with no blood loss and no time pressures. For end-to-end repairs, one clamp will be needed on each side, ideally at least 1 cm away from the cut lines since the vein wall retracts to the clamp more than expected. The tumor and vein can be cut off quickly. The vein reconstruction can be running with an air knot for "growth" or interrupted sutures for guaranteed alignment. For interposition grafts, we use the internal jugular vein (usually the left since many patients have their ports on the right side), while others have reported using the left renal vein or non-native grafts (cadaveric or bovine pericardium). With no valves in an IJ graft, there is no concern about the direction. We typically sew the trickier end first. After reconstruction, the heparin is not reversed. We use prophylactic low molecular weight heparin as our standard plus an 81 mg aspirin for vein resection.

If margins for the pancreatic neck and CBD are positive on frozen section, they can be re-cut if safely feasible. There is debate [53] about the oncologic value of this, and thus we never convert a positive margin into a total pancreatectomy. However, if an additional centimeter-wide piece of pancreas can be safely mobilized off the splenic vein while not hitting the splenic artery, then we will often send this extra piece for permanent section.

Reconstruction

Reconstruction Step 1 is the pancreaticojejunostomy. We typically recommend a 2-layer modified Blumgart technique in which a 3-0 polypropylene straightened needle is used to wrap the bowel around the cut end of the pancreas to sandwich it around the inner duct-to-mucosa reconstruction. The inner layer is created using interrupted 5-0 polydioxanone suture (or similar) in a symmetric, radial arrangement to allow easy alignment and reproducibility for trainees.

Reconstruction Step 2 is the hepaticojejunostomy. Good blood supply at the tip of the cut bile duct is confirmed before a single layer 5-0 polydioxanone suture anastomosis is created about 10cm distal to the pancreatic anastomosis. The key is symmetry as in a clock face. We tuck the falciform flap between the pancreatic and biliary anastomoses, sometimes tying it down, to protect the GDA stump.

Reconstruction Step 3 is the gastrojejunostomy which is performed either with a handsewn technique when open and stapler when minimally invasive. Of note, the Pittsburgh group has used video analyses to suggest a large (4.5 cm), handsewn, angle anastomosis for ideal DGE mitigation [54]. Otherwise, there is no international standard on this final reconstruction [51].

Finally, as a group, we placed a drain over the anastomoses. The drain fluid amylase is measured on postoperative days 1 and 3, and we will remove them as early as possible, ideally by day 3 [55]. This follows the international consensus that a drain, if placed, should be removed in a timely fashion by day 3 when feasible [56, 57].

Distal Pancreatectomy

The goals of a distal pancreatectomy include a safe resection and recovery, negative margins, and nodal clearance. One can choose direction for dissection: either lateral to medial or medial to lateral. BR tumor anatomy often dictates vein resection to be done as the final step, which is similar to hanging the pancreatic head on the SMV-PV during a PD with vein resection.

Gaining access to the lesser sac is similar to Step 1 of a PD. Exposure of the pancreas and spleen, including seeing the inferior border of the pancreas and the lower pole of the spleen, helps define the boundaries of the resection. This was accomplished by taking down the splenic flexure and allowing gravity to relax the transverse mesocolon and left colon out of the pancreatic resection bed. The stomach can be retracted after using an energy device to go through the omentum between the stomach and spleen. The gastroepiploic arcade should be carefully preserved until the short gastrics to save collateral gastric blood flow.

Sometimes due to tumor encasement of the splenic vein, there is sinistral (left-sided) hypertension. To prevent variceal bleeding during the operation, the splenic artery can be tied off early in the operation at any place where it is visible. Often for neck and body tumors, access to the proximal splenic artery and celiac is not safely seen early in the case. In these situations, a simple tie or figure-8 ligation of the distal splenic artery in the pancreatic tail can decompress the spleen and varices.

To find the splenic artery, remove the station 8 (CHA) node, follow the CHA to its base, and see the celiac trifurcation and the splenic artery takeoff. Once an adequate splenic artery stump is dissected, double ligation can be accomplished as with the GDA in the PD. A stapler can be used if the splenic artery is large enough for enough staples to land on the stump.

If AR with no vein resection, the SMV-PV tunnel can be made, and the neck is transected using cautery or stapler with the caveat that the stapler should not be used in neck tumors with close margins because the stapler (and its reinforcement) uses up several millimeters of margin. Then the splenic vein can be ligated at its insertion to the SMV-PV. If there is narrowing right at the confluence, a side-biting clamp can be used to cut the splenic vein stump and repair the side wall of the PV. The rest of the dissection is medial to lateral, taking the retroperitoneal tissue and the lymphatic tissue above the splenic artery as part of the nodal clearance. For BR tumors, it may be easier to go lateral to medial and leave the last part attached to the PV-SMV.

For a pancreatic neck which was transected with cautery, we use direct suture ligation of a visible duct (6-0 polypropylene) with pledget-reinforced U-stitches to tamponade the cut edge of the pancreas. Despite no international consensus [58], drain placement is routine with postoperative days 1 and 3 drain amylases checked per our published thresholds [55].

Histopathological Assessment

Margin status is evaluated by frozen section intraoperatively and then by permanent section using College of American Pathologist (CAP) and American Joint Committee on Cancer (AJCC) guidelines [30]. The SMA margin, or retroperitoneal margin, along with pancreatic neck margin and the bile duct transection margin forms the three standardized margins that should be checked in a PD [45]. The pancreatic neck and bile duct transection margin are considered positive if tumor cells are present at the ink. Because of the perceived risk of injuring the SMA, some surgeons use only palpation to feel and not see the SMA and then use energy devices to seal the peri-adventitial tissue or even staple or cut through uncinate tissue to avoid skeletonizing the dissection plane directly on the bare white adventitia. However, dissecting along the plane will ensure the optimal tumor clearance and find all pancreatic branches to tears on the SMA. The SMA margin should be standardly sectioned to note the actual distance from the cut surface, with tumor cells present <1 mm of inked edge considered R1 resections [59].

Adjuvant Therapy

In patients who receive surgery upfront, adjuvant therapy is the standard of care. However, the benefit of additional postoperative therapy remains debated. In one large retrospective study, receiving postoperative therapy had a positive effect in anatomically and borderline resectable PDAC patients who had been treated with chemotherapy [60]. Prospective trials that randomize patients after resection to additional postoperative therapy vs. surveillance are required to answer the question of additional therapy after neoadjuvant therapy. Until then, this decision will depend on patient and provider biases.

Postoperative Management

Enhanced Recovery

At MDACC since July 2011, all patients who undergo a pancreatectomy are prospectively monitored for adverse events for at least 90 days [61]. We initiated our Risk Stratified Pancreatectomy Clinical Pathways for pancreas surgery in 2016 which immediately led to a reduction in our postoperative length of stay (LOS) to 6 days from 9 days (similar to national databases) [62]. Three separate pathways were created to fast-track patients according to their postoperative complications risk determined by histology, BMI (Body Mass Index), and pancreatic duct diameter. We review our data systemically and have continued iterative changes to reduce usage of nasogastric tube, earlier drain removal, and substantially decreasing our total and discharge opioid usage [63–65]. Current updates continue to reduce LOS and opioid use further and incorporating pathways for minimally invasive surgeries [66].

Postoperative pancreatic fistula (POPF) is the most commonly studied complication due to its high downstream morbidity and mortality despite decades of work to mitigate its risk [67]. Despite the creation and validation of risk scores, excellent surgical technique remains the ideal mitigation technique. Even a randomized trial that showed reduction of POPF from use of pasireotide has not been externally validated and was limited by its original cohort of high and low risk patients and definitions of POPF which were different than international guidelines [68, 69]. Our group stopped using pasireotide following internal analysis showing no changes in our outcome, especially in our low risk "Green" pathway patients [70].

Blood transfusions and major postoperative complications may have sequelae beyond worse short-term surgical outcomes and impact quality of life and oncological outcomes [71, 72]. Retrospective data have shown associations with worse survival in patients after blood transfusions and major complications, especially patients treated with upfront surgery. Whether this is due to delays or omissions of adjuvant therapy and/or immunological effects due to untreated micro-metastatic disease is unknown [73, 74]. A "successful" operation is not judged solely on the pathology report, but rather the conduct of the operation itself and avoiding complications.

Quality Measures

Surgeons play an integral role in ensuring a quality outcome. While current quality metrics are pathology based, we are working towards future metrics involving patient-centered outcomes such as return to baseline function and intended oncologic therapy.

As with other gastrointestinal cancers such as colon and stomach, pancreatectomy has recommended lymph node harvest rates based on PD ($\geq$15) vs. distal pancreatectomy ($\geq$10) [75]. Obviously, nodal harvest rates do not tell the whole story regarding surgical quality, but as with other cancers, it is used as a surrogate for regional clearance.

Future Directions

Systematic improvements must be continually made to increase the proportion of patients who are optimized before undertaking a pancreatic resection. Centralization or regionalization to high-volume centers seems ideal in theory, although this is unrealistic in a free choice healthcare system and a wide geographic area as we have in the United States [76]. Finally, outcomes need to be iteratively studied at each center and within each state and region so that surgeons can have feedback for individual improvement through a learning health system model.

References

1. Siegel RL, Miller KD, Wagle NS, Jemal A. Cancer statistics, 2023. CA Cancer J Clin. 2023;73(1):17–48.
2. Oettle H, Post S, Neuhaus P, et al. Adjuvant chemotherapy with gemcitabine vs observation in patients undergoing curative-intent resection of pancreatic cancer: a randomized controlled trial. JAMA. 2007;297(3):267–77.
3. Conroy T, Hammel P, Hebbar M, et al. FOLFIRINOX or gemcitabine as adjuvant therapy for pancreatic cancer. N Engl J Med. 2018;379(25):2395–406.
4. Cloyd JM, Katz MH, Prakash L, et al. Preoperative therapy and pancreatoduodenectomy for pancreatic ductal adenocarcinoma: a 25-year single-institution experience. J Gastrointest Surg. 2017;21(1):164–74.
5. Katz MH, Ahmad S, Nelson H. Borderline resectable pancreatic cancer: pushing the technical limits of surgery. Bull Am Coll Surg. 2013;98(1):61–3.
6. Katz MH, Pisters PW, Evans DB, et al. Borderline resectable pancreatic cancer: the importance of this emerging stage of disease. J Am Coll Surg. 2008;206(5):833–46; discussion 846-838.
7. Tzeng CW, Fleming JB, Lee JE, et al. Defined clinical classifications are associated with outcome of patients with anatomically resectable pancreatic adenocarcinoma treated with neoadjuvant therapy. Ann Surg Oncol. 2012;19(6):2045–53.
8. Isaji S, Mizuno S, Windsor JA, et al. International consensus on definition and criteria of borderline resectable pancreatic ductal adenocarcinoma 2017. Pancreatology. 2018;18(1):2–11.
9. Hayasaki A, Isaji S, Kishiwada M, et al. Survival analysis in patients with pancreatic ductal adenocarcinoma undergoing chemoradiotherapy followed by surgery according to the international consensus on the 2017 definition of borderline resectable cancer. Cancer. 2018;10(3):65.
10. Tzeng CW, Katz MH, Fleming JB, et al. Morbidity and mortality after pancreaticoduodenectomy in patients with borderline resectable type C clinical classification. J Gastrointest Surg. 2014;18(1):146–55; discussion 155–146.
11. Newhook TE, Vreeland TJ, Griffin JF, et al. Prognosis associated with CA19-9 response dynamics and normalization during neoadjuvant therapy in resected pancreatic adenocarcinoma. Ann Surg. 2023;277(3):484–90.
12. Tzeng CW, Balachandran A, Ahmad M, et al. Serum carbohydrate antigen 19-9 represents a marker of response to neoadjuvant therapy in patients with borderline resectable pancreatic cancer. HPB. 2014;16(5):430–8.

13. Satoi S, Murakami Y, Motoi F, et al. Reappraisal of peritoneal washing cytology in 984 patients with pancreatic ductal adenocarcinoma who underwent margin-negative resection. J Gastrointest Surg. 2015;19(1):6–14; discussion 14.
14. Suker M, Beumer BR, Sadot E, et al. FOLFIRINOX for locally advanced pancreatic cancer: a systematic review and patient-level meta-analysis. Lancet Oncol. 2016;17(6):801–10.
15. van Veldhuisen E, van den Oord C, Brada LJ, et al. Locally advanced pancreatic cancer: work-up, staging, and local intervention strategies. Cancer. 2019;11(7):976.
16. Katz MH, Fleming JB, Bhosale P, et al. Response of borderline resectable pancreatic cancer to neoadjuvant therapy is not reflected by radiographic indicators. Cancer. 2012;118(23):5749–56.
17. Jimenez RE, Warshaw AL, Rattner DW, Willett CG, McGrath D, Fernandez-del CC. Impact of laparoscopic staging in the treatment of pancreatic cancer. Arch Surg. 2000;135(4):409–14; discussion 414-405.
18. Gourgou-Bourgade S, Bascoul-Mollevi C, Desseigne F, et al. Impact of FOLFIRINOX compared with gemcitabine on quality of life in patients with metastatic pancreatic cancer: results from the PRODIGE 4/ACCORD 11 randomized trial. J Clin Oncol. 2013;31(1):23–9.
19. Perri G, Prakash L, Katz MHG. Defining and treating borderline resectable pancreatic cancer. Curr Treat Options in Oncol. 2020;21(9):71.
20. Denbo JW, Bruno ML, Cloyd JM, et al. Preoperative chemoradiation for pancreatic adenocarcinoma does not increase 90-day postoperative morbidity or mortality. J Gastrointest Surg. 2016;20(12):1975–85.
21. Conroy T, Desseigne F, Ychou M, et al. FOLFIRINOX versus gemcitabine for metastatic pancreatic cancer. N Engl J Med. 2011;364(19):1817–25.
22. Von Hoff DD, Ervin T, Arena FP, et al. Increased survival in pancreatic cancer with nab-paclitaxel plus gemcitabine. N Engl J Med. 2013;369(18):1691–703.
23. Tempero MA, Malafa MP, Al-Hawary M, et al. Pancreatic adenocarcinoma, version 2.2021, NCCN clinical practice guidelines in oncology. J Natl Compr Cancer Netw. 2021;19(4):439–57.
24. Perri G, Prakash LR, Katz MHG. Response to preoperative therapy in localized pancreatic cancer. Front Oncol. 2020;10:516.
25. Ferrone CR, Marchegiani G, Hong TS, et al. Radiological and surgical implications of neoadjuvant treatment with FOLFIRINOX for locally advanced and borderline resectable pancreatic cancer. Ann Surg. 2015;261(1):12–7.
26. Blazer M, Wu C, Goldberg RM, et al. Neoadjuvant modified (m) FOLFIRINOX for locally advanced unresectable (LAPC) and borderline resectable (BRPC) adenocarcinoma of the pancreas. Ann Surg Oncol. 2015;22(4):1153–9.
27. Eisenhauer EA, Therasse P, Bogaerts J, et al. New response evaluation criteria in solid tumours: revised RECIST guideline (version 1.1). Eur J Cancer. 2009;45(2):228–47.
28. Eshmuminov D, Aminjonov B, Palm RF, et al. FOLFIRINOX or gemcitabine-based chemotherapy for borderline resectable and locally advanced pancreatic cancer: a multi-institutional, patient-level, meta-analysis and systematic review. Ann Surg Oncol. 2023;30(7):4417–28.
29. Wong W, Raufi AG, Safyan RA, Bates SE, Manji GA. BRCA Mutations in pancreas cancer: spectrum, current management, challenges and future prospects. Cancer Manag Res. 2020;12:2731–42.
30. Prakash LR, Katz MHG. Multimodality management of borderline resectable pancreatic adenocarcinoma. Chin Clin Oncol. 2017;6(3):27.
31. Jang JY, Han Y, Lee H, et al. Oncological benefits of neoadjuvant chemoradiation with gemcitabine versus upfront surgery in patients with borderline resectable pancreatic cancer: a prospective, randomized, open-label, multicenter phase 2/3 trial. Ann Surg. 2018;268(2):215–22.
32. Versteijne E, Suker M, Groothuis K, et al. Preoperative chemoradiotherapy versus immediate surgery for resectable and borderline resectable pancreatic cancer: results of the Dutch randomized phase III PREOPANC trial. J Clin Oncol. 2020;38(16):1763–73.
33. Cloyd JM, Crane CH, Koay EJ, et al. Impact of hypofractionated and standard fractionated chemoradiation before pancreatoduodenectomy for pancreatic ductal adenocarcinoma. Cancer. 2016;122(17):2671–9.

34. Katz MH, Wang H, Balachandran A, et al. Effect of neoadjuvant chemoradiation and surgical technique on recurrence of localized pancreatic cancer. J Gastrointest Surg. 2012;16(1):68–78; discussion 78-69.
35. Stokes JB, Nolan NJ, Stelow EB, et al. Preoperative capecitabine and concurrent radiation for borderline resectable pancreatic cancer. Ann Surg Oncol. 2011;18(3):619–27.
36. Mukherjee S, Hurt CN, Bridgewater J, et al. Gemcitabine-based or capecitabine-based chemoradiotherapy for locally advanced pancreatic cancer (SCALOP): a multicentre, randomised, phase 2 trial. Lancet Oncol. 2013;14(4):317–26.
37. Cameron JL, He J. Two thousand consecutive pancreaticoduodenectomies. J Am Coll Surg. 2015;220(4):530–6.
38. Winter JM, Brennan MF, Tang LH, et al. Survival after resection of pancreatic adenocarcinoma: results from a single institution over three decades. Ann Surg Oncol. 2012;19(1):169–75.
39. Bassi C, Marchegiani G, Dervenis C, et al. The 2016 update of the International Study Group (ISGPS) definition and grading of postoperative pancreatic fistula: 11 years after. Surgery. 2017;161(3):584–91.
40. van Hilst J, de Rooij T, Bosscha K, et al. Laparoscopic versus open pancreatoduodenectomy for pancreatic or periampullary tumours (LEOPARD-2): a multicentre, patient-blinded, randomised controlled phase 2/3 trial. Lancet Gastroenterol Hepatol. 2019;4(3):199–207.
41. Nassour I, Winters SB, Hoehn R, et al. Long-term oncologic outcomes of robotic and open pancreatectomy in a national cohort of pancreatic adenocarcinoma. J Surg Oncol. 2020;122(2):234–42.
42. Bilimoria KY, Bentrem DJ, Lillemoe KD, Talamonti MS, Ko CY. Assessment of pancreatic cancer care in the United States based on formally developed quality indicators. J Natl Cancer Inst. 2009;101(12):848–59.
43. Bilimoria KY, Bentrem DJ, Ko CY, et al. Multimodality therapy for pancreatic cancer in the U.S.: utilization, outcomes, and the effect of hospital volume. Cancer. 2007;110(6):1227–34.
44. Bilimoria KY, Bentrem DJ, Ko CY, Stewart AK, Winchester DP, Talamonti MS. National failure to operate on early stage pancreatic cancer. Ann Surg. 2007;246(2):173–80.
45. Katz MH, Lee JE, Pisters PW, Skoracki R, Tamm E, Fleming JB. Retroperitoneal dissection in patients with borderline resectable pancreatic cancer: operative principles and techniques. J Am Coll Surg. 2012;215(2):e11–8.
46. Kim BJ, Prakash L, Narula N, et al. Contemporary analysis of complications associated with biliary stents during neoadjuvant therapy for pancreatic adenocarcinoma. HPB. 2019;21(6):662–8.
47. Parker NH, Basen-Engquist K, Rubin ML, et al. Factors influencing exercise following pancreatic tumor resection. Ann Surg Oncol. 2020;28:2299–309.
48. Parker NH, Lee RE, O'Connor DP, et al. Supports and barriers to home-based physical activity during preoperative treatment of pancreatic cancer: a mixed-methods study. J Phys Act Health. 2019;16(12):1113–22.
49. Cloyd JM, Nogueras-Gonzalez GM, Prakash LR, et al. Anthropometric changes in patients with pancreatic cancer undergoing preoperative therapy and pancreatoduodenectomy. J Gastrointest Surg. 2018;22(4):703–12.
50. Ngo-Huang A, Holmes HM, des Bordes JKA, et al. Association between frailty syndrome and survival in patients with pancreatic adenocarcinoma. Cancer Med. 2019;8(6):2867–76.
51. Klaiber U, Probst P, Strobel O, et al. Meta-analysis of delayed gastric emptying after pylorus-preserving versus pylorus-resecting pancreatoduodenectomy. Br J Surg. 2018;105(4):339–49.
52. Liu L, Katz MH, Lee SM, et al. Superior mesenteric artery margin of posttherapy pancreaticoduodenectomy and prognosis in patients with pancreatic ductal adenocarcinoma. Am J Surg Pathol. 2015;39(10):1395–403.
53. Kooby DA, Lad NL, Squires MH 3rd, et al. Value of intraoperative neck margin analysis during Whipple for pancreatic adenocarcinoma: a multicenter analysis of 1399 patients. Ann Surg. 2014;260(3):494–501; discussion 501-493.
54. Jung JP, Zenati MS, Dhir M, et al. Use of video review to investigate technical factors that may be associated with delayed gastric emptying after pancreaticoduodenectomy. JAMA Surg. 2018;153(10):918–27.

55. Newhook TE, Vega EA, Vreeland TJ, et al. Early postoperative drain fluid amylase in risk-stratified patients promotes tailored post-pancreatectomy drain management and potential for accelerated discharge. Surgery. 2020;167(2):442–7.
56. Beane JD, House MG, Ceppa EP, Dolejs SC, Pitt HA. Variation in drain management after pancreatoduodenectomy: early versus delayed removal. Ann Surg. 2019;269(4):718–24.
57. Fagenson AM, Gleeson EM, Lau KKN, Karachristos A, Pitt HA. Early drain removal after hepatectomy: an underutilized management strategy. HPB. 2020;22(10):1463–70.
58. Ecker BL, McMillan MT, Allegrini V, et al. Risk factors and mitigation strategies for pancreatic fistula after distal pancreatectomy: analysis of 2026 resections from the International, Multi-institutional Distal Pancreatectomy Study Group. Ann Surg. 2019;269(1):143–9.
59. Vreeland TJ, Katz MHG. Pancreatoduodenectomy: superior mesenteric artery dissection. American College of Surgeons. 2020. https://www.facs.org/quality-programs/cancer/acs-crp/oscs/video. Accessed 14 September 2020.
60. Perri G, Prakash L, Qiao W, et al. Postoperative chemotherapy benefits patients who received preoperative therapy and pancreatectomy for pancreatic adenocarcinoma. Ann Surg. 2020;271(6):996–1002.
61. Schwarz L, Bruno M, Parker NH, et al. Active surveillance for adverse events within 90 days: the standard for reporting surgical outcomes after pancreatectomy. Ann Surg Oncol. 2015;22(11):3522–9.
62. Denbo JW, Bruno M, Dewhurst W, et al. Risk-stratified clinical pathways decrease the duration of hospitalization and costs of perioperative care after pancreatectomy. Surgery. 2018;164(3):424–31.
63. Ayabe RI, Prakash LR, Bruno ML, et al. Differential gains in surgical outcomes for high-risk vs low-risk pancreatoduodenectomy with successive refinements of risk-stratified care pathways. J Am Coll Surg. 2023;237(1):4–12.
64. Newton AD, Newhook TE, Bruno ML, et al. Iterative changes in risk-stratified pancreatectomy clinical pathways and accelerated discharge after pancreaticoduodenectomy. J Gastrointest Surg. 2022;26(5):1054–62.
65. Arango NP, Prakash LR, Chiang YJ, et al. Risk-stratified pancreatectomy clinical pathway implementation and delayed gastric emptying. J Gastrointest Surg. 2021;25(9):2221–30.
66. Witt RG, Hirata Y, Prakash LR, et al. Comparative analysis of opioid use between robotic and open pancreatoduodenectomy. J Hepatobiliary Pancreat Sci. 2023;30(4):523–31.
67. Bassi C, Dervenis C, Butturini G, et al. Postoperative pancreatic fistula: an international study group (ISGPF) definition. Surgery. 2005;138(1):8–13.
68. Allen PJ, Gonen M, Brennan MF, et al. Pasireotide for postoperative pancreatic fistula. N Engl J Med. 2014;370(21):2014–22.
69. Liu X, Pausch T, Probst P, et al. Efficacy of pasireotide for prevention of postoperative pancreatic fistula in pancreatic surgery: a systematic review and meta-analysis. J Gastrointest Surg. 2020;24(6):1421–9.
70. Denbo JW, Slack RS, Bruno M, et al. Selective perioperative administration of pasireotide is more cost-effective than routine administration for pancreatic fistula prophylaxis. J Gastrointest Surg. 2017;21(4):636–46.
71. Sutton JM, Kooby DA, Wilson GC, et al. Perioperative blood transfusion is associated with decreased survival in patients undergoing pancreaticoduodenectomy for pancreatic adenocarcinoma: a multi-institutional study. J Gastrointest Surg. 2014;18(9):1575–87.
72. Tzeng CW, Tran Cao HS, Lee JE, et al. Treatment sequencing for resectable pancreatic cancer: influence of early metastases and surgical complications on multimodality therapy completion and survival. J Gastrointest Surg. 2014;18(1):16–24; discussion 24-15.
73. Wu W, He J, Cameron JL, et al. The impact of postoperative complications on the administration of adjuvant therapy following pancreaticoduodenectomy for adenocarcinoma. Ann Surg Oncol. 2014;21(9):2873–81.
74. Merkow RP, Bilimoria KY, Tomlinson JS, et al. Postoperative complications reduce adjuvant chemotherapy use in resectable pancreatic cancer. Ann Surg. 2013;275(5):979–84.

75. Tol JA, Gouma DJ, Bassi C, et al. Definition of a standard lymphadenectomy in surgery for pancreatic ductal adenocarcinoma: a consensus statement by the International Study Group on Pancreatic Surgery (ISGPS). Surgery. 2014;156(3):591–600.
76. Birkmeyer JD, Finlayson SR, Tosteson AN, Sharp SM, Warshaw AL, Fisher ES. Effect of hospital volume on in-hospital mortality with pancreaticoduodenectomy. Surgery. 1999;125(3):250–6.

Radiation Therapy for Pancreatic Cancer: Current and Evolving Paradigms

3

Gohar Shahwar Manzar, Joseph Abi Jaoude,
Cullen M. Taniguchi, Albert C. Koong, Eugene J. Koay,
and Ethan B. Ludmir

Background

Ionizing radiation therapy (RT) uses high-energy rays or subatomic particles to impart DNA damage to decrease cell multiplicity and survival. RT is a component of treatment for 50% of all patients diagnosed with cancer and, together with surgery and systemic therapy, forms a pillar of cancer treatment [1]. External beam RT has been utilized for various indications in the treatment of pancreatic cancer, with evolving paradigms that potentiate both curative and palliative intent in both neoadjuvant and adjuvant settings. Across these disease states, RT may be beneficial as curative preoperative therapy, consolidative local therapy for locally advanced pancreatic cancer (LAPC), a palliative modality, and potentially even to consolidate oligometastatic disease in well-selected patients on clinical trials.

Gohar Shahwar Manzar and Joseph Abi Jaoude contributed equally with all other contributors.

G. S. Manzar · J. A. Jaoude
Department of Radiation Oncology, The University of Texas MD Anderson Cancer Center, Houston, TX, USA

C. M. Taniguchi · A. C. Koong · E. J. Koay
Department of Gastrointestinal Radiation Oncology, The University of Texas MD Anderson Cancer Center, Houston, TX, USA

E. B. Ludmir (✉)
Department of Gastrointestinal Radiation Oncology, The University of Texas MD Anderson Cancer Center, Houston, TX, USA

Department of Biostatistics, The University of Texas MD Anderson Cancer Center, Houston, TX, USA
e-mail: ebludmir@mdanderson.org

S. Pant (ed.), *Pancreatic Cancer*, https://doi.org/10.1007/978-3-031-38623-7_3

While only 15% of patients with pancreatic cancer are deemed to have resectable disease at upfront staging, up to 50% of patients harbor localized disease that is not yet metastatic [2]. Even for the considerable proportion of patients with metastatic disease, patients often succumb to or suffer from complications of local progression [3]. Local progression from pancreatic tumors may lead to severe morbidity and compromises quality of life from pain, biliary obstruction, associated infection, or invasion of adjacent luminal tissues. In this regard, especially for non-metastatic disease, RT is commonly used to optimize local control and limits the morbidity and mortality from local disease recurrence or progression. Neoadjuvant RT offers improved clinical outcomes in patients eligible for surgery and is associated with higher rates of negative surgical margins. RT is also useful in patients presenting with tumors that are difficult to resect surgically, as local treatment with RT often downstages tumors enough to allow for surgical resection.

While RT is typically delivered in the neoadjuvant setting in combination with chemotherapy, choice of radiation modality, dose, and fractionation across clinical contexts remains challenging owing to lack of clear consensus within the pancreatic cancer radiation oncology community and diverse choice of doses and fractionation schemes in prospective trials. In this chapter, we offer an overview of the literature on radiation therapy across stages and states of pancreatic cancer (Fig. 3.1). We present technological considerations in RT delivery for pancreatic cancer, along with future directions as the role for RT continues to evolve.

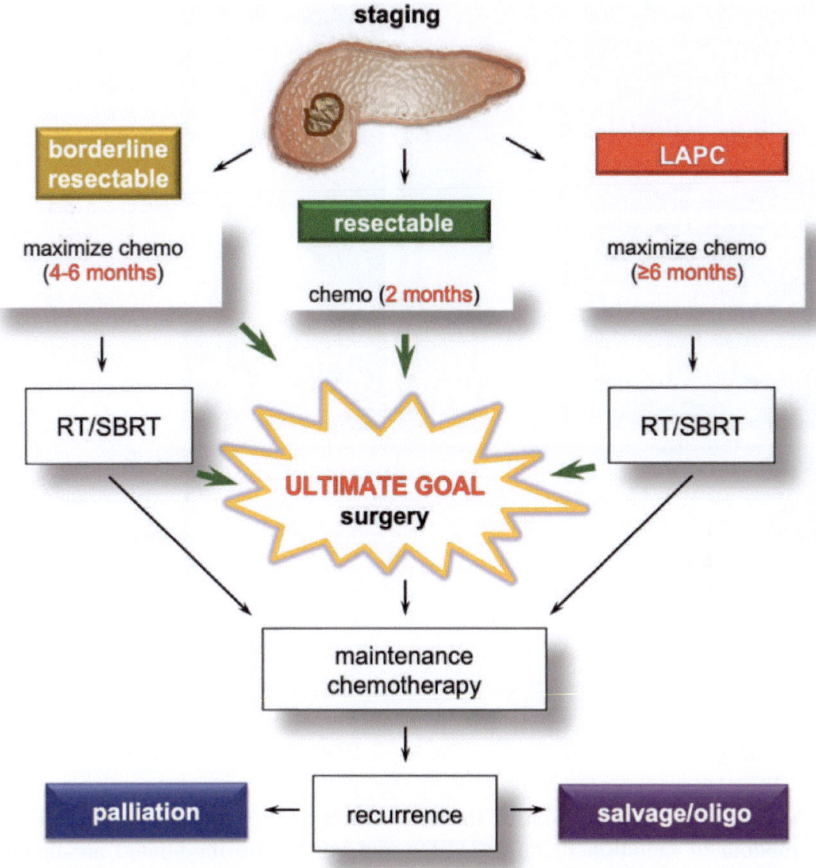

Fig. 3.1 Treatment paradigm incorporating multimodality management of pancreatic cancer across different stages of disease

Primer on Modern Radiotherapy

External beam radiation therapy is generated by a linear accelerator, which delivers ionizing beams of RT conformally shaped to target areas of disease and avoid normal tissues [4]. While some RT effects are due to direct DNA damage, most RT manifests DNA damage through indirect generation of free radicals in an oxygen-dependent process. These ionizing beams may consist of high energy photon rays more commonly, or mass-bearing particles. Within the arena of photon therapy, a primitive form is known as 3D radiation, which involves straight beams of radiation directed in various angles by the gantry, allowing for concentration of dose where the beams intersect at the target [5].

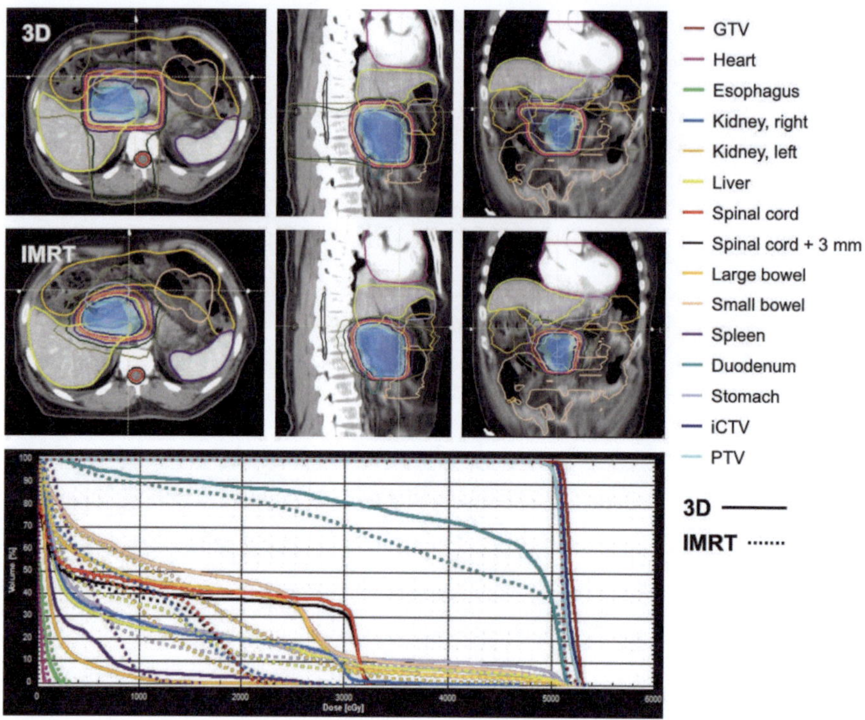

Fig. 3.2 Sample treatment plan comparison of 3D vs. IMRT for pancreatic cancer

Building on this, photon-based therapies that are more advanced include intensity modulated radiation therapy (IMRT) and volumetric modulated arc therapy (VMAT). IMRT utilizes photon energy and delivers treatment using multiple radiation beams at varying intensities and discrete angles, with multi-leaf collimation at each angle to allow for change of the shape as the gantry turns [6]. This modality is particularly valuable when treating targets with complex shapes, rendering it suitable to treat pancreatic tumors (Fig. 3.2) [7].

VMAT is a state-of-the-art photon-based radiation modality that also utilizes photon energy but allows for continuous modulation of the multi-leaf collimation across a high number of radiation beams delivered across an uninterrupted arc in a relatively short period [8]. While data regarding VMAT is relatively limited, one dosimetric study comparing VMAT, IMRT, and 3D RT showed that VMAT could achieve adequate treatment planning, while having better sparing of organs at risk (OARs), particularly the duodenum and small bowel [9]. In this study, VMAT was also associated with fewer cases of grade 3+ gastrointestinal toxicity [9]. 3D RT, IMRT, or VMAT in conventional doses is typically given in 1.8–2 Gy equivalents per day, rendering fractionation schedules that can span up to 5.5 weeks of daily weekday treatment. On occasion, these fractions can be abbreviated with higher doses per fraction, a term called hypofractionation, which has been investigated with some promise in pancreatic cancer.

To this end, more exaggerated hypofractionation has its own classification as a unique therapeutic modality known as stereotactic body radiation therapy (SBRT). SBRT is an advanced radiation modality that delivers highly conformal radiation with significant dose escalation to ≥5 Gy per fraction, compared to conventional fractionation with ≤3 Gy per dose [10]. Owing to the higher doses per fraction, SBRT allows for treatment delivery in a shorter fractionation schedule, typically consisting of 1–5 fractions. However, the high doses per fraction with SBRT limit the role of this modality in patients for whom distance between disease and organs at risk is adequate to avoid severe radiation-induced toxicity. As such, treatment planning with SBRT is similar to that of IMRT, but necessitates smaller margins and higher fidelity, complex image-guidance while delivering treatment. As we will discuss below, studies in BR pancreatic cancer and LAPC show some promising signals with SBRT, but progress is needed to (1) clarify its impact on patient outcomes, (2) optimize patient selection, and (3) refine the indications for treatment with this modality.

Finally, a different form of ionizing radiation involves the use of particles, such as protons, neutrons, or carbon ions, which have a higher relative biological effectiveness compared to photons [11]. These beams manifest radiation with minimal or no exit dose due to targeted fall-off of radiation beams at precise distances, enabling dose escalation to the target while minimizing dose to normal tissue beyond the target [11]. Proton and carbon beams also create a "Bragg peak" with high dose at the distal end of the radiation beam. A disadvantage with these types of RT is uncertainty of the "hot" beam edge, which may be precarious in the setting of pancreatic cancer treatment due to the sensitivity of lumen in neighboring bowel.

Resectable and Borderline Resectable Pancreatic Cancer

One-fourth of all patients with pancreatic cancer present with resectable or borderline resectable (BR) disease (Fig. 3.3) [12].

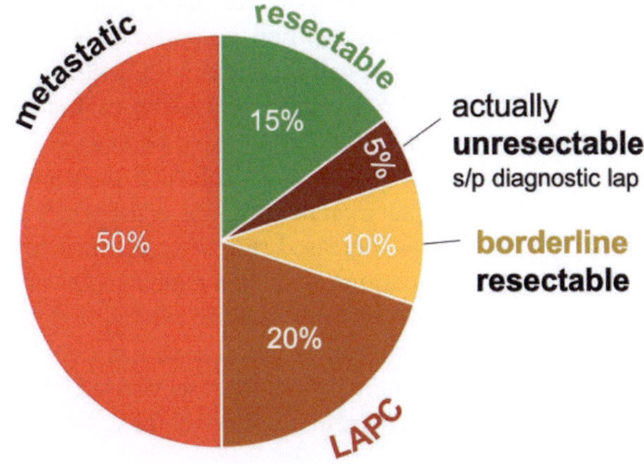

Fig. 3.3 Proportion of pancreatic cancer in staging categories at diagnosis

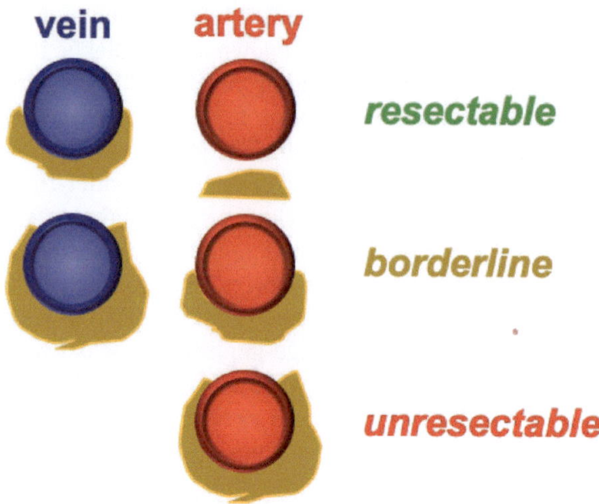

Fig. 3.4 Degree of vessel involvement by pancreatic cancer defines resectability

While TNM staging has been devised for pancreatic cancer, patient disposition to treatment is primarily guided by CT-guided delineation of resectability [13]. While definitions vary across regional sites of the oncology community, resectable disease generally denotes disease that does not involve surrounding arteries, with a tumor-vessel interface (TVI) that does not exceed 180° (Fig. 3.4). BR pancreatic cancer describes a tumor confined to the pancreas, with limited encirclement of adjacent vasculature (<180° encirclement of the SMA or celiac trunk), and in situations where vascular reconstruction is feasible. The concept of BR pancreatic cancer has emerged in the past decade to encompass a distinct spectrum of disease for which resection is relatively more likely to yield a microscopic positive margin (R1 resection), ascribed to the relationship between the pancreatic cancer and neighboring blood vessels [13].

Other key factors that influence the disposition of patients include features that signify a higher risk for the presence of occult metastatic disease. This includes patients with elevated CA 19-9 (>100 U/mL) levels or symptomatic patients with extreme pain or weight loss [14]. Advanced disease may also be noted on imaging with a tumor larger than 3 cm or the presence of suspicious lymph nodes. These factors may suggest optimal treatment with neoadjuvant systemic therapy prior to consideration of surgery to ensure that a surgical outcome is worthwhile.

Surgery is widely considered the sole potentially curative modality for patients with pancreatic cancer who can achieve a margin-negative resection [14]. The potential of positive surgical margins has consistently portended poorer overall survival (OS), as well as increased risk of tumor recurrence and progression [15]. In ESPAC-1, positive margins conferred a median OS of 11 months vs. 17 months in patients with negative margins [16]. Similarly, a single-institution report of 1175 patients with pancreatic cancer found a median OS of 14 months with margin-positive resection vs. 20 months with R0 resection [17]. Microscopic tumor at resection margins offered a detriment to survival to a similar extent as grossly positive

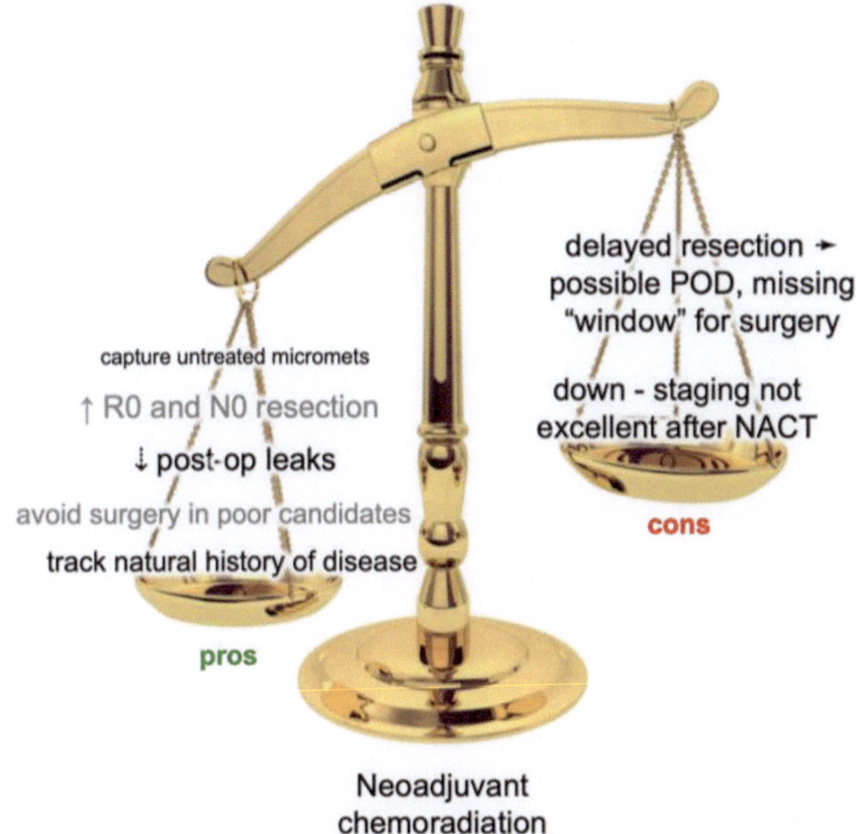

Fig. 3.5 Proposed and observed benefits with the neoadjuvant chemoradiation approach for the treatment of pancreatic cancer

margins [15]. The importance of negative margins in determining post-resection survival has spurred investigation of preoperative therapy, including RT, for patients with resectable and borderline resectable pancreatic cancer. The aims of this approach are to optimize the odds of margin-negative resection, decrease the risk of postoperative relapse, and improve the likelihood of longer-term disease control (Fig. 3.5).

The safety and feasibility of neoadjuvant RT was assessed in a 1997 prospective aggregate analysis comparing clinical outcomes and toxicity between preoperative and postoperative chemoradiation in patients with resectable disease. This trial demonstrated that preoperative RT was safe and associated with similar outcomes to postoperative treatment [18]. Another single center trial included patients with resectable pancreatic cancer treated with preoperative chemoradiation with 5-fluorouracil [19]. Patients who did not progress 1 month after treatment underwent surgical resection with intraoperative RT [19]. The trial showed that

Table 3.1 Summary of outcomes with modern neoadjuvant chemoradiation (CRT) optimizing the resectability and survival of patients with pancreatic cancer

PREOPANC	Surgery ($n = 127$)	Neoadjuvant CRT ($n = 119$)	p-value
Resection rate	72%	61%	0.065
R0 resection rate	40%	71%	<0.001
Serious adverse events	41%	62%	0.28
5-year OS	6.5% (95% CI: 3.1–13.7)	20.5% (95% CI: 14.2–29.8)	0.025
Hazard ratio	0.73 (95% CI: 0.56–0.96)		
Jang et al. [21]	Surgery ($n = 18$)	Neoadjuvant CRT ($n = 17$)	p-value
Resection rate	78.3%	63%	>0.05
R0 resection rate	26.1%	51.8%	0.01
Grade ≥ 3 adverse events	11.1%	7.7%	0.643
2-year OS	40.7%	26.1%	0.028
ESPAC-5F1	Surgery ($n = 32$)	Neoadjuvant CRT ($n = 56$)	p-value
Resection rate	62%	55%	0.668
R0 resection rate	15%	23%	0.721
Adverse events	–	17.6%	0.28
1-year OS	40% (95% CI: 26–62%)	77% (95% CI: 66–89%)	<0.001
Hazard atio	0.27 (95% CI: 0.13–0.55)		

neoadjuvant RT was safe and associated with minimal toxicity, with only 9% of patients experiencing grade 3 toxicity [19].

More recently, the PREOPANC trial was a phase III randomized controlled trial that included patients with resectable or BR pancreatic cancer [20], generating significant support for the neoadjuvant treatment approach (Table 3.1). In this well-balanced multicenter intention-to-treat trial, patients were randomized at diagnosis to either receive preoperative chemoradiotherapy followed by surgery and adjuvant gemcitabine or undergo upfront surgery followed by similar adjuvant therapy [20]. RT was delivered with 36 Gy in 15 fractions. Of note, resectability in this trial was defined according to the Dutch criteria, which are more stringent and thus may exclude patients that may be considered resectable or borderline resectable by conventional understanding in the United States. In the PREOPANC trial, resectable disease was defined as $\leq 90°$ involvement of the superior mesenteric vein (SMV) or portal vein (PV) and no contact of the superior mesenteric artery (SMA). Borderline resectable pancreatic cancer was defined as $\leq 270°$ involvement of the SMV or PV, and $\leq 90°$ involvement of the celiac axis, hepatic artery, or SMA. Other exclusion criteria included T1 tumors.

With the primary endpoint of OS in the long-term follow-up report, neoadjuvant chemoradiation followed by surgery demonstrated improvement compared to upfront surgery, with a 5-year OS of 20% vs. 6% ($p < 0.001$). In the initial report, the OS benefit was only seen in the per-protocol analysis as well as in patients with BR pancreatic cancer. Significantly, patients who received neoadjuvant chemoradiation had improved rates of R0 resections (71% vs. 40% for patients treated with upfront surgery, $p < 0.001$) [20]. Moreover, the addition of preoperative RT was also associated with improved local-regional control and disease-free survival [20].

These results favoring neoadjuvant RT were supported by a multicenter phase II/III randomized controlled trial published in 2018 by Jang et al. [21]. This study randomized patients with BR pancreatic cancer to receive either neoadjuvant gemcitabine-based chemoradiation followed by surgery or upfront surgery [21]. The trial showed that patients receiving neoadjuvant therapy had improved 2-year survival rates, with a median survival of 21 months vs. 12 months in the upfront surgery arm, and higher 2-year survival at 40.7% vs. 26.1% [21]. Patients in the neoadjuvant chemoradiation arm also had double the rate of R0 resection compared to patients treated with upfront surgery at 52% vs. 26% [21].

The evidence discussed thus far highlights the compelling role for preoperative chemoradiation in treating patients with resectable or BR pancreatic cancer. However, the aforementioned trials did not compare neoadjuvant chemoradiation to chemotherapy alone. The Alliance A021501 trial included 126 patients with BR pancreatic cancer and randomized them to either neoadjuvant mFOLFIRINOX alone for 8 cycles, or neoadjuvant mFOLFIRINOX for 7 cycles followed by high-dose, specialized RT preceding surgery in patients without disease progression, followed by adjuvant mFOLFOX6. The RT used in this trial consisted of either SBRT to 33–40 Gy in 5 fractions or hypofractionated RT to a dose of 25 Gy in 5 fractions in other patients [22]. This supremely conformal, focused, and high-dose radiation treatment was used for its potential to achieve sharper dose fall-off gradients to normal tissue, deliver higher doses to areas at elevated risk for R1 resection, and decrease the time to resection.

This phase II trial paradoxically showed—considering the other work noted above—that patients receiving chemoradiation had worse 18-month OS and surgical outcomes compared to patients treated with chemotherapy alone [23]. The radiation treatment arm of this trial was closed prematurely at the interim futility analysis based on stopping rules rooted on a concerningly high margin-positive resection rate observed in the preoperative RT arm. As a result, statistical requirements to conclude efficacy were unable to be met, and there was inadequate power for comparison. Nevertheless, the trial included two patients that showed pathologic complete response, and both of those patients were in the radiation arm. The suggestion from the Alliance trial was that not all patients with BR pancreatic cancer would benefit from local treatment with neoadjuvant SBRT.

Notably, this Alliance trial randomized patients at the start of all preoperative therapy, not after the initial mFOLFIRNOX. Thus, there were imbalances between the two arms by the time these patients came to SBRT vs. undergoing one more cycle of mFOLFIRNOX. The design of this trial was counterintuitive to the treatment paradigm generally instituted, in which local therapy with curative intent, such as surgery, is offered only to thoughtfully selected patients who have no disease progression or signs of distant failure. Similar to how surgical resection is not typically a treatment that these mutable patients are blindly randomized to, highly conformal SBRT may not offer a favorable outcome if patients are not carefully chosen and thus poised to benefit from such a local treatment modality. In other words, "routine" disposition of patients to SBRT is not meant to be done, and patients undergoing such therapy must be carefully selected. Additionally, the participating trial institutions had varying comfort levels with this highly specialized form of RT. The allowance for an inadequate RT dose of 25 Gy in 5 fractions rendered

Table 3.2 Summary of outcomes with adjuvant chemotherapy or radiation in patients with pancreatic cancer

Trial	*n*	Postoperative regimens	R1 status (%)	LN "+" (%)	Median OS
GITSG 91-73 [26]	43	Observation *vs.* 5-FU + RT → maintenance 5-FU	0	28	11 *vs.* 20 mos
EORTC 40891 [27]	218	Observation *vs.* bolus 5-FU + RT	22	50	12.6 *vs.* 17.1 mos
ESPAC-1 [16]	541	Observation *vs.* bolus 5-FU *vs.* 5-FU + RT *vs.* 5-FU + RT + consolidative 5-FU	18	54	16.9 (obs) *vs.* 21.6 (chemo only) *vs.* 19.9 (CRT) *vs.* 14.2 mos (CRT + chemo)
RTOG 9704 [28]	442	5-FU → CRT (5-FU) → 5-FU *vs.* gem → CRT (5-FU) → gem	34	66	16.7 (5-FU) *vs.* 18.8 mos (gem)
ECOG-FFCD [25]	74	Gem vs. gem → gem + RT	3	70	9.2 *vs.* 11.1 mos

potential subtherapeutic variability that may have compromised treatment outcomes. Ultimately, this trial underscores the crucial need for a close multidisciplinary approach between radiologists, radiation, surgical, and medical oncologists to select which patients to treat with RT and also highlights the need for prognostic biomarkers to aid in optimal patient selection.

Historical efforts to supplement surgery with multimodality treatment involved adjuvant combinations of chemotherapy or RT [24], which lacked the benefit of prognostication and optimal patient selection that is apparent with a neoadjuvant approach described above. Mixed results were seen in the adjuvant setting, with several trials showing minimal improvement in OS when comparing chemoradiation with chemotherapy alone (ECOG-FFCD [25]) or observation (GITSG 91-73 [26], EORTC 40891 [27]), detailed in Table 3.2. The ESPAC-1 trial published in 2001 remains among the most well-known adjuvant therapy trials but is widely criticized for its methodology [16]. It demonstrated a benefit of adjuvant chemotherapy alone (median OS 15.5 months with observation vs. 21 months with chemotherapy) and suggested a surprising detriment to survival with adjuvant chemoradiation (median OS 15.9 months with chemoradiation vs. 17.9 months with chemotherapy alone). These findings require contextualization considering several trial shortcomings, including lack of loyalty to protocol assignment, with incomplete chemotherapy in 50% of the patients, subtherapeutic RT in 33% of the patients, and 33% of patients in observation and chemotherapy alone arms who unexpectedly underwent RT [16]. There was also selection bias in treatment choice, with physician input incorporated into randomization and background therapy, inconsistent RT dose, and no central quality assurance of RT. Thus, it is challenging to appreciate the true value or lack thereof regarding adjuvant RT based on these trials. The ongoing Phase III trial RTOG 0848 may address this open-ended question [28, 29], but notably does not utilize modern systemic therapy.

Overall, in contrast to neoadjuvant chemoradiation, postoperative RT appears to be more toxic due to anastomoses and bowel falling into the radiation field [30]. Chemotherapy may be given before the RT to avoid the additional toxicity of concurrent treatment. Ultimately, indications for postoperative radiation therapy in pancreatic cancer are rare and typically include a positive margin at the time of surgery in a patient for whom there is no evidence of relapse or increasing CA-19-9 after the completion of the adjuvant chemotherapy. We hold a relatively high threshold to offer adjuvant RT and instead attempt to reserve RT as an option in the future in the event of localized local or regional relapse.

As a result of the above evidence, ASTRO has issued conditional recommendations [31] for neoadjuvant treatment of BR pancreatic cancer with 45–50.4 Gy in 180–200 cGy fractions, or dose escalation with SBRT to 30–33 Gy in 6–6.6 Gy fractions with a consideration for a simultaneous integrated boost of up to 40 Gy to the tumor vessel interface. However, in light of the Alliance trial results described above [23], our practice has not involved dose escalation for neoadjuvant RT in the treatment of BR pancreatic cancer.

In practice, RT dosing and fractionation in resectable and BR pancreatic cancer is decided on a case-by-case basis with multidisciplinary discussion, prognostication, and physician preference (Fig. 3.6a).

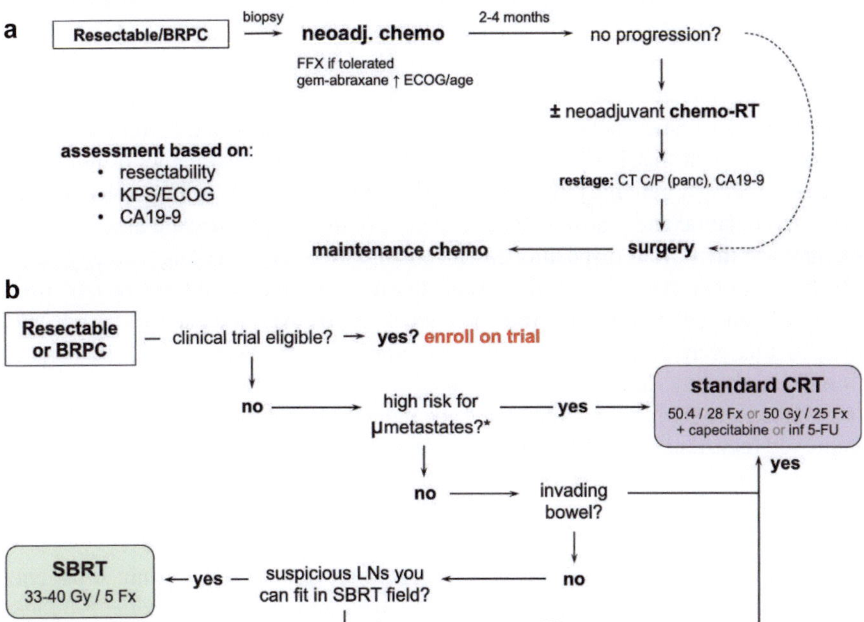

Fig. 3.6 Treatment approach for the management of resectable or borderline resectable pancreatic cancer. (**a**) Resectable and BR pancreatic cancer via biopsy. (**b**) Resectable and BR pancreatic cancer clinical trail

Within this treatment paradigm, we consider radiation regimens based on the expected biology and anatomy of disease (Fig. 3.6b). A preoperative radiation regimen that may be considered for patients who are deemed almost certain surgical candidates involves 3D radiation or intensity modulated radiation therapy (IMRT) delivered to a dose of 30 Gy in 10 fractions [32]. A more standard approach is to deliver 50 Gy in 25 fractions with IMRT. For high-risk patients, prognostication for the risk of micrometastases affords the possibility that surgery may not transpire. High-risk disease is defined by the presence of elevated CA 19-9 levels, symptoms, or features of advanced disease on imaging. For these patients, treatment is favored with long-course concurrent chemoradiation to 50–50.4 Gy in 180–200 cGy fractions, as opposed to highly conformal SBRT that is suboptimal by itself by way of its narrow treatment field. SBRT would also be contraindicated in patients with tumor invading bowel, or for whom the proximity of tumor to luminal structures is ≤1 cm.

Locally Advanced Pancreatic Cancer

Patients with locally advanced pancreatic cancer (LAPC) present with localized disease that has extensive involvement of major neighboring vessels, making surgical resection infeasible. For LAPC patients, both systemic therapy and RT tend to be utilized. Systemic therapy is typically delivered first, allowing for a "test of biology" to address both the primary tumor while assessing risk of distant metastatic disease progression or development, since this is the primary driving pattern of spread for pancreatic ductal adenocarcinoma [30]. Typically, the current treatment paradigm is such that LAPC patients are treated with approximately 6 months of systemic therapy, generally with multi-agent regimens, such as FOLFIRINOX or gemcitabine/abraxane. Those without evidence of distant progression after systemic therapy are then often dispositioned to consolidative RT [33]. This strategy helps identify patients that have occult distant disease and that would not benefit from RT. Krishnan et al. published a retrospective series of over 300 patients with LAPC in 2007 that were either treated with chemoradiation or gemcitabine-based induction chemotherapy followed by RT, with 85% of patients treated to a dose of 30 Gy in 10 fractions [33]. Patients treated with induction chemotherapy before RT had improved recurrence patterns and overall survival, suggesting that induction chemotherapy could help identify patients with rapid distant progression and exclude those from receiving additional unnecessary and potentially harmful local treatment [33]. The benefit of RT in addition to chemotherapy in patients with LAPC was also suggested in another retrospective study by Huguet et al., which examined patients enrolled on the GERCOR studies and divided them into two cohorts: patients treated with chemotherapy alone or chemoradiation to a dose of 55 Gy in 30 fractions as well as a conedown 10 Gy boost over 8 fractions delivered in the last 2 weeks of treatment [34]. Results of this study showed that adding RT after disease control with initial chemotherapy leads to improved progression-free and overall survival [34].

Promising results from those two studies were later tested in the LAP07 phase III randomized controlled trial [35]. The trial included patients with LAPC that were treated with 4 months of chemotherapy and showed stable disease. After successful induction chemotherapy, patients were randomized to continue chemotherapy alone or receiving chemoradiation to a dose of 54 Gy in 30 fractions. While the trial did not show any difference in overall survival between the two arms, patients treated with additional RT had lower rates of local progression (32% vs. 46% in the chemotherapy-only arm), without having a significant increase in grade 3+ toxicity [35]. The decrease in local progression with chemoradiation was not correlated to quality of life, which was not examined in this cohort, unfortunately. Other notable limitations of the trial included the presence of RT deviations in 60% of the chemoradiation arm, 20% of the chemotherapy arm undergoing RT, and the use of gemcitabine, which was later found to be inferior to FOLFIRINOX.

One of the main challenges in treating LAPC is that pancreatic adenocarcinoma is often very radioresistant, and hence higher doses of RT are needed to achieve proper local control [36]. However, dose escalation can be very challenging with LAPC owing to potential toxicity to nearby organs at risk, particularly the duodenum. One of the first studies to analyze dose escalation in LAPC was a study by Krishnan et al., which included patients treated with induction chemotherapy followed by IMRT [36]. The study compared clinical outcomes between patients receiving RT with biologically effective dose (BED) higher or lower than 70 Gy, demonstrating that a BED >70 Gy was associated with improved overall survival and local-regional control. Furthermore, the study showed that treatment with BED >70 Gy was safe, as no additional toxicity was noted in this cohort of patients [36]. A more recent study by Reyngold et al. assessed the role of ablative RT in LAPC. Patients in this study were treated with a BED of 98 Gy and showed promising overall survival (median OS from diagnosis: 26.8 months, median OS from RT: 18.4 months) and local-regional failure rates (12-month: 17.6%, 24-month: 32.8%), while still showing tolerable treatment toxicity [37]. Results from those studies show safe and promising clinical outcomes for dose escalation in LAPC [38]. A phase I/II trial is currently assessing the role of radiomodulation with GC4419 in LAPC to allow for further dose escalation with SBRT [39]. Patients on this trial are treated with 50–55 Gy in 5 fractions in the hope of achieving stronger local control and better overall survival rates, while still showing tolerable toxicity. Conceptually, results suggest that currently, these dose-escalated regimens potentially confer some advantage over conventional doses. However, this remains driven primarily by nonrandomized data, and these observations should be interpreted with caution.

For LAPC, we employ a management schema that considers the array of possible RT regimens specified by anatomical considerations and coverage goals (Fig. 3.7). There are a variety of approaches in terms of dose-fractionation, ranging from conventional fractionation to 50.4 Gy in 28 fractions, or dose escalation with either SBRT to a dose of 50–55 Gy in 5 fractions, or hypofractionated ablative RT to 67.5 Gy in 15 fractions, or ablative RT consisting of 75 Gy in 25 fractions. Ultimately,

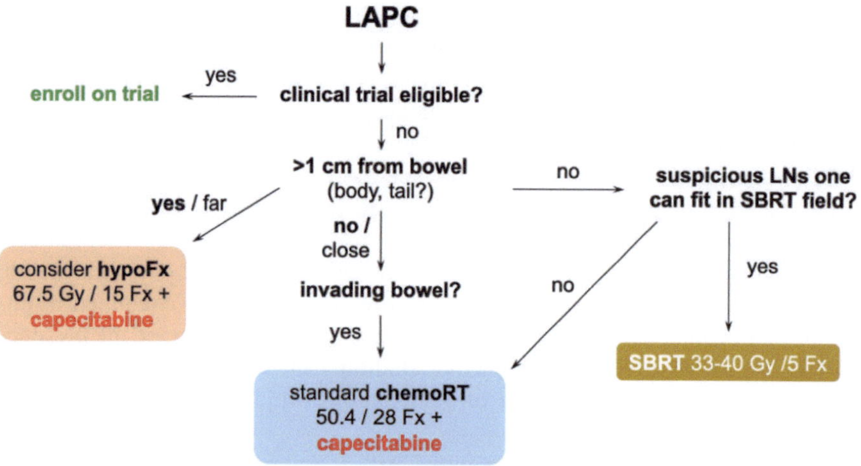

Fig. 3.7 Treatment approach for the management of locally advanced pancreatic cancer

while further progress is needed to demonstrate overarching benefits of dose-escalated RT for LAPC compared to no radiation or conventional RT, the strategy appears promising.

Palliative Radiation Therapy

Palliative RT is occasionally offered to patients with pancreatic cancer presenting with poor performance status or metastatic pancreatic cancer. Patients may present with celiac artery compression syndrome, which may manifest as a constellation of symptoms, including epigastric pain shooting to the back, "gnawing" abdominal pain, or nausea and emesis [40]. The main aim in such patients would be to alleviate abdominal or epigastric pain caused by the tumor compressing upon the celiac artery or plexus. Nevertheless, limited data exist on the effectiveness of palliative RT in patients with advanced pancreatic cancer.

A small retrospective study in Poland analyzed the role of palliative RT in 31 patients with unresectable pancreatic cancer, where 26 (84%) had M0, and 5 (16%) had M1 disease, and the median ECOG performance status was 2 [41]. Patients in this study were treated with 6–30 Gy delivered over 1–10 fractions. Treatment was overall well-tolerated, with no finding of treatment interruptions or hospitalization due to toxicity. Only mild early toxicity was noted in 30% of patients, and no grade 3+ early or late toxicity was seen in the study. The study also analyzed pain intensity associated with pancreatic cancer prior to RT, and 1 month after treatment. Approximately half of the patients (55%) achieved good pain control after palliative RT with no pharmacological therapy, and 40% of patients reduced their analgesic requirements [41]. In another prospective study, Tian et al. enrolled 31 patients with stage III or IV pancreatic cancer and treated them with palliative RT using 40–42 Gy over 7–10 fractions [42]. The trial was designed to assess quality of life using patient reported outcomes and showed that a considerable proportion of patients showed improvements in pain following therapy [42]. According to the BPI, 57% of patients had significant improvement in abdominal symptoms 1 month after therapy, and 43% of patients reported improvement in daily life parameters such as mood, sleep, walking, and work [42].

As noted above, the radioresistance of pancreatic ductal adenocarcinoma may mean that even palliative approaches require dose escalation to optimally palliate patients. A recent single-arm phase II trial was published in 2022 that assessed the use of single-fraction celiac plexus radiosurgery in patients with upper abdominal cancers (including pancreatic cancer), who presented with moderate to severe retro-peritoneal pain [43]. The study evaluated 18 patients that were treated with a single fraction of 25 Gy to the entire retroperitoneal celiac plexus. Results from this trial show that single-fraction radiosurgery was safe and tolerable with only mild grade 1–2 toxicity noted. Moreover, 84% of patients reported pain improvement 3 weeks after therapy, with median pain level decreased from 6/10 at baseline to 3/10. Further improvements were noted 6 weeks post-RT, with median pain level at 2.8/10 on the pain scale and 4 patients with complete pain eradication [43]. This study offers very promising results for the use of single-fraction radiosurgery as an option for celiac plexus pain palliation, especially compared to nerve block, which is an invasive procedure with a variable success rate and complication risks, including hypotension.

Future Directions and Promising Technologies

Recent interest has emerged in the use of particle therapy to treat pancreatic cancer. More specifically, proton and carbon therapy both show promising results in treat-ing localized pancreatic cancer. Proton therapy enables the delivery of radiation with minimal or no exit dose, allowing for target dose escalation, while minimizing radiation side effects to normal tissue beyond the target [11]. A phase I/II trial by Terashima et al. assessed the role of proton therapy in patients with LAPC using either 50 Gy in 25 fractions, 67.5 Gy in 25 fractions, or 70.2 Gy in 26 fractions and demonstrated similar clinical outcomes to historical data with minimal grade 3+ toxicity [44, 45]. Carbon therapy is a rarer form of particle-based therapy that has shown promising results in many disease sites, including pancreatic cancer. The use of carbon ions offers some advantages over proton- and photon-based RT [46]. Carbon ions have a higher relative biological effectiveness and less lateral scatter-ing. Moreover, carbon ion therapy has a relatively lower oxygen enhancement ratio, signifying that the tumor-killing effect of carbon ions is independent of tumor oxy-genation [47]. This property of carbon therapy is particularly desirable in pancreatic malignancies, owing to the hypoxic and radioresistant tumor environments of pan-creatic cancer. Despite some data showing the effectiveness of carbon therapy, the major limitation of this therapy is its limited availability in cancer centers, with only a few centers offering this modality across the world. The CIPHER trial is an ongoing phase III trial comparing the use of IMRT to carbon therapy in patients with LAPC, and will help oncologists better understand the role of carbon therapy in pancreatic cancer (NCT03536182) [48].

Lastly, FLASH-RT is a modern advanced radiation modality that delivers ultra-high doses of radiation to the tumor target, while sparing neighboring normal tissue, a phenomena being dubbed the FLASH effect [49]. While conventional radiation modalities deliver radiation at rates smaller than 0.1 Gy/s, radiation delivery with FLASH-RT is typically higher than 40 Gy/s [50, 51]. FLASH therapy has been studied in preclinical models with promising results in multiple disease sites, and FLASH-RT could potentially be well-suited to treat pancreatic cancer owing to its highly radioresistant tumor environment and close proximity of organs at risk [52]. Currently, IntraOp Medical has developed an electron-based FLASH LINAC that has recently been approved for use in preclinical and human studies and will hopefully be tested in future clinical trials, but will likely be focused on treatment of dermal malignancies initially due to its shallow penetration [53]. Future studies could include intraoperative FLASH but that is speculative at this time. Proton FLASH studies are ongoing. Higher energies may allow for treatment of deep-seated tumors, including possibly pancreatic cancer.

To bolster the therapeutic ratio, combinatorial approaches are being investigated that use either radiosensitizers to amplify radiation target effects or radioprotectors to fortify adjacent normal tissue, including the stomach or duodenum. As introduced above, a phase I/II trial is determining if radioprotection by GC4419 may enable dose escalation with SBRT in LAPC [39]. Furthermore, non-SBRT courses of RT are routinely delivered in our practice with concurrent radiosensitization with capecitabine. Nanoparticles are also being developed to support these aims, with taggable cargo that may influence the therapeutic ratio by synergizing with radiation to enhance target sensitivity [54].

Finally, there is dynamic evolution in our traditional understanding of metastatic disease as being incurable [55]. A frontier of investigation is devoted to the potential conversion of patients with a few sites of metastatic disease into a curable state. The EXTEND trial is an ongoing phase II trial at the MD Anderson Cancer Center that will assess the role of RT in patients with solid tumors, including pancreatic cancer, presenting with oligometastatic disease, and will hopefully shed light on the role of consolidative RT in the oligometastatic setting (NCT03599765) [56].

Summary

RT is a common modality in pancreatic cancer regardless of disease stage. Neoadjuvant therapy is commonly employed in patients with resectable or BR pancreatic cancer, with the principal goal of sterilizing surgical margins after resection and, by doing so, limiting tumor recurrence after surgery. Patients with LAPC also benefit from local treatment with RT to delay or abrogate local progression, especially since surgical resection is often not feasible in those patients. Owing to the aggressive nature of LAPC, dose escalation is typically needed to achieve proper local control and improve survival rates. Limited data exist on the effectiveness of palliative RT in advanced pancreatic cancer. However, owing to promising results from small retrospective and prospective studies, this approach could be considered to alleviate pain in patients with LAPC or metastatic pancreatic cancer. Lastly, while photon-based therapy has shown positive results in the past, modern therapies including particle-based RT and FLASH-RT are being studied. Cutting edge ongoing investigation may help identify the role of these modern therapies in the treatment of pancreatic cancer.

References

1. Baskar R, Lee KA, Yeo R, Yeoh KW. Cancer and radiation therapy: current advances and future directions. Int J Med Sci. 2012;9:193–9.
2. Coveler AL, Herman JM, Simeone DM, Chiorean EG. Localized pancreatic cancer: multidisciplinary management. Am Soc Clin Oncol Educ Book. 2016;35:217–26.
3. Iacobuzio-Donahue CA, Fu B, Yachida S, et al. DPC4 gene status of the primary carcinoma correlates with patterns of failure in patients with pancreatic cancer. J Clin Oncol. 2009;27:1806–13.
4. Berman AT, Plastaras JP, Vapiwala N. Radiation oncology: a primer for medical students. J Cancer Educ. 2013;28:547–53.
5. Prasad S, Cambridge L, Huguet F, et al. Intensity modulated radiation therapy reduces gastrointestinal toxicity in locally advanced pancreas cancer. Pract Radiat Oncol. 2016;6:78–85.
6. Taylor A, Powell ME. Intensity-modulated radiotherapy–what is it? Cancer Imaging. 2004;4:68–73.
7. Intensity Modulated Radiation Therapy Collaborative Working G. Intensity-modulated radiotherapy: current status and issues of interest. Int J Radiat Oncol Biol Phys. 2001;51:880–914.
8. Manzar GS, Lester SC, Routman DM, et al. Comparative analysis of acute toxicities and patient reported outcomes between intensity-modulated proton therapy (IMPT) and volumetric modulated arc therapy (VMAT) for the treatment of oropharyngeal cancer. Radiother Oncol. 2020;147:64–74.
9. Jin L, Wang R, Jiang S, et al. Dosimetric and clinical toxicity comparison of critical organ preservation with three-dimensional conformal radiotherapy, intensity-modulated radiotherapy, and RapidArc for the treatment of locally advanced cancer of the pancreatic head. Curr Oncol. 2016;23:41–8.
10. Abi Jaoude J, Kouzy R, Nguyen ND, et al. Radiation therapy for patients with locally advanced pancreatic cancer: evolving techniques and treatment strategies. Curr Probl Cancer. 2020;44:100607.
11. Paganetti H. Relative biological effectiveness (RBE) values for proton beam therapy. Variations as a function of biological endpoint, dose, and linear energy transfer. Phys Med Biol. 2014;59:419–72.
12. Perri G, Prakash LR, Katz MHG. Response to preoperative therapy in localized pancreatic cancer. Front Oncol. 2020;10:516.
13. Toesca DAS, Koong AJ, Poultsides GA, et al. Management of borderline resectable pancreatic cancer. Int J Radiat Oncol Biol Phys. 2018;100:1155–74.
14. Takagi C, Kikuchi Y, Shirakawa H, et al. Predictive factors for elevated postoperative carbohydrate antigen 19-9 levels in patients with resected pancreatic cancer. Anticancer Res. 2019;39:3177–83.
15. Arrington AK, Hsu CH, Schaefer KL, O'Grady CL, Khreiss M, Riall TS. Survival after margin-positive resection in the era of modern chemotherapy for pancreatic cancer: do patients still benefit? J Am Coll Surg. 2021;233:100–9.

16. Neoptolemos JP, Dunn JA, Stocken DD, et al. Adjuvant chemoradiotherapy and chemotherapy in resectable pancreatic cancer: a randomised controlled trial. Lancet. 2001;358:1576–85.

17. Winter JM, Cameron JL, Campbell KA, et al. 1423 pancreaticoduodenectomies for pancreatic cancer: a single-institution experience. J Gastrointest Surg. 2006;10:1199–210. discussion 210-1

18. Spitz FR, Abbruzzese JL, Lee JE, et al. Preoperative and postoperative chemoradiation strategies in patients treated with pancreaticoduodenectomy for adenocarcinoma of the pancreas. J Clin Oncol. 1997;15:928–37.

19. Pisters PW, Abbruzzese JL, Janjan NA, et al. Rapid-fractionation preoperative chemoradiation, pancreaticoduodenectomy, and intraoperative radiation therapy for resectable pancreatic adenocarcinoma. J Clin Oncol. 1998;16:3843–50.

20. Versteijne E, Suker M, Groothuis K, et al. Preoperative chemoradiotherapy versus immediate surgery for resectable and borderline resectable pancreatic cancer: results of the Dutch randomized phase III PREOPANC trial. J Clin Oncol. 2020;38:1763–73.

21. Jang JY, Han Y, Lee H, et al. Oncological benefits of neoadjuvant chemoradiation with gemcitabine versus upfront surgery in patients with borderline resectable pancreatic cancer: a prospective, randomized, open-label, multicenter phase 2/3 trial. Ann Surg. 2018;268:215–22.

22. Katz MHG, Ou FS, Herman JM, et al. Alliance for clinical trials in oncology (ALLIANCE) trial A021501: preoperative extended chemotherapy vs. chemotherapy plus hypofractionated radiation therapy for borderline resectable adenocarcinoma of the head of the pancreas. BMC Cancer. 2017;17:505.

23. Katz MHG, Shi Q, Meyers JP, et al. Alliance A021501: Preoperative mFOLFIRINOX or mFOLFIRINOX plus hypofractionated radiation therapy (RT) for borderline resectable (BR) adenocarcinoma of the pancreas. J Clin Oncol. 2021;39:377.

24. Sultana A, Cox T, Ghaneh P, Neoptolemos JP. Adjuvant therapy for pancreatic cancer. Recent Results Cancer Res. 2012;196:65–88.

25. Loehrer PJ Sr, Feng Y, Cardenes H, et al. Gemcitabine alone versus gemcitabine plus radiotherapy in patients with locally advanced pancreatic cancer: an Eastern Cooperative Oncology Group trial. J Clin Oncol. 2011;29:4105–12.

26. Kalser MH, Ellenberg SS, Pancreatic cancer. Adjuvant combined radiation and chemotherapy following curative resection. Arch Surg. 1985;120:899–903.

27. Klinkenbijl JH, Jeekel J, Sahmoud T, et al. Adjuvant radiotherapy and 5-fluorouracil after curative resection of cancer of the pancreas and periampullary region: phase III trial of the EORTC gastrointestinal tract cancer cooperative group. Ann Surg. 1999;230:776–82; discussion 82-4.

28. Gemcitabine hydrochloride with or without erlotinib hydrochloride followed by the same chemotherapy regimen with or without radiation therapy and capecitabine or fluorouracil in treating patients with pancreatic cancer that has been removed by surgery. https://ClinicalTrials.gov/show/NCT01013649.

29. Regine WF, Winter KW, Abrams R, et al. RTOG 9704 a phase III study of adjuvant pre and post chemoradiation (CRT) 5-FU vs. gemcitabine (G) for resected pancreatic adenocarcinoma. J Clin Oncol. 2006;24:(Suppl 18):4007.

30. Goodman KA, Hajj C. Role of radiation therapy in the management of pancreatic cancer. J Surg Oncol. 2013;107:86–96.

31. Palta M, Godfrey D, Goodman KA, et al. Radiation therapy for pancreatic cancer: executive summary of an ASTRO clinical practice guideline. Pract Radiat Oncol. 2019;9:322–32.

32. Cloyd JM, Crane CH, Koay EJ, et al. Impact of hypofractionated and standard fractionated chemoradiation before pancreatoduodenectomy for pancreatic ductal adenocarcinoma. Cancer. 2016;122:2671–9.

33. Krishnan S, Rana V, Janjan NA, et al. Induction chemotherapy selects patients with locally advanced, unresectable pancreatic cancer for optimal benefit from consolidative chemoradiation therapy. Cancer. 2007;110:47–55.

34. Huguet F, Andre T, Hammel P, et al. Impact of chemoradiotherapy after disease control with chemotherapy in locally advanced pancreatic adenocarcinoma in GERCOR phase II and III studies. J Clin Oncol. 2007;25:326–31.

35. Hammel P, Huguet F, van Laethem JL, et al. Effect of chemoradiotherapy vs chemotherapy on survival in patients with locally advanced pancreatic cancer controlled after 4 months of gemcitabine with or without erlotinib: The LAP07 randomized clinical trial. JAMA. 2016;315:1844–53.
36. Krishnan S, Chadha AS, Suh Y, et al. Focal radiation therapy dose escalation improves overall survival in locally advanced pancreatic cancer patients receiving induction chemotherapy and consolidative chemoradiation. Int J Radiat Oncol Biol Phys. 2016;94:755–65.
37. Reyngold M, O'Reilly EM, Varghese AM, et al. Association of ablative radiation therapy with survival among patients with inoperable pancreatic cancer. JAMA Oncol. 2021;7:735–8.
38. Colbert LE, Rebueno N, Moningi S, et al. Dose escalation for locally advanced pancreatic cancer: how high can we go? Adv Radiat Oncol. 2018;3:693–700.
39. Moser EC, Hoffe SE, Frakes J, et al. Adaptive dose optimization trial of stereotactic body radiation therapy (SBRT) with or without GC4419 (avasopasem manganese) in pancreatic cancer. J Clin Oncol. 2020;38:4670.
40. Yang F, Jin C, Fu D. Celiac axis compression syndrome and pancreatic head cancer. Pancreatology. 2014;14:310–1.
41. Wolny-Rokicka E, Sutkowski K, Grzadziel A, et al. Tolerance and efficacy of palliative radiotherapy for advanced pancreatic cancer: a retrospective analysis of single-institutional experiences. Mol Clin Oncol. 2016;4:1088–92.
42. Tian Q, Zhang F, Wang Y. Clinical assessment of palliative radiotherapy for pancreatic cancer. Cancer Radiother. 2018;22:778–83.
43. Hammer L, Hausner D, Ben-Ayun M, et al. Single-fraction celiac plexus radiosurgery: a preliminary proof-of-concept phase 2 clinical trial. Int J Radiat Oncol Biol Phys. 2022;113:588–93.
44. Takatori K, Terashima K, Yoshida R, et al. Upper gastrointestinal complications associated with gemcitabine-concurrent proton radiotherapy for inoperable pancreatic cancer. J Gastroenterol. 2014;49:1074–80.
45. Terashima K, Demizu Y, Hashimoto N, et al. A phase I/II study of gemcitabine-concurrent proton radiotherapy for locally advanced pancreatic cancer without distant metastasis. Radiother Oncol. 2012;103:25–31.
46. Durante M, Loeffler JS. Charged particles in radiation oncology. Nat Rev Clin Oncol. 2010;7:37–43.
47. Loeffler JS, Durante M. Charged particle therapy—optimization, challenges and future directions. Nat Rev Clin Oncol. 2013;10:411–24.
48. Trial of carbon ion versus photon radiotherapy for locally advanced, unresectable pancreatic cancer. 2019. https://ClinicalTrials.gov/show/NCT03536182.
49. Wilson JD, Hammond EM, Higgins GS, Petersson K. Ultra-high dose rate (FLASH) radiotherapy: silver bullet or fool's gold? Front Oncol. 2019;9:1563.
50. Favaudon V, Caplier L, Monceau V, et al. Ultrahigh dose-rate FLASH irradiation increases the differential response between normal and tumor tissue in mice. Sci Transl Med. 2014;6:245ra93.
51. Schuler E, Acharya M, Montay-Gruel P, Loo BW Jr, Vozenin MC, Maxim PG. Ultra-high dose rate electron beams and the FLASH effect: from preclinical evidence to a new radiotherapy paradigm. Med Phys. 2022;49:2082–95.
52. Okoro CM, Schuler E, Taniguchi CM. The therapeutic potential of FLASH-RT for pancreatic cancer. Cancer. 2022;14(5):1167.
53. Moeckli R, Goncalves Jorge P, Grilj V, et al. Commissioning of an ultra-high dose rate pulsed electron beam medical LINAC for FLASH RT preclinical animal experiments and future clinical human protocols. Med Phys. 2021;48:3134–42.
54. Manoharan D, Chang LC, Wang LC, et al. Synchronization of Nanoparticle Sensitization and Radiosensitizing Chemotherapy through Cell Cycle Arrest Achieving Ultralow X-ray Dose Delivery to Pancreatic Tumors. ACS Nano. 2021;15:9084–100.
55. Palma DA, Olson R, Harrow S, et al. Stereotactic ablative radiotherapy versus standard of care palliative treatment in patients with oligometastatic cancers (SABR-COMET): a randomised, phase 2, open-label trial. Lancet. 2019;393:2051–8.
56. Systemic therapy with or without local consolidative therapy in treating patients with oligometastatic solid tumor. https://ClinicalTrials.gov/show/NCT03599765.

Therapy for Metastatic Pancreatic Cancer

Benjamin Musher and Huili Zhu

Introduction

Pancreatic ductal adenocarcinoma (PDAC) is the third leading cause of cancer-related mortality in the United States [1]. About 50% of patients present with metastatic disease, which carries a dismal 5-year survival of <5% [2]. Despite better understanding of the pathogenesis underlying PDAC and the emergence of more effective combination chemotherapy regimens, effective options for systemic therapy remain limited, due to a dearth of known actionable molecular targets and resistance to readily available immunotherapeutic agents.

First-Line Systemic Therapy

Until the 2000s, the mainstay of systemic treatment for metastatic PDAC (mPDAC) was single-agent chemotherapy. In 1997, Burris et al. [3] reported the results of a pivotal trial randomizing patients with locally advanced or mPDAC to weekly gemcitabine or bolus 5-fluorouracil (5-FU). When compared to 5-FU, gemcitabine yielded superior "clinical benefit" (a composite measure of pain, performance status [PS], and weight), median overall survival (OS) (5.65 vs 4.41 months, $P = 0.0025$), and 12-month survival (18% vs 2%, P value not reported). Despite its modest survival benefit and an objective response rate of only 5.4%, single-agent gemcitabine became the standard regimen for treating advanced PDAC.

Over the next decade, numerous gemcitabine-based combinations showed promise in single-arm Phase II trials, but subsequent randomized-controlled trials adding cytotoxic agents (e.g., capecitabine, S1) to gemcitabine failed to demonstrate

B. Musher (✉) · H. Zhu
Dan L. Duncan Comprehensive Cancer Center, Baylor College of Medicine,
Houston, TX, USA
e-mail: blmusher@bcm.edu; huili.zhu@bcm.edu

S. Pant (ed.), *Pancreatic Cancer*, https://doi.org/10.1007/978-3-031-38623-7_4

improved outcomes over gemcitabine alone. In 2009, Cunningham et al. reported that their Phase III trial comparing gemcitabine/capecitabine (GEM-CAP) to gemcitabine in patients with advanced PDAC narrowly missed its primary endpoint of OS (HR 0.86; 95% CI 0.72–1.02; $P = 0.08$). In the same paper, they combined their results with two similar studies, yielding a statistically significant benefit of GEM-CAP over gemcitabine (HR 0.86; 95% CI 0.75–0.98; $P = 0.02$).

Following the approval of targeted therapies for other cancers, clinical trials investigating biologic agents with various mechanisms of action (e.g., cetuximab [4], bevacizumab [5], axitinib [6], and sorafenib [7]) in patients with mPDAC yielded negative results until Moore et al. reported the results of NCIC CTG PA.3, in which 569 patients with locally advanced unresectable or mPDAC were randomized to gemcitabine plus erlotinib or gemcitabine alone [8]. The experimental arm yielded a statistically significant improvement in median progression-free survival (PFS) (HR 0.77; $P = 0.004$), median OS (6.24 vs 5.91 months, HR 0.82; $P = 0.038$), and 1-year OS (23% v 17%; $P = 0.023$), but no improvement in response rate (8.6% vs 8.0%) or disease control rate (57.0% vs 49.2%, $P = 0.07$). Of note, the presence of a treatment-related rash was associated with longer median OS and a higher 1-year survival rate, but no tissue biomarker predictive of response to erlotinib was ever identified. The modest clinical benefit (albeit statistically significant) of gemcitabine/erlotinib, combined with its low response rate and the absence of a predictive biomarker, tempered practitioners' enthusiasm and therefore compromised its widespread use.

In 2011, a major shift in the treatment paradigm for mPDAC occurred when the results of the PRODIGE [9] trial were reported. This landmark Phase III randomized controlled trial (RCT) compared FOLFIRINOX (biweekly infusional 5-FU, irinotecan, and oxaliplatin) to gemcitabine among patients with mPDAC who were ≤75 years old with an ECOG PS of 0–1. When compared to gemcitabine, FOLFIRINOX demonstrated a superior overall response rate (ORR) (31.6% vs 9.4%, $P < 0.001$), median PFS (6.4 vs 3.3 months, HR 0.47; $P < 0.001$), and median OS (11.1 vs 6.8 months, HR 0.57; $P < 0.001$). Common grade 3/4 toxicities associated with FOLFIRINOX included neutropenia (45.7%; but only 5.4% febrile neutropenia), fatigue (23.6%), vomiting (14.5%), diarrhea (12.7%), and sensory neuropathy (9.0%). Despite these toxicities, patients in the FOLFIRINOX arm experienced better quality of life (QOL) at 6 months by the Global Health Status and Quality of Life scales (HR 0.47; 95% CI 0.30 to 0.70; $P < 0.001$) and demonstrated improved QOL and a slower deterioration of QOL. This pivotal study changed the standard of care for managing mPDAC in patients ≤75 years old with preserved ECOG PS and became widely adopted in academic centers and the community alike. To reduce the myelosuppression induced by FOLFIRINOX, modified versions of this regimen with the addition of growth factor support were tested in single-arm studies and yielded comparable efficacy with less neutropenia and better tolerability [10].

Unlike PRODIGE, which was conducted in French academic centers and excluded patients older than 75 and with an ECOG PS > 1, the Phase III MPACT ABI-007 trial [11] was conducted in 193 sites across three continents, had no specified age limit for inclusion, and required a Karnofsky performance status (KPS) ≥70 (thus enrolling some patients with an ECOG PS 2). In this RCT reported by Von Hoff et al. in 2013, the combination of nab-paclitaxel and gemcitabine (nPG) yielded a superior ORR (23% vs 7%, P < 0.001), PFS (5.5 vs 3.7 months, HR 0.69; P < 0.001), OS (8.5 vs 6.7 months, HR 0.72; P < 0.001), and 1-year OS (35% vs 22%, P < 0.001) over single-agent gemcitabine. The most common grade 3/4 adverse events in the nPG arm were neutropenia (38%), fatigue (17%), and neuropathy (17%). Of note, grade 3/4 diarrhea occurred in only 6% and grade 3/4 nausea and/or vomiting in <5% of patients received nPG. To date, there has been no RCT comparing FOLFIRINOX and nPG in untreated mPDAC. As such, one has not been proven to be superior, and both are considered standard options for untreated mPDAC. Keeping in mind the pitfalls of cross-trial comparison, FOLFIRINOX yielded numerically superior treatment-related outcomes (ORR, PFS, OS, and 1-year OS) than nPG. On the other hand, nPG was associated with numerically less myelosuppression and GI toxicity and was tested in a more inclusive patient population (sites throughout the world, KPS ≥70, no limit on age). Thus, when discussing these two regimens with patients, clinicians should consider efficacy, toxicity, age, performance status, and logistical factors (a biweekly regimen that includes a 46-h 5-FU infusion pump versus a weekly that does not contain an infusion pump) when helping patients to weigh their options.

Results of NAPOLI-3 [12], a randomized, global, Phase III study comparing NALIRIFOX [13] (liposomal irinotecan, 5-FU, and oxaliplatin) to nPG in patients with treatment-naïve mPDAC, were presented at the 2023 ASCO Gastrointestinal Symposium. At a median follow-up of 16.1 months, the trial met its primary endpoint of median OS (11.1 with NALIRIFOX vs 9.2 month with nPG, HR 0.84; 95% CI 0.71 to 0.99, P = 0.04) and its secondary endpoint of PFS (7.4 with NALIRIFOX vs 5.6 month with nPGs, HR 0.70; 95% CI 0.59 to 0.84, P = 0.0001). Grade 3/4 gastrointestinal treatment-related adverse events (diarrhea, nausea, and hypokalemia) were more common with NALIRFOX, while grade 3/4 anemia and neutropenia were more common with nPG. Although these results support consideration of NALIRIFOX as a new reference regimen for first-line treatment of metastatic PDAC, it is unclear whether NALIRIFOX is superior to standard FOLFIRINOX or sequential administration of doublet regimens (e.g., nPG followed by 5FU/liposomal irinotecan or nPG followed by FOLFIRINOX).

Second-Line Systemic Therapy

Unfortunately, many patients who progress on first-line therapy are not eligible for additional treatment due to decline in organ function and overall performance status. Of those who are medically appropriate for additional therapy, standard options are limited. Only a handful of randomized trials have investigated second-line systemic therapy for mPDAC. In 2009, Yoo et al. [14] reported the results of a single-center, randomized Phase II trial comparing FOLFIRI (biweekly 5-FU, leucovorin, and irinotecan) and mFOLFOX (biweekly 5-FU, leucovorin, and oxaliplatin) in patients with gemcitabine-refractory advanced PDAC. Median OS was 16.6 and 14.9 weeks in the FOLFIRI and FOLFOX arms, respectively, and both regimens were tolerated with expected and manageable side effects.

The combination of 5-FU and oxaliplatin was subsequently reported in two larger trials. The German CONKO-study group conducted a Phase III trial [15] that randomized patients with advanced PDAC whose disease had progressed on gemcitabine to the OFF regimen (5-FU, folinic acid, and oxaliplatin) or best supportive care (BSC). The trial terminated prematurely due to poor accrual, but even with its limited numbers showed improved median PFS and OS with OFF compared to BSC. The follow-up CONKO-003 trial [16] showed that, when compared to FF (5-FU and folinic acid), OFF improved median OS (5.9 vs 3.3 months, HR 0.66; 95% CI 0.48–0.91; $P = 0.010$) and time to progression (2.9 vs 2.0 months, HR 0.68; 95% CI 0.50–0.94; $P = 0.019$). Contrary to these findings, the PANCREOX trial [17] demonstrated inferior survival and more toxicity in patients receiving mFOLFOX6 compared to 5-FU and folinic acid (median OS 6.1 vs 9.9 months, HR 1.78; 95% CI 1.08–2.93; $P = 0.024$). While difficult to explain, the conflicting results of these two trials may have been related to differences in chemotherapy dosing and inclusion criteria. Nevertheless, PANCREOX called into question the benefit of 5-FU and oxaliplatin as second-line therapy for mPDAC.

To date, the only well-powered RCT that has shown a clear survival benefit with combination chemotherapy in refractory mPDAC is NAPOLI-1 [18], a Phase III study that compared infusional 5-FU/leucovorin (LV) plus nanoliposomal irinotecan (Nal-Iri) to 5-FU/LV in patients whose disease had progressed on gemcitabine-based therapy. In this landmark study, 5-FU/LV plus Nal-Iri yielded superior median OS (6.1 vs 4.2 months, HR 0.67; 95% CI 0.49–0.92; $P = 0.012$) over 5-FU/LV. As expected, the most common grade 3/4 adverse events in the combination arm were neutropenia (27%), diarrhea (13%), vomiting (11%), and fatigue (14%). Since, to date, no RCT has investigated FOLFIRINOX as a second-line regimen for patients whose disease has progressed on gemcitabine, NAPOLI-1 established the combination of 5-FU/LV and Nal-Iri as the most evidence-based chemotherapy option for gemcitabine-refractory PDAC.

Targeted Therapy

Comprehensive profiling of PDAC has revealed common alterations in *KRAS, TP53, CDKN2A,* and *SMAD4,* but targeting these genes has not yielded positive results in clinical trials [19, 20]. The most common PDAC molecular alterations to be successfully targeted are germline mutations in *BRCA1* and *BRCA2,* which are present in 4–7% of patients with PDAC [21–23]. In the Phase III POLO trial [24], 154 patients with mPDAC who harbored a germline *BRCA* mutation and whose disease was stable or responding after at least 16 weeks of platinum-based chemotherapy were randomized in a 3:2 ratio to the PARP inhibitor olaparib or placebo. Compared to placebo, olaparib maintenance yielded superior median PFS (7.4 vs 3.8 months; HR 0.53, 95% CI 0.35–0.82; $P = 0.004$), but no improvement in median

OS (18.9 vs 18.0 months; HR 0.91, 95% CI 0.56–1.46, $P = 0.68$). A final analysis of OS reported by Kindler et al. [25] confirmed that maintenance olaparib did not improve median OS (19.0 vs 19.2 months, HR 0.83; 95% CI 0.56–1.22; $P = 0.3487$). However, the Kaplan Meier survival curves separated at 24 months, and 3-year survival was higher in the maintenance olaparib arm when compared to placebo (33.9% vs 17.8% with placebo). Furthermore, maintenance olaparib delayed reintroduction of cytotoxic chemotherapy and was well-tolerated, with the most common grade 3/4 side effects being anemia (11%), fatigue (5%), and decreased appetite (3%). In light of these data, olaparib was approved by the FDA for maintenance therapy after response to or stability on platinum-based therapy for PDAC associated with germline *BRCA* mutation.

Multiple Phase I and II trials have demonstrated benefit of *NTRK* inhibitors across various tumor types harboring *NTRK* gene fusions, resulting in the FDA's approval of larotrectinib (2018) and entrectinib (2019) for *NTRK* fusion-positive tumors, regardless of tissue of origin. *NTRK* gene fusions can be found in <1% of PDACs so data on the efficacy of *NTRK* inhibitors in PDAC are limited to case reports and small case series that have shown responses lasting up to 6 months.

Pancreatic cancer cells harbor relatively few somatic mutations, which limits expression of potentially immunogenic epitopes, and these cells live in a microenvironment characterized by high concentrations of myeloid-derived suppressor cells, T-regulatory cells, and immunosuppressive cytokines. As a result, immunotherapy has not proven effective for the vast majority of PDAC. KEYNOTE 158 [26] showed impressive activity of pembrolizumab in a cohort of patients with microsatellite unstable (or deficient mismatch repair) non-colorectal cancers. However, among the 22 patients with PDAC (9.4% of the study population), the ORR (18%), median PFS (2.1 months), median OS (4.0 months), and median duration of response (13.4 months) were considerably lower than the corresponding results for the entire cohort (34.3%, 4.1 months, 23.5 months, and not reached, respectively), indicating that checkpoint immunotherapy may not be particularly effective in the vanishingly small proportion (<1%) of PDAC that are microsatellite unstable.

Future Directions

The 5-year survival rate of PDAC has increased from 5% to 11% in the past three decades, largely due to advances in systemic therapy [27]. Nevertheless, mPDAC remains universally lethal, and even those patients who are fit enough for multiple lines of systemic therapy survive an average of 12–18 months [28]. Newer combinations of cytotoxic chemotherapy as well as novel agents targeting tumor-specific molecular alterations, the tumor microenvironment, and the host immune response are being investigated in clinical trials of all phases.

Targeting the intracellular GTPase *KRAS* remains an important research initiative since >95% of PDACs harbor *KRAS* mutations. Sotorasib, a *KRAS* inhibitor targeting the G12C mutation, was recently approved for *KRAS* G12C-mutated non-squamous non-small cell lung cancer based on a Phase II trial published by Skoulidis et al. [29] showing an ORR of 33%, disease control rate of 88%, and median PFS of 6.8 months in that population. *KRAS* G12C mutations are found in only 3% of PDACs, but agents targeting this particular mutation as well as more common *KRAS* mutations are currently being investigated. For example, adagrasib (MRTX849) also targets the *KRAS* G12C mutation and has demonstrated early efficacy in advanced solid tumors [30], including two patients with pancreatic cancer. NCT04185883 is an ongoing international, multicentered, multi-armed Phase Ib/II clinical trial studying combinations of *KRAS* inhibitors with trametinib (MEK inhibitor), AMG 404 (anti-PD-1 monoclonal antibody in NCT04185883), RMC-4630 (SHP2 inactivator), afatinib (EGFR inhibitor), pembrolizumab (anti-PDL1), and panitumumab (EGFR inhibitor) with or without chemotherapy in advanced solid malignancy with *KRAS* G12C mutation.

PDAC's complex tumor microenvironment (TME), which consists of myofibroblast-like cells that create a mechanical barrier to the delivery of chemotherapy [31] and infiltration of cytotoxic immune cells, has become an important focus of clinical research. On the heels of promising results reported in mouse models and early phase human trials, stromal targets have not improved tumor-related outcomes when combined with standard therapy in RCTs. A Phase Ib/II trial showed that adding the hyaluronidase PEGPH20 to FOLFIRINOX actually reduced OS when compared to FOLFIRINOX alone [32]. Although HALO 202 [33], a randomized Phase II comparing PEGPH20 plus PG to nPG alone showed that the combination led to longer PFS and OS in a subset of hyaluronan-high tumors, a follow-up study in hyaluronan-high tumors only (HALO 109-301 [34]) showed increased ORR in the experimental group without any improvement in PFS or OS. Similarly, the hedgehog inhibitor vismodegib yielded encouraging results in early-phase studies, but did not improve ORR, PFS, nor OS when added to standard gemcitabine in a small randomized study [35]. With PEGPH20 and vismodegib having failed to improve outcomes in mPDAC, newer agents targeting the PDAC stroma, including sibrotuzumab (anti-fibroblast activating protein [FAP]), talabostat (FAP inhibitor), marimastat/tanomastat (multi-matrix metalloproteinase inhibitors), and pamrevlumab (connective tissue growth factor inhibitor), are being investigated in combination with chemotherapy and novel immunotherapy. Additionally, targeting cancer cell metabolism may have direct apoptotic effects on cancer cells while remodeling the TME [33]. For example, SM88 [36], an oral tyrosine derivative that dysregulates metabolism via the Warburg Effect and oxidative stress—and CPI 613 [37], a lipoate analog that induces apoptosis by hyper-stimulating an endogenous redox mechanism, has advanced to randomized trials after demonstrating activity in early phase studies.

Finally, immunotherapy continues to be an active area of PDAC research. As our understanding of the various mechanisms that induce resistance to anti-tumor immunity has deepened, immunotherapeutic agents have evolved from simple protein-based vaccines to more sophisticated immunostimulatory antibodies (e.g., CD40 agonists), oncolytic viruses, tumor-specific CAR T-cells, checkpoint inhibitors, and combinations thereof [38]. Researchers hope that, in the upcoming years, immunotherapy will improve outcomes in PDAC as much as it has in other malignancies.

Progress will not occur without cutting-edge basic research and forward-thinking, innovative clinical trials. For a variety of reasons, only ~5% of patients with PDAC enroll in clinical trials despite clear recommendations in all national and society guidelines. In order to improve outcomes for patients inflicted with PDAC, every effort must be made to translate existing scientific knowledge into clinical application and encouraging all patients to consider participating in clinical research. In addition to serving as a valuable resource to patients with PDAC seeking clinical trial enrollment, the Pancreatic Cancer Action Network (PanCAN) has created the Precision Promise adaptive clinical trial program to expedite bench-to-bedside translation of promising therapeutic agents in a consortium of academic centers.

Conclusion

PDAC remains a difficult cancer to treat. Compared to the early days of gemcitabine monotherapy, newer systemic therapies are producing more favorable results in metastatic PDAC, but overall outcomes remain guarded and grim. A more sophisticated understanding of the molecular underpinnings of PDAC, the complex tumor microenvironment, and its mechanisms of immunoresistance have spurred the emergence of promising novel agents that will hopefully yield more significant progress in the not-too-distant future.

References

1. Surveillance, epidemiology, and end results (SEER) program. Cancer stat facts: pancreatic cancer. [Cited 2022 July 10]. Available from www.seer.cancer.gov.
2. Siegel Rebecca L, et al. Cancer statistics, 2021. CA Cancer J Clin. 2021;71(1):7–33.
3. Burris H, Moore MJ, Andersen J, Green MR, Rothenberg ML, Modiano MR, Christine Cripps M, Portenoy RK, Storniolo AM, Tarassoff P. Improvements in survival and clinical benefit with gemcitabine as first-line therapy for patients with advanced pancreas cancer: a randomized trial. J Clin Oncol. 1997;15(6):2403–13.
4. Philip PA, Benedetti J, Corless CL, Wong R, O'Reilly EM, Flynn PJ, Rowland KM, Atkins JN, Mirtsching BC, Rivkin SE, Khorana AA. Phase III study comparing gemcitabine plus cetuximab versus gemcitabine in patients with advanced pancreatic adenocarcinoma: Southwest Oncology Group–directed intergroup trial S0205. J Clin Oncol. 2010;28(22):3605.
5. Kindler HL, Niedzwiecki D, Hollis D, Sutherland S, Schrag D, Hurwitz H, Innocenti F, Mulcahy MF, O'Reilly E, Wozniak TF, Picus J. Gemcitabine plus bevacizumab compared with gemcitabine plus placebo in patients with advanced pancreatic cancer: phase III trial of the Cancer and Leukemia Group B (CALGB 80303). J Clin Oncol. 2010;28(22):3617.
6. Kindler HL, Ioka T, Richel DJ, Bennouna J, Létourneau R, Okusaka T, Funakoshi A, Furuse J, Park YS, Ohkawa S, Springett GM. Axitinib plus gemcitabine versus placebo plus gemcitabine in patients with advanced pancreatic adenocarcinoma: a double-blind randomised phase 3 study. Lancet Oncol. 2011;12(3):256–62.
7. Kindler HL, Wroblewski K, Wallace JA, Hall MJ, Locker G, Nattam S, Agamah E, Stadler WM, Vokes EE. Gemcitabine plus sorafenib in patients with advanced pancreatic cancer:

a phase II trial of the University of Chicago Phase II Consortium. Investig New Drugs. 2012;30(1):382–6.

8. Moore MJ, Goldstein D, Hamm J, Figer A, Hecht JR, Gallinger S, Au HJ, Murawa P, Walde D, Wolff RA, Campos D. Erlotinib plus gemcitabine compared with gemcitabine alone in patients with advanced pancreatic cancer: a phase III trial of the National Cancer Institute of Canada Clinical Trials Group. J Clin Oncol. 2007;25(15):1960–6.

9. Conroy T, Desseigne F, Ychou M, Bouché O, Guimbaud R, Bécouarn Y, Adenis A, Raoul JL, Gourgou-Bourgade S, de la Fouchardière C, Bennouna J. FOLFIRINOX versus gemcitabine for metastatic pancreatic cancer. N Engl J Med. 2011;364(19):1817–25.

10. Stein SM, James ES, Deng Y, Cong X, Kortmansky JS, Li J, Staugaard C, Indukala D, Boustani AM, Patel V, Cha CH. Final analysis of a phase II study of modified FOLFIRINOX in locally advanced and metastatic pancreatic cancer. Br J Cancer. 2016;114(7):737–43.

11. Von Hoff DD, Ervin T, Arena FP, Chiorean EG, Infante J, Moore M, Seay T, Tjulandin SA, Ma WW, Saleh MN, Harris M. Increased survival in pancreatic cancer with nab-paclitaxel plus gemcitabine. N Engl J Med. 2013;369(18):1691–703.

12. Wainberg ZA, et al. NAPOLI-3: a randomized, open-label phase 3 study of liposomal irinotecan+ 5-fluorouracil/leucovorin+ oxaliplatin (NALIRIFOX) versus nab-paclitaxel+ gemcitabine in treatment-naïve patients with metastatic pancreatic ductal adenocarcinoma (mPDAC). J Clin Oncol. 2023;41:661.

13. Wainberg ZA, et al. First-line liposomal irinotecan with oxaliplatin, 5-fluorouracil and leucovorin (NALIRIFOX) in pancreatic ductal adenocarcinoma: a phase I/II study. Eur J Cancer. 2021;151:14–24.

14. Yoo C, Hwang JY, Kim JE, Kim TW, Lee JS, Park DH, Lee SS, Seo DW, Lee SK, Kim MH, Han DJ. A randomised phase II study of modified FOLFIRI. 3 vs modified FOLFOX as second-line therapy in patients with gemcitabine-refractory advanced pancreatic cancer. Br J Cancer. 2009;101(10):1658–63.

15. Pelzer U, Schwaner I, Stieler J, Adler M, Seraphin J, Dörken B, Riess H, Oettle H. Best supportive care (BSC) versus oxaliplatin, folinic acid and 5-fluorouracil (OFF) plus BSC in patients for second-line advanced pancreatic cancer: a phase III-study from the German CONKO-Study Group. Eur J Cancer. 2011;47(11):1676–81.

16. Oettle H, Riess H, Stieler JM, Heil G, Schwaner I, Seraphin J, Görner M, Mölle M, Greten TF, Lakner V, Bischoff S. Second-line oxaliplatin, folinic acid, and fluorouracil versus folinic acid and fluorouracil alone for gemcitabine-refractory pancreatic cancer: outcomes from the CONKO-003 trial. J Clin Oncol. 2014;32(23):2423–9.

17. Gill S, Ko YJ, Cripps C, Beaudoin A, Dhesy-Thind S, Zulfiqar M, Zalewski P, Do T, Cano P, Lam WY, Dowden S. PANCREOX: a randomized phase III study of fluorouracil/leucovorin with or without oxaliplatin for second-line advanced pancreatic cancer in patients who have received gemcitabine-based chemotherapy. J Clin Oncol. 2016;34(32):3914–20.

18. Wang-Gillam A, Li CP, Bodoky G, Dean A, Shan YS, Jameson G, Macarulla T, Lee KH, Cunningham D, Blanc JF, Hubner RA. Nanoliposomal irinotecan with fluorouracil and folinic acid in metastatic pancreatic cancer after previous gemcitabine-based therapy (NAPOLI-1): a global, randomised, open-label, phase 3 trial. Lancet. 2016;387(10018):545–57.

19. Al Baghdadi T, Halabi S, Garrett-Mayer E, Mangat PK, Ahn ER, Sahai V, Alvarez RH, Kim ES, Yost KJ, Rygiel AL, Antonelli KR. Palbociclib in patients with pancreatic and biliary cancer with CDKN2A alterations: results from the targeted agent and profiling utilization registry study. JCO Precis Oncol. 2019;1:1–8.

20. Zeitouni D, Pylayeva-Gupta Y, Der CJ, Bryant KL. KRAS mutant pancreatic cancer: no lone path to an effective treatment. Cancer. 2016;8(4):45.

21. Ghiorzo P. Genetic predisposition to pancreatic cancer. World J Gastroenterol. 2014;20(31):10778.

22. Holter S, Borgida A, Dodd A, Grant R, Semotiuk K, Hedley D, Dhani N, Narod S, Akbari M, Moore M, Gallinger S. Germline BRCA mutations in a large clinic-based cohort of patients with pancreatic adenocarcinoma. J Clin Oncol. 2015;33(28):3124–9.

23. Friedenson B. BRCA1 and BRCA2 pathways and the risk of cancers other than breast or ovarian. Medscape Gen Med. 2005;7(2):60.
24. Golan T, Hammel P, Reni M, Van Cutsem E, Macarulla T, Hall MJ, Park JO, Hochhauser D, Arnold D, Oh DY, Reinacher-Schick A. Maintenance olaparib for germline BRCA-mutated metastatic pancreatic cancer. N Engl J Med. 2019;381(4):317–27.
25. Kindler HL, Hammel P, Reni M, Van Cutsem E, Macarulla T, Hall MJ, Park JO, Hochhauser D, Arnold D, Oh DY, Reinacher-Schick A. Overall survival results from the POLO trial: a phase III study of active maintenance olaparib versus placebo for germline BRCA-mutated metastatic pancreatic cancer. J Clin Oncol. 2022;40:34.
26. Marabelle A, Le DT, Ascierto PA, Di Giacomo AM, De Jesus-Acosta A, Delord JP, Geva R, Gottfried M, Penel N, Hansen AR, Piha-Paul SA. Efficacy of pembrolizumab in patients with noncolorectal high microsatellite instability/mismatch repair–deficient cancer: results from the phase II KEYNOTE-158 study. J Clin Oncol. 2020;38(1):1.
27. National Cancer Institute. Cancer stat facts: pancreatic cancer. https://seer.cancer.gov/statfacts/html/pancreas.html. Accessed 7 July 2022.
28. Yu KH, Hendifar AE, Alese OB, Draper A, Abdelrahim M, Burns E, Khan G, Cockrum P, Bhak RH, Nguyen C, DerSarkissian M. Clinical outcomes among patients with metastatic pancreatic ductal adenocarcinoma treated with liposomal Irinotecan. Front Oncol. 2021;11:2704.
29. Skoulidis F, Li BT, Dy GK, Price TJ, Falchook GS, Wolf J, Italiano A, Schuler M, Borghaei H, Barlesi F, Kato T. Sotorasib for lung cancers with KRAS p. G12C mutation. N Engl J Med. 2021;384(25):2371–81.
30. Johnson ML, Ou SH, Barve M, Rybkin II, Papadopoulos KP, Leal TA, Velastegui K, Christensen JG, Kheoh T, Chao RC, Weiss J. KRYSTAL-1: activity and safety of adagrasib (MRTX849) in patients with colorectal cancer (CRC) and other solid tumors harboring a KRAS G12C mutation. Eur J Cancer. 2020;138:S2.
31. Ho WJ, Jaffee EM, Zheng L. The tumour microenvironment in pancreatic cancer—clinical challenges and opportunities. Nat Rev Clin Oncol. 2020;17(9):527–40.
32. Ramanathan RK, McDonough SL, Philip PA, Hingorani SR, Lacy J, Kortmansky JS, Thumar J, Chiorean EG, Shields AF, Behl D, Mehan PT. Phase IB/II randomized study of FOLFIRINOX plus pegylated recombinant human hyaluronidase versus FOLFIRINOX alone in patients with metastatic pancreatic adenocarcinoma: SWOG S1313. J Clin Oncol. 2019;37(13):1062.
33. Hingorani SR, Zheng L, Bullock AJ, Seery TE, Harris WP, Sigal DS, Braiteh F, Ritch PS, Zalupski MM, Bahary N, Oberstein PE. HALO 202: randomized phase II study of PEGPH20 plus nab-paclitaxel/gemcitabine versus nab-paclitaxel/gemcitabine in patients with untreated, metastatic pancreatic ductal adenocarcinoma. J Clin Oncol. 2018;36(4):359–66.
34. Van Cutsem E, Tempero MA, Sigal D, Oh DY, Fazio N, Macarulla T, Hitre E, Hammel P, Hendifar AE, Bates SE, Li CP. Randomized phase III trial of pegvorhyaluronidase alfa with nab-paclitaxel plus gemcitabine for patients with hyaluronan-high metastatic pancreatic adenocarcinoma. J Clin Oncol. 2020;38(27):3185.
35. Catenacci DV, Junttila MR, Karrison T, Bahary N, Horiba MN, Nattam SR, Marsh R, Wallace J, Kozloff M, Rajdev L, Cohen D. Randomized phase Ib/II study of gemcitabine plus placebo or vismodegib, a hedgehog pathway inhibitor, in patients with metastatic pancreatic cancer. J Clin Oncol. 2015;33(36):4284.
36. Noel MS, Wang-Gillam A, Ocean AJ, Chawla SP, Del Priore G, Picozzi VJ. Phase II trial of SM-88 in patients with metastatic pancreatic cancer: preliminary results of the first stage. J Clin Oncol. 2021;39:437.
37. Alistar A, Morris BB, Desnoyer R, Klepin HD, Hosseinzadeh K, Clark C, Cameron A, Leyendecker J, D'Agostino R, Topaloglu U, Boteju LW. Safety and tolerability of the first-in-class agent CPI-613 in combination with modified FOLFIRINOX in patients with metastatic pancreatic cancer: a single-centre, open-label, dose-escalation, phase 1 trial. Lancet Oncol. 2017;18(6):770–8.
38. Neoptolemos JP, Kleeff J, Michl P, Costello E, Greenhalf W, Palmer DH. Therapeutic developments in pancreatic cancer: current and future perspectives. Nat Rev Gastroenterol Hepatol. 2018;15(6):333–48.

Targeted Therapies for Pancreatic Cancer

5

Michael S. Lee and Shubham Pant

Introduction

Pancreatic cancer is the third highest cause of cancer death in the United States, causing an estimated 49,830 deaths in 2022 [1]. Only 13% of patients diagnosed with pancreatic cancer have localized disease, while 47% have incurable disease with distant metastases [1]. For patients with metastatic pancreatic cancer with adequate performance status, first-line multiagent combinations of conventional chemotherapy, such as FOLFIRINOX [2] or gemcitabine/nab-paclitaxel [3], are the current standard of care; however, median overall survival (OS) with these regimens is only 11.1 or 8.5 months, respectively. More recently, treatment with personalized targeted therapies selected using predictive biomarkers to identify rational vulnerabilities in patients' tumors is an important approach. Guidelines now recommend that pancreatic cancers are tested for germline mutations, somatic mutations and fusions, and microsatellite instability/mismatch repair deficiency [4] to optimize selection of standard or investigational therapies.

M. S. Lee (✉)
Department of Gastrointestinal Medical Oncology, The University of Texas MD Anderson Cancer Center, Houston, TX, USA
e-mail: mslee2@mdanderson.org

S. Pant
GI Medical Oncology, The University of Texas MD Anderson Cancer Center, Houston, TX, USA
e-mail: spant@mdanderson.org

© The Author(s), under exclusive license to Springer Nature Switzerland AG 2023
S. Pant (ed.), *Pancreatic Cancer*, https://doi.org/10.1007/978-3-031-38623-7_5

Germline and Somatic Mutations Impairing DNA Damage Repair Pathways

From 4 to 10% of pancreatic cancer, patients harbor a pathogenic germline mutation [5–9], and some single-center analyses with higher rates of germline *BRCA1/2* mutations have rates as high as 19.8% [10]. Up to half of pancreatic cancer patients with a pathogenic germline mutation did not have a suspicious family history [8, 10]; consequently, national guidelines recommend that all patients with pancreatic adenocarcinoma undergo germline testing [4]. The most commonly found germline mutations are *BRCA1/2* (3–5%), *ATM* (1.7–3.3%), *PALB2* (0.6%), and *CDKN2A*, *TP53*, and DNA mismatch repair (MMR) genes (*MLH1*, *MSH2*, *MSH6*, and *PMS2*).

BRCA1, *BRCA2*, and *PALB2* germline mutations cause homologous recombination defects (HRD), which lead to increased mutagenesis and carcinogenesis, with consequent increased risk of developing several cancer types including pancreatic cancer. Carriers with pathogenic *BRCA1/2* variants have a relative risk of developing pancreatic cancer of 2.36–3.34 and have an absolute risk of 2.3–3.0% of developing pancreatic cancer by age 80 [11]. It is important to recognize patients whose cancers have HRD, as these cancers are highly susceptible to cytotoxic therapies like platinum agents that cause double-stranded DNA breaks requiring homologous recombination for repair. For example, in a prospective phase II trial of gemcitabine + cisplatin backbone chemotherapy in patients with metastatic pancreatic cancer with HRD germline mutations, response rate was 70% [12], which is dramatically higher than response rate to FOLFIRINOX or gemcitabine/nab-paclitaxel in all-comers with metastatic pancreatic cancer. Additionally, retrospective data demonstrates that treatment with first-line platinum-based chemotherapy regimens like FOLFIRINOX yields superior progression-free survival compared to non-platinum-based regimens in patients with HRD pancreatic cancers [13].

Cancers with germline mutations causing HRD, like *BRCA1/2* mutations, also have synthetic lethality when treated with inhibitors of DNA damage repair (DDR) mechanisms, particularly poly (ADP-ribose) polymerase (PARP) inhibitors. These cancers are particularly reliant on alternative mechanisms of DNA damage repair to prevent mitotic catastrophe and cell death. PARP inhibitors block the repair of single-strand DNA breaks and also contribute to additional double-strand DNA breaks by trapping their PARP substrate on the DNA strand, causing further cytotoxicity [14]. In the phase III POLO trial, the PARP inhibitor olaparib was proven to be an effective maintenance therapy in patients with metastatic pancreatic cancer with germline *BRCA1/2* mutations after receiving 4–6 months of induction platinum chemotherapy. Maintenance with olaparib significantly improved median PFS compared to placebo, with hazard ratio of 0.53 (95% CI 0.35–0.82), with improvement in median PFS from 3.8 months to 7.4 months [15]. Importantly, there was no significant difference in time to deterioration in health-related quality of life or in physical functioning scores between patients who received maintenance olaparib versus placebo [16], indicating that olaparib was tolerated with manageable side effects. Though median OS was not significantly different at 19.0 vs 19.2 months (HR 0.83, 95% CI 0.56–1.22), there was a trend toward improved 36-months survival with olaparib (33.9% vs 17.8%) [17]. These data also demonstrate the better prognosis of patients with *BRCA1/2* germline mutated pancreatic cancer, as median OS with standard therapies in unselected metastatic pancreatic cancer patients is under 12 months. Given the results of the POLO trial, olaparib maintenance therapy is now FDA approved for patients with metastatic pancreatic adenocarcinoma with germline *BRCA1/2* mutation after at least 16 weeks of first-line platinum-based chemotherapy. *PALB2* germline mutations also appear to be predictive for susceptibility to PARP inhibitors, with small numbers of patients with germline PALB2 mutations with breast or prostate cancer benefiting from PARP inhibitors [18–20]. A phase II trial of maintenance therapy with the PARP inhibitor rucaparib in patients with germline HRD mutations showed that 2/2 patients with *PALB2* mutations had response to rucaparib [21], suggesting that similar susceptibility to platinum chemotherapy and PARP inhibitors is likely with *PALB2* germline mutations. However, patients with germline *PALB2* mutations were not included in the POLO trial and are not included in the FDA approval for olaparib maintenance.

There is emerging preclinical and early phase clinical trial data for novel combinations of PARP inhibitors with additional therapies, especially immune checkpoint inhibitors. In *BRCA1/2*-deficient cancer models, PARP inhibition increased expression of interferon-stimulated genes and the STING pathway, triggering innate and adaptive immune responses, with enhancement of immune responses with addition of anti-PD-1 therapy [22, 23]. *BRCA1/2* mutant pancreatic cancers also had higher tumor mutation burden and were more likely to have PD-L1 expression [24]. The SWOG S2001 trial is enrolling patients who would be eligible for maintenance olaparib to be randomized to either olaparib alone vs olaparib + pembrolizumab (NCT04548752). More recent data from a phase II trial of maintenance niraparib combined with either the anti-PD1 therapy nivolumab or the anti-CTLA4 therapy ipilimumab showed that niraparib + nivolumab ($n = 44$) showed median PFS of only 1.9 (95% CI 1.4–2.3) with 6-mo PFS rate of 20.6% (95% CI 8.3–32.9). However, niraparib + ipilimumab had a promising median PFS of 8.1 months (95% CI 5.5–10.6) with 6-months PFS rate of 59.6% (95% CI 44.3–74.9) [25]. These data, while not definitive, hint that immune checkpoint inhibitors other than anti-PD1 therapies may be more effective when combined with PARP inhibitors. Multiple additional DNA damage repair inhibitors are in development, and clinical trials of combinations of these inhibitors are underway.

Besides germline *BRCA1/2* mutations, somatic *BRCA1/2* mutations are found in approximately 2% of pancreatic cancers [13]. Though the POLO trial only enrolled patients with germline *BRCA1/2* mutations, patients whose cancers have somatic *BRCA1/2* mutations may also benefit from PARP inhibitors. For example, in a study of rucaparib in patients with either germline or somatic *BRCA1/2* mutation, among three patients who had somatic *BRCA2* mutations, one had a complete response and one had a partial response [26]. Meta-analysis pooling results from multiple cancer types showed comparable response rates with PARP inhibitor therapy with somatic *BRCA1/2* mutations (55.8%) and germline mutations (43.9%) [27]. Clinical trials for pancreatic cancer patients including those with somatic *BRCA1/2* or *PALB2* mutations are ongoing, including niraparib combined with the PD-1 antibody dostarlimab (NCT04493060), or olaparib plus pembrolizumab (NCT04666740). Additionally, the randomized APOLLO clinical trial is assessing the efficacy of adjuvant olaparib compared to placebo in patients with resected pancreatic cancer with germline or somatic *BRCA1/2* or *PALB2* mutation (NCT04858334).

From 1.7% to 3.3% of pancreatic cancers arise in patients with germline *ATM* mutations [28, 29], and carriers of *ATM* germline mutations have a relative risk of developing pancreatic cancer in their lifetime of 6.5 (95% CI 4.5–9.5) [30]. Somatic *ATM* mutations also arise in pancreatic cancers, and in total, 4–5% of pancreatic cancers harbor a somatic or germline *ATM* mutation [13, 31]. Optimal strategies for targeting *ATM* mutated pancreatic cancers are still being investigated. Preclinical studies suggested that PARP inhibitors and topoisomerase-1 inhibitors, like irinotecan, may be effective in *ATM*-mutated cancers [29, 32]. However, maintenance therapy with PARP inhibitors did not demonstrate activity in case reports in *ATM*-mutated pancreatic cancers [33, 34], suggesting that PARP inhibitors alone are not sufficient for synergistic lethality. As evidence of this, PARP inhibitor therapy, while cytostatic, was not tumoricidal in *ATM*-deficient pancreatic cancer cell models [35]. Targeted DDR inhibitors including ATM inhibitors, ATR inhibitors, and CHK1 inhibitors [36] or combinations of these therapies [29] have shown more preclinical efficacy. Indeed, only patients with cancers with *ATM* loss or mutation had response in a phase I trial of the ATR inhibitor BAY1895344 [37]. There are early phase clinical trials of these strategies in *ATM*-mutated pancreatic cancer ongoing [38].

Immune Checkpoint Inhibitors in Microsatellite Unstable Cancers

Microsatellite instability (MSI-High) or deficient mismatch repair is found in 1–2% of pancreatic ductal adenocarcinoma [39, 40]. While MSI-High pancreatic cancers are significantly enriched for medullary or mucinous/colloid histology, the majority of MSI-High pancreatic cancers (68%) still have conventional adenocarcinoma histology [39]. MSI-High pancreatic cancers can arise through germline mutations in the MMR genes *MLH1*, *MSH2*, *MSH6*, or *PMS2* causing Lynch syndrome; patients with Lynch syndrome have an 8.6-fold (95% CI 4.7–15.7) increased risk of developing pancreatic cancer compared to the general population [41]. In patients with MSI-High cancers of multiple different cancer types, the programmed cell death protein 1 (PD-1) antibody pembrolizumab has been shown to be effective. In early clinical trials, 2/8 (25%) of patients with MSI-High pancreatic cancer had complete response with pembrolizumab, and 3/8 (37%) had partial response [42]. With more patients treated with pembrolizumab in the KEYNOTE-158 trial, 4/22 patients with MSI-High pancreatic cancer had an objective response (18.2%, 95% CI 5.2–40.3), with median duration of response of 13.4 months (ranging from 8.1 to 16.0+ months) [43]. This response rate was lower than other that seen in other MSI-High cancer types within KEYNOTE-158; however, other studies have shown higher response rates with immune checkpoint inhibitors. For example, a retrospective case series showed 7/9 (77%) of patients with MSI-H pancreatic cancer treated with immune checkpoint inhibitors showed response [44]. Additionally, in the GARNET trial, 5/11 patients (45.5%; 95% CI 16.7–76.6) with MSI-High pancreatic cancer treated with dostarlimab had response, which was comparable to the 43.1% response rate observed in all non-endometrial MSI-High cancers [45]. Ultimately, given the potential for durable and/or complete responses, immunotherapy is an important strategy for treatment of the rare subgroup of MSI-High or deficient MMR pancreatic cancers. Both pembrolizumab and dostarlimab received FDA accelerated approval for patients with MSI-High and/or deficient mismatch repair solid cancers refractory to prior therapy.

Additionally, the FDA approved pembrolizumab for solid tumors with a tumor mutation burden (TMB) of ≥ 10 mutations per megabase, but it remains debatable whether high TMB is a reliable predictive biomarker in microsatellite stable (MSS) pancreatic cancer. In KEYNOTE-158, in 9 cancer types with high TMB, there was a response rate of 29% (95% CI 21–39), compared to a response rate of 6% (95% CI 5–8) in cancers without high TMB [46]; however, pancreatic cancer was not one of the nine studied tumor types, and there is a lack of data for high TMB as a predictive biomarker for immune checkpoint inhibitors in pancreatic cancer. Of course, high TMB is expected in MSI-High cancers, and a recent meta-analysis showed 19/32 (59.4%) of TMB-high pancreatic cancers were MSI-High (with TMB definitions varying in each included study [47]. It remains unproven if high TMB in MSS pancreatic cancer is predictive of response to immune checkpoint inhibitors. On one hand, a recent study showed 12/161 (7.5%) of resected MSS pancreatic adenocarcinomas were TMB-high (≥ 10 mutations/Mb), and these TMB-high cancers had highest T-cell density and upregulation of immune pathways [48], suggesting immune checkpoint inhibitors could indeed be rational. However, a pan-cancer analysis conversely showed that pancreatic cancer, among many other immune-cold cancers, does not have a significant correlation between CD8 T-cell infiltration and neoantigen load, and in these cancers, TMB-High fails to predict for response to immune checkpoint inhibitors [49]. Indeed, in a recent retrospective cohort study, only 2/36 (6%) of MSS pancreatic cancers had TMB ≥ 10 mutations/Mb, and 0/2 of these patients had a response to anti PD-1 or PD-L1 therapy [50]. Thus, at this time, there is limited to no data for the efficacy of immune checkpoint inhibitors in the small subgroup of TMB-High MSS pancreatic cancer.

KRAS Mutation Inhibitors

Activating *KRAS* mutations occur in 90–93% of pancreatic cancers [31, 51, 52], and *KRAS* is the most commonly mutated oncogene in pancreatic cancer. KRAS is a small GTPase switch, cycling between an inactive GDP-bound state and an active GTP-bound state. When receptor tyrosine kinases (RTKs), like the epidermal growth factor receptor (EGFR) and the related family members ERBB2 (HER2), ERBB3 (HER3), and ERRB4 (HER4), are activated by ligand binding, they trigger activation of KRAS by exchanging GDP for GTP, with this exchange is catalyzed by guanine exchange factors (GEFs) like SOS1. GTP-bound KRAS remains active until GTP is hydrolyzed to GDP; while KRAS has intrinsic GTP hydrolytic activity, GTPase-activating proteins (GAPs) catalyze GTP hydrolysis to promote inactivation of KRAS signaling. Multiple effector pathways, including importantly the RAF-MEK-ERK MAPK signaling cascade, transduce signaling from the activated KRAS node downstream to the nucleus to alter gene expression and promote cell cycle progression and cell division. Oncogenic *KRAS* mutations cause significant decreases in GTP hydrolysis or accelerate GDP-GTP exchange, causing accumulation of active GTP-bound KRAS and constitutive activation of mitogenic signaling [53, 54]. Several activating mutations arise within *KRAS*; in pancreatic cancer, the most common mutant alleles are G12D, G12V, and G12R (Fig. 5.1) [53].

There have historically been multiple challenges in developing direct KRAS inhibitors. Because the KRAS GTP binding site has picomolar affinity for GTP, competitive inhibitors to the GTP binding pocket have not been possible. Due to the KRAS protein surface lacking obvious pockets for drug binding, developing allosteric KRAS inhibitors has also been challenging [54]. However, further

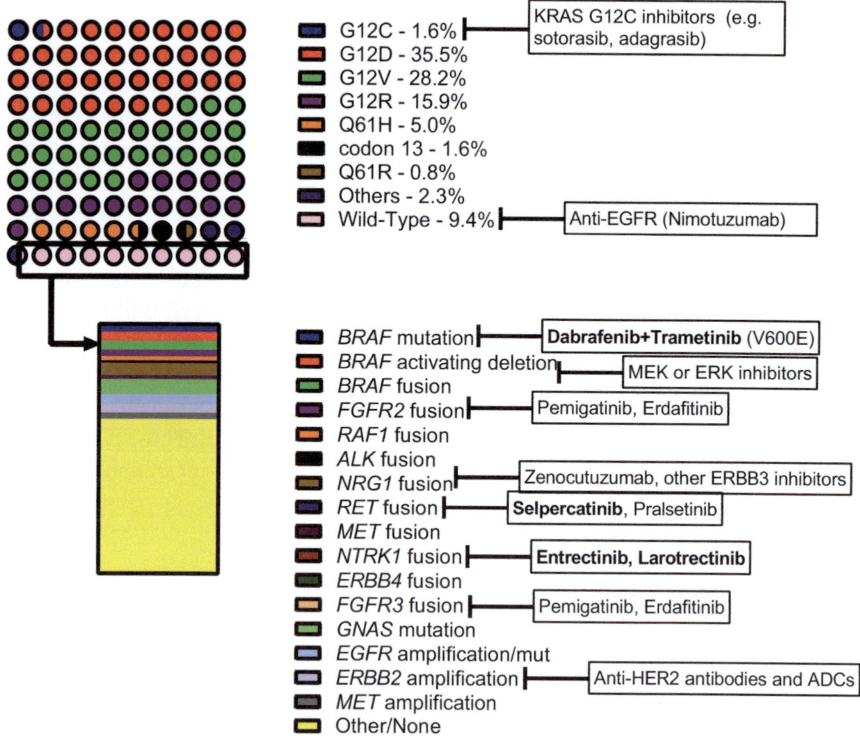

Fig. 5.1 Frequency of KRAS and other selected mutations and genomic aberrations in pancreatic cancer and selected potential targeted therapies with evidence of activity from clinical trials or case reports [55]. Therapies that are now FDA approved for pancreatic cancer or tumor-agnostic indications are in bold

understanding of the structure of various KRAS mutant proteins and their conformation in binding to GAPs and GEFs have enabled development of new mutant allele-specific inhibitors and new drugs targeting GEF binding. Modern strategies to target KRAS either focus on mutation-specific strategies selectively targeting specific mutant proteins or focus on pan-KRAS therapies that have broad activity across a range of mutations [56].

KRAS G12C Inhibitors

KRAS G12C mutation is found in only 1% of pancreatic cancers [31], but direct KRAS G12C inhibitors have been developed and are furthest in clinical investigation at this time. KRAS G12C inhibitors bind to a surface pocket on the mutant KRAS protein and covalently bind to the reactive G12C cysteine residue [57, 58]. Sotorasib (AMG510) is a G12C inhibitor that has a high response rate of 32% in *KRAS* G12C mutant NSCLC [59], leading to FDA approval as a monotherapy in NSCLC. Sotorasib also has shown a promising response rate as a single agent in *KRAS* G12C mutant pancreatic cancer in the CodeBreaK100 phase I/II trial, where 8/38 patients had confirmed partial response with sotorasib monotherapy (ORR 21.1%, 95% CI 9.6–37.3), and disease control rate was 32/38 (84.2%, 95% CI 68.8–94.0) [60]. While these data are promising, the durability of response and improvements in survival remain to be determined; median PFS was 4.0 months (95% CI 2.8–5.6) with median OS 6.9 months (95% CI 5.0–9.1) and median DOR 2.8 months (ranging from 1.4 months to 5.8 months) [60]. Adagrasib (MRTX849), another KRAS G12C inhibitor, had a high response rate in *KRAS* G12C mutant NSCLC of 45% [61], and early data from 12 pancreatic cancer patients showed 5/10 (50%) evaluable patients had partial responses, with 10/10 (100%) having disease control, and median PFS was 6.6 months (95% CI 1.0–9.7) [62]. While these G12C inhibitors have compelling response rate, ultimately resistance does emerge. Mechanisms of acquired resistance to KRAS G12C inhibitor monotherapy observed in other *KRAS* G12C mutant cancer types include acquisition of new subclonal *KRAS* mutations or amplification, activating mutations in other MAPK pathway genes, or novel oncogenic fusions [63, 64]. Novel combinations of various targeted therapies with KRAS G12C inhibitors in colorectal cancer and NSCLC have been studied preclinically [65, 66], and multiple combinations are now in clinical trials. The CodeBreaK-101 trial has multiple additional arms combining sotorasib with new agents including MEK inhibitor, PD1 inhibitor, SHP2 inhibitor, pan-ERBB inhibitor, PD-L1 inhibitor, CDK inhibitor, or mTOR inhibitor (NCT04185883), and the KRYSTAL-1 trial has added additional arms combining adagrasib with novel agents, particularly the anti-EGFR antibody cetuximab (NCT03785249). Multiple additional G12C inhibitors are also in clinical development.

Additional Direct Inhibitors of Mutant *KRAS*

Direct small molecular inhibitors of additional *KRAS* mutant alleles besides KRAS G12C are in development. These are particularly critical for pancreatic cancer, where *KRAS* G12C is uncommon; the most common *KRAS* mutant alleles found in pancreatic cancer are G12D, G12V, and G12R. With further discoveries in the biochemistry and structure of these mutant proteins, novel drugs have been engineered to noncovalently bind to mutant KRAS proteins and inhibit signaling. For example, MRTX1133 is a potent, noncovalently binding inhibitor of KRAS G12D that successfully impaired tumor growth of *KRAS* G12D models in vitro and in vivo, including in 8/11 pancreatic adenocarcinoma mouse models and in orthotopic pancreatic cancer models [67, 68]. Further development of KRAS G12D inhibitors is highly anticipated. RMC-6236 is a small molecule inhibitor that binds the chaperone protein cyclophilin A, which forms a binary complex that can then covalently bind to active GTP-bound RAS and disrupt effector signaling [69]. RMC-6236 caused tumor regression in 12/17 in vivo *KRAS* codon 12 mutant pancreatic adenocarcinoma models [70], and phase I clinical trials have now started (NCT05379985). Additional more selective drugs with more activity via formation of the inhibitory tri-complex with specific KRAS mutant proteins are also in development, including drugs targeting KRAS G12C (RMC-6291) [71], G12D (RMC-9805) [72], and G13C (RMC-8839), and the G12C inhibitor is now in phase I clinical trials (NCT05462717).

SOS1 Inhibitors

SOS1 is a GEF that promotes KRAS activation by catalyzing GDP exchange for GTP loading, and thus drug compounds that block the SOS1-KRAS interaction impair KRAS-mediated signaling [73]. These SOS1 inhibitors are predicted to synergize with MAPK pathway inhibitors. Phosphorylation of SOS1 by the MAPK effector pathway causes feedback inhibition of SOS1 activity; MAPK pathway inhibition with MEK or ERK inhibitors de-represses SOS1 activity to enable reactivation of KRAS activation to promote alternative signaling to drive resistance. Preclinical studies showed that addition of SOS1 inhibitors to MEK or ERK inhibitors is synergistic [74]. Several SOS1 inhibitors are in development for RAS-mutated cancers and show promise for treatment of cancers with KRAS codon 12 or 13 mutations, primarily in combination with MEK or ERK inhibitors. However, different KRAS mutant isoforms have different dependencies on SOS1. For example, KRAS G12R does not interact with SOS1 [75], and codon 61 mutant KRAS has lower intrinsic GTPase activity [76], and thus these isoforms are not expected to be as susceptible to SOS1 inhibition. In preclinical models, treatment with a SOS1 inhibitor significantly decreased GTP loading of mutant KRAS and thus decreased proliferation in most *KRAS* codon 12 and 13 mutant isoforms, though not in *KRAS* G12R or in codon 61 mutant models [77]. The SOS1 inhibitor BI1701963 is a clinical drug candidate that synergized with MEK inhibitor and had in vivo efficacy [78].

BI1701963 is being studied in clinical trials in *KRAS* mutant cancers (NCT04111458) [79]. Additionally, SOS1 inhibitors also have been shown preclinically to synergize with KRAS G12C inhibitors in preclinical models [73, 77, 80]. MRTX0902 is a potent SOS1:KRAS inhibitor [80], and clinical trials of MRTX0902 with adagrasib are in development (NCT05578092).

SHP2 Inhibitors in *KRAS* Codon 12 Mutant Isoforms

SHP2 (*PTPN11*) is a non-receptor protein tyrosine phosphatase that is recruited by myriad activated receptor tyrosine kinases to potentiate SOS1-dependent GEF function and GTP-loading and activation of KRAS [81]. When KRAS mutant cells are treated with MAPK pathway inhibitors, feedback activation of upstream RTKs mediates reactivation of signaling dependent on SHP2. Given this, impairing SHP2 signaling may relieve these resistance-mediating feedback activation mechanisms. Indeed, SHP2 activity is indispensable for oncogenic *KRAS* mutations to drive carcinogenesis in mouse models, and SHP2 inhibitors synergize with MEK inhibitors in *KRAS* mutant cancer models in vivo [82]. Multiple SHP2 inhibitors are in development for *KRAS* mutant cancers; however, similar to SOS1 inhibitors, KRAS mutant isoform does impact efficacy of SHP2 inhibition. For example, monotherapy with the allosteric SHP2 inhibitor RMC-4550 successfully impaired activation of multiple codon 12 mutated *KRAS* proteins, but was ineffective against codon 13 and codon 61 *KRAS* mutations [81]. SHP2 inhibitors will likely be most effective when given in combination with direct RAS inhibitors or other downstream effector inhibitors. For example, combinations of SHP2 inhibitor and MEK inhibitor more effectively blocked feedback reactivation of the MAPK pathway than either single agent in *KRAS* codon 12 mutant models [83–85]. SHP2 inhibitor and KRAS G12C inhibitor combinations also were synergistic in preclinical models, including in pancreatic cancer models [86]. Clinical trials of SHP2 inhibitors are early in development, but early reports from phase I trials of TNO155 showed the drug is reasonably tolerated, with modest monotherapy activity, with stable disease noted in 22% of patients [87]. Multiple SHP2 inhibitors are currently in clinical trials enrolling patients with *KRAS* mutant pancreatic or other cancers, either with SHP2 inhibitor monotherapy or in combination with MEK inhibitors, ERK inhibitors, or KRAS G12C inhibitors.

KRAS Mutation-Targeting Vaccine and Cellular Therapies

KRAS mutations produce cancer-specific neoepitopes that could be targeted through an adaptive immune response. Algorithms to predict HLA classes that could potentially present specific epitopes determined that HLA-A*11:01 are capable of presenting mutant *KRAS* epitopes, and T cells reactive to *KRAS* G12V and G12D could indeed be produced in vivo in mouse models [88]. HLA-A*11:01 restricted peripheral T cells against KRAS G12V were indeed detectable in blood samples of cancer patients [89], and human T-cell receptors specific to KRAS G12D peptides presented via HLA-A*11 have been described and facilitate selective killing of KRAS G12D expressing cancer cells [90]. Additionally, tumor-infiltrating lymphocytes identifying the KRAS G12D epitope were expanded ex vivo from a patient with metastatic colorectal cancer, and infusion of these HLA-C*08:02-restricted CD8+ T cells caused significant tumor regression [91]. The specificity of the HLA-C*08:02 restricted T-cell receptor against KRAS G12D has been described, with nanomolar to low micromolar affinity [92]. A clinical trial of chimeric antigen receptor-T (CAR-T) cell therapy is underway in patients with HLA-A*11:01 class with metastatic *KRAS* G12V or G12D mutant cancers refractory to standard therapies; peripheral blood lymphocytes will be harvested through leukapheresis, expanded ex vivo, transduced with anti-KRAS G12V recombinant murine T-cell receptors, and then reinfused after preceding lymphodepletion (NCT03190941, NCT03745326). Additionally, a trial of CAR-T cells of HLA-C*08:02 restricted T cells engineered to express KRAS G12D targeting T-cell receptors resulted in a case of a patient with metastatic *KRAS* G12D mutant pancreatic cancer who had a partial response of metastases persisting for over 6 months [93] (NCT04520711). Given these exciting early demonstrations of activity, additional predictive algorithms for HLA restricted mutant KRAS epitopes are ongoing, and additional work demonstrates additional potential targets may include G12V/HLA-A*03:01, G12V/HLA-A*11:01, and G12R/HLA-B*07:02 [94].

Additional clinical trials have sought to develop cancer vaccines that can facilitate a de novo immune response against common mutant KRAS epitopes. mRNA-5671/V941 is a tetravalent mRNA vaccine targeting *KRAS* G12D, G12V, G13D, and G12C mutations, and results from a phase I clinical trial as a monotherapy or in combination with pembrolizumab are pending (NCT03948763) [95]. Additionally, a pooled mutant KRAS-targeted long peptide vaccine is being combined with nivolumab and ipilimumab in patients with colorectal or pancreatic cancer harboring *KRAS* G12C, G12V, G12D, G12A, G13D, or G12R mutation (NCT04117087). Additional approaches seek to improve targeting of KRAS antigens and vaccine adjuvants to draining lymph nodes by conjugation to albumin-binding lipids, facilitating trafficking to lymph nodes to generate stronger immune responses [96]. Initial clinical trials of a bivalent product targeting KRAS G12D and G12R are ongoing, with plans to expand to a heptavalent vaccine in the AMPLIFY-201 trial (NCT04853017).

KRAS Mutation-Specific Oligonucleotide Therapies

Antisense oligonucleotide therapies induce destruction of target mRNA sequences and thus may enable specific gene silencing of driver oncogenes if effectively delivered to target cells. However, there have been several challenges in developing oligonucleotide therapies, such as ensuring delivery to target tissues and oligonucleotide specificity to prevent off-target effects, and so potential therapies need to be engineered for optimal drug delivery [97]. siG12D LODER is a therapeutic comprised of a small interfering RNA (siRNA) targeting KRAS G12D embedded in a biodegradable polymer matrix, which can be directly injected intratumorally into locally advanced *KRAS* G12D mutant pancreatic cancers [98], and was well tolerated in phase 1/2a clinical trial [99]; the PROTACT phase 2 clinical trial is ongoing (NCT01676259). Additional *KRAS* mutation-specific oligonucleotide therapies are in development [100–102]. Anti-mutant *KRAS* siRNA can also be packaged within exosomes, extracellular vesicles containing protective membrane-anchored proteins like CD47, which helps prevent phagocytosis and increases circulating half-life. iExosomes are anti-*KRAS* G12D siRNA encapsulated within exosomes, and preclinical studies showed improvement in overall survival in *KRAS* G12D mutated pancreatic cancer mouse models treated with iExosomes compared to controls treated with gemcitabine [100]. A clinical trial of iExosomes in *KRAS* G12D mutant pancreatic cancers is ongoing [103] (NCT03608631).

Additional Strategies Targeting Effector Pathway Signaling

Generally, therapies targeting mutant *KRAS* effector pathway signaling have not proven effective to date. The primary pathway that has been targeted is the RAF-MEK-ERK pathway. Multiple clinical trials of MEK inhibitors have shown lack of activity in patients with pancreatic cancer [104–106]. *KRAS* G12R-mutated pancreatic cancers were predicted to be more sensitive to MEK or ERK inhibitors due to the incapability of KRAS G12R protein to activate the PI3K-AKT pathway with consequent greater reliance on MAPK signaling [75], but a clinical trial of selumetinib in *KRAS* G12R mutant pancreatic cancer was halted early for futility after none of eight patients had a response, though three patients did have stable disease for over 6 months [107]. In another study, among 6 patients with chemorefractory *KRAS* G12R-mutated pancreatic cancer who received cobimetinib and gemcitabine, 1/6 patients had a partial response and 6/6 patients had disease control, with median PFS of 6.0 months (95% CI 3–9.3) [108]. These results demonstrate that for effector pathway modulation to be effective, novel combination therapies guided by specific mutation-specific biochemistry are needed, along with newer generation MAPK inhibiting drugs.

Additional clinical trials of MAPK pathway inhibitor combinations selecting for *KRAS* mutant pancreatic cancer patients are ongoing. Selected trials are described in Table 5.1. Of interest, preclinical studies found that MEK or ERK inhibition results in an increase in autophagic flux which mitigates cytotoxicity, and inhibition of autophagy with therapies like hydroxychloroquine synergizes with MEK or ERK inhibitors [109, 110]. Anecdotes have described patients with *KRAS* mutant cancers who had response with MEK inhibitors combined with chloroquine or hydroxychloroquine [110, 111], and prospective clinical trials are ongoing (see Table 5.1).

Table 5.1 Selected MEK or ERK inhibitor-based combination clinical trials in pancreatic cancer

Therapies	Biomarker criterion	Clinicaltrials. gov
MEK inhibitor + autophagy inhibitor (binimetinib + hydroxychloroquine)	Any *KRAS* mutation on tumor or liquid biopsy	NCT04132505
MEK inhibitor + autophagy inhibitor (trametinib + hydroxychloroquine)	Unselected	NCT03825289
MEK inhibitor + autophagy inhibitor + anti-PD-L1 (cobimetinib + hydroxychloroquine + atezolizumab)	Any *KRAS* mutation	NCT04214418
MEK inhibitor + asparaginase inhibitor (Cobimetinib + Calaspargase pegol-mknl)	Unselected	NCT05034627
MEK inhibitor + anti-PD-L1 (selumetinib + durvalumab) – randomized against FOLFIRI	Any *KRAS* mutation	NCT04348045
MEK inhibitor + JAK1/2 inhibitor (trametinib + ruxolitinib)	Any *KRAS* mutation	NCT04303403
MEK inhibitor + JAK/STAT inhibitor + anti-PD1 (Trametinib + Ruxolitinib + Retifanlimab)	Unselected	NCT05440942
MEK inhibitor + CDK4/6 inhibitor neoadjuvantly (Binimetinib + Palbociclib)	Any *KRAS* mutation	NCT04870034
MEK inhibitor + CDK4/6 inhibitor (binimetinib + palbociclib)	Any *KRAS*, *NRAS*, or *HRAS* mutation	NCT05554367
ERK inhibitor + CDK4/6 inhibitor (ulixertinib + palbociclib)	Unselected	NCT03454035
ERK inhibitor +/− autophagy inhibitor (LY3214996 +/− hydroxychloroquine)	Unselected	NCT04386057
ERK inhibitor + SHP2 inhibitor (LY3214996 + RMC-4630)	Any *KRAS* mutation	NCT04916236

KRAS Wild-Type Tumors Are Enriched for Other Targetable Aberrations

KRAS wild-type status is found in 7–10% of pancreatic cancers in Western populations [31, 51] and tends to occur more commonly in younger patients under age 50 [55, 112]. *KRAS* wild-type disease may be more common in other populations, like in China, where up to 17% of patients were *KRAS* wild-type [113]. Patients with *KRAS* wild-type cancers tend to have superior overall survival compared to those who are *KRAS* mutant [114]. Moreover, *KRAS* wild-type pancreatic adenocarcinomas have distinct mutation and gene expression patterns compared to *KRAS* mutant cancers, suggesting these cancers are a distinct molecular entity [115]. For example, *KRAS* wild-type pancreatic cancers were more likely to harbor germline mutations ($p = 0.027$), like in *ATM* or *PRSS1* (which causes familial pancreatitis) [51]. Additional somatic gene mutations and fusions more likely found in *KRAS* wild-type pancreatic cancers include *BRAF* activating missense mutations, *BRAF* activating in-frame intragenic deletions, *BRAF* kinase fusions, *NRG1* fusions, HER2 amplification, MET amplification, *FGFR2* fusions, *RAF1* fusions, and *ALK* fusions; other rare fusions occurring in less than 1% of KRAS wild-type pancreatic cancers involve *RET, MET, NTRK1, ERBB4,* and *FGFR3* [55, 116, 117]. Overall, 38% of the *KRAS* WT tumors had other driver mutations or fusions activating the RAS-MAPK pathway [55], many of which are potentially actionable (Fig. 5.1). Clinical trials have assessed the efficacy of the anti-EGFR antibody nimotuzumab in *KRAS* wild-type pancreatic cancers, and in a randomized phase II trial, treatment with the combination of gemcitabine + nimotuzumab resulted in improved 12-months OS rate compared to gemcitabine + placebo in the subgroup of patients who were *KRAS* wild-type (53.8% vs 15.8%, HR 0.32 (95% CI 0.13–0.84)) [118]. Subsequently, a prospective phase III randomized controlled trial enrolling 92 patients with *KRAS* wild-type pancreatic cancers to receive gemcitabine + nimotuzumab or gemcitabine + placebo was performed in China and showed gemcitabine + nimotuzumab resulted in significant improvement in OS (median 10.9 vs 8.5 months, HR 0.50 (95% CI 0.06–0.94)) and PFS (median 4.2 months vs 3.6 months, HR 0.56 (95% CI 0.12–0.99)) [119]. Additional studies of EGFR targeted therapies are needed in Western populations and using doublet chemotherapy backbones which are considered standard of care, but this data does provide evidence for activity of anti-EGFR therapy in *KRAS* wild-type pancreatic cancer.

NRG1 Fusions

NRG1 encodes neuregulin, a ligand of the EGFR receptor family which promotes heterodimerization of ERBB2 and ERBB3 receptors and downstream activation of the RAS-RAF-MAPK and other effector pathways. *NRG1* fusions are recurrent oncogenic events in multiple cancer types and are enriched in *KRAS* wild-type pancreatic cancers. In these fusion proteins, a chimeric protein is generated with a transmembrane domain from the fusion partner and preservation of the ERBB2/3 binding domain of NRG1, causing constitutive oncogenic signaling through ERBB2/3 [116, 120]. Given this mechanism of oncogenesis, targeted agents against ERBB family members, particularly ERBB2 or ERBB3, appear effective across *NRG1* fusion cancers of multiple cancer types, including the pan-ERBB inhibitor afatinib and the ERBB2xERBB3 bispecific antibody zenocutuzumab [121–123]. In *NRG1* fusion pancreatic cancers, afatinib treatment caused responses in 2/3 patients in a prospective case series [116]. Another study showed 2/3 patients with *NRG1* fusion pancreatic cancers responded to ERBB family-directed treatments (1 of afatinib, 1 of erlotinib + pertuzumab) [112]. Recent prospective clinical trials have shown encouraging response rates with zenocutuzumab, with 8/19 (42%; 95% CI 20–67%) patients with *NRG1* fusion pancreatic cancer having an objective response; among responders on the study across tumor types, the median duration of response was 9.1 months (95% CI 7.4-NR) [124]. Multiple ongoing prospective basket trials of targeted ERBB family inhibitors in patients with *NRG1* fusion cancers are ongoing, including afatinib on TAPUR (NCT02693535), zenocutuzumab (NCT02912949), and the anti-ERBB3 antibody seribantumab (NCT04383210)

Activating BRAF Mutations and In-Frame Deletions

Activating *BRAF* mutations, including both missense mutations and in-frame deletions, are among the most common driver mutations found in *KRAS* wild-type pancreatic cancers [55]. *BRAF* V600E comprises over half of *BRAF* point mutations, with the remainder of the mutations comprised of atypical *BRAF* mutations including D594G, G469V, and G469S [55]. Case reports or trials with pancreatic cancer cohorts describe partial responses with vemurafenib [125, 126] and improvement in CA19-9 [127] or near complete response [128] with dabrafenib + trametinib in *BRAF* V600E mutant pancreatic cancer. A retrospective study of patients with *BRAF* V600E mutations showed that 2/3 patients had a response with BRAF + MEK inhibitor therapy, particularly dabrafenib + trametinib [129]. Notably, a patient treated with dabrafenib and trametinib had ongoing survival exceeding 20 months and PFS exceeding 6 months [128]. Recently, the US FDA granted accelerated approval for dabrafenib and trametinib in patients with *BRAF* V600E mutant solid cancers refractory to prior therapy.

BRAF non-V600 mutations have more heterogeneous effects on MAPK signaling, which impacts optimal choice of targeted therapy. *BRAF* mutations comprise 3 classes [130]: class 1 consists of V600E mutation, causing constitutive signaling; class 2 *BRAF* mutations, like G469V/S, also cause constitutive signaling, which may be targeted with downstream effector inhibitors like MEK inhibitors; and class 3 mutations, like D594G, have deficient kinase activity but active upstream RTKs and RAS and thus increase MAPK pathway signaling, which could be optimally targeted with MEK inhibitors combined with RTK inhibitors [131, 132]. Trials assessing responses to targeted therapies of atypical *BRAF* mutations must account for the class of mutation, and optimal targeting strategies are still being determined. For example, in the MATCH clinical trial, in 31 patients with various cancer types (though none with pancreatic cancer) with class 2 or 3 non-V600 *BRAF* mutations who were treated with the MEK inhibitor trametinib, there was only a 3% response rate and a 34% disease control rate [133]. Thus, single-agent MEK inhibitor is likely insufficient for high response rate in patients with these mutations.

Activating in-frame *BRAF* deletions, most commonly ΔN486_P490 (ΔNVTAP), occur in 3.6% of *KRAS* WT pancreatic cancers [55]. The ΔNVTAP deletion in *BRAF* locks the mutant protein into an active conformation [134, 135], causing constitutive activation of *BRAF* with activation of downstream signaling, independent of homodimerization or heterodimerization with CRAF [134]. Notably, this conformational change impedes binding of several drugs, particularly vemurafenib, to the mutant BRAF protein; indeed, cell line models harboring the ΔNVTAP *BRAF* mutation were resistant to vemurafenib, partially sensitive to GDC-0879 and dabrafenib, and sensitive to AZ-628 [134]. A case report of a patient with *BRAF* ΔNVTAP-mutated pancreatic cancer described a partial response and clinical improvement with dabrafenib therapy [136]. A series of 5 patients with *BRAF* ΔNVTAP-mutated pancreatic cancer showed that 1 patient treated with trametinib had partial response, another had stable disease exceeding 16 weeks treatment duration, and another two had progression; additionally, a patient treated with a pan-RAF inhibitor had progression [129]. Thus, while some drugs are likely to be effective, the likelihood of efficacy depends on whether the specific drug compound can successfully bind the mutant BRAF protein. Clinical trials are enrolling patients with *BRAF* non-V600E mutations or other *BRAF* aberrations (including activating deletions), including trials of the ERK inhibitor ulixertinib (NCT04488003, NCT02465060).

BRAF and RAF1 Fusions

Activating *BRAF* fusions occur in 3.1% of *KRAS* WT pancreatic adenocarcinomas, most commonly fused with SND1, but with many other fusion partners described. Interestingly, BRAF or RAF1 fusions are more commonly found in pancreatic acinar cell carcinomas (23% of PACCs have *BRAF* or *RAF1* fusions) [137]. BRAF fusions can have heterogeneous effects that depend on the breakpoint and the fusion partner. For example, melanoma cell lines with various *BRAF* fusions had heterogeneous responses to BRAF inhibitors in vitro—but all cell lines were resistant to vemurafenib and dabrafenib, and some fusion partner genes had dimerization domains that actually promoted paradoxical activation of MAPK signaling pathways upon treatment with classical RAF inhibitors [138]. The impact of these preclinical observations on clinical efficacy of BRAF inhibitors remains unclear, but different inhibitors are likely to have varying effectiveness in different *BRAF* fusions. A patient with *CUX1-BRAF* fusion pancreatic cancer who received vemurafenib did experience a partial response in the MyPathway basket trial [139]. Patients with *MBNL2-BRAF* fusion had a partial response with trametinib lasting 73 weeks, while 2 patients with *SND1-BRAF* fusion had stable disease with trametinib [129]. The MATCH trial is currently enrolling patients with *BRAF* fusions to receive ulixertinib (NCT02465060).

RAF1 fusions occur in about 1.6% of KRAS WT pancreatic cancers. Preclinical studies suggest that *RAF1* fusion cancers may respond to MEK inhibitors like trametinib [140]. Case reports describe exceptional response with improved survival in a patient with *AKAP9-RAF1* fusion treated with the multikinase inhibitor apatinib [141]. Another case of a patient with *KANK4-RAF1* fusion described partial response lasting over 21 weeks with treatment with trametinib [129].

NTRK1/2/3 Fusions

NTRK1/2/3 fusions occur in <1% of pancreatic cancers [142, 143], but are important to recognize as there are FDA-approved TRK inhibitors, entrectinib, and larotrectinib, available. Across all NTRK1/2/3 fusion tumors, entrectinib treatment resulted in ORR 61.2% (95% CI 51.9–69.9) including 16% complete responses and median DOR of 20.0 months (95% CI 13.0–38.2), and 3/4 pancreatic cancer patients had a response with median DOR 12.9 months [144, 145]. Larotrectinib treatment yielded ORR 69% (95% CI 63–75) including 26% complete responses and median

DOR 32.9 months (95% CI 27.3–41.7) [146–148], including 1/1 pancreatic cancer patients having a partial response. Additional published case reports describe a patient with *CTRC-NTRK1* fusion pancreatic cancer achieving partial response with larotrectinib [149] and two patients with *TPR-NTRK1* fusion pancreatic cancers achieving partial response or clinical benefit with entrectinib [150].

RET Fusions

RET fusions are also found in *KRAS* WT pancreatic cancer and are now an actionable target. Selpercatinib treatment in *RET* fusion positive non-lung or thyroid cancers showed a response rate of 43.9% (95% CI 28.5–60.3), including 6/11 response rate in pancreatic cancer (ORR 55%, 95% CI 23–83) [151, 152]. Pralsetinib treatment resulted in 4/4 responses in *RET* fusion pancreatic cancer, including 1 complete response lasting over 33 months in a patient with *RET-TRIM33* and *RET-JMJD1C* fusions [153, 154]. Selpercatinib received FDA accelerated approval for refractory metastatic solid tumors with RET fusions in September 2022.

FGFR1/2/3 Fusions

FGFR1-3 fusions or rearrangements are also occasionally found in pancreatic cancers. In the FIGHT-101 phase I/II basket trial, a patient with pancreatic cancer with *FGFR2-USP33* fusion had a response with pemigatinib lasting 10.7 months [155]. Case reports of treatment with erdafitinib showed a partial response in a pancreatic cancer harboring an *FGFR2* rearrangement in intron 17 [156], a response lasting over 12 months in another patient with intron 17 *FGFR2* rearrangement cancer [157], and a complete response in a patient with *FGFR2-TACC2* fusion [158].

Additional Rare Fusions and Amplifications

ALK rearrangements arise in <0.2% of pancreatic adenocarcinomas [159], and cases suggest activity of ALK inhibitors in these patients. Three out of four patients with *ALK* fusion pancreatic cancers had disease control, response, or clinical benefit with treatment with ALK inhibitors like crizotinib or ceritinib [159]. Another case report of a patient with *PPFIBP1-ALK* translocation pancreatic cancer described stable disease with alectinib treatment, with acquisition of the *ALK* resistance mutations G1202R and V1180L upon progression, followed by disease control with treatment with the newer generation ALK inhibitor lorlatinib [160]. Another case report describes a patient with *EML4-ALK* fusion treated with crizotinib with partial response lasting for 8 months, who then developed brain metastasis but had further response with alectinib [161].

MET and *ROS1* fusions are also rarely found in *KRAS* WT pancreatic cancer. A case report found a patient with *RDX-MET* fusion pancreatic cancer treated with crizotinib had a durable complete response for over 12 months [156]. Another case of a *SLC4A4-ROS1* fusion pancreatic cancer patient treated with entrectinib showed disease control with clinical benefit lasting for 7 months [150].

HER2 Amplification

HER2 amplification appears to be an actionable driver event in a subset of pancreatic cancers, particularly in *KRAS* wild-type cancers, where it is found in 3.4% of cases [55]. In the MyPathway trial, treatment with trastuzumab+pertuzumab resulted in a response rate of 1/10 among all pancreatic cancers, but the only responder was *KRAS* wild-type, and among *KRAS* wild-type pancreatic cancers, the response rate was 1/3 [162]. One patient with HER2 amplified pancreatic cancer enrolled in the phase I trial of the antibody-drug conjugate trastuzumab deruxtecan and had just over 30% reduction in size of target lesions [163].

Additional Targetable Biomarkers

TP53 Targeted Therapies

TP53 is a key tumor suppressor gene that functions by detecting cell stressors threatening genomic stability and responding either by invoking cell cycle arrest and DNA repair or by invoking cell death [164]. *TP53* is mutated in 66–72% of pancreatic cancers [31, 51] and missense *TP53* mutations drive metastasis in vivo [165, 166]. Despite the clear driver role of *TP53* mutations in oncogenesis, identifying targeted therapies against mutant *TP53* has been particularly challenging, due to the difficulty restoring lost function of a tumor suppressor and the presence of multiple heterogeneous *TP53* mutations that alter protein function and structure in multiple ways [164]. Multiple attempts at targeting *TP53* have been studied preclinically and in clinical trials previously, though none have yet resulted in approved therapies in pancreatic cancer [164]; however, research and clinical trials are ongoing. *TP53* Y220C mutation is found in 1.4% of pancreatic cancers, and PC14586 is a novel small molecule that binds selectively to mutant p53 Y220C protein to stabilize the protein in wild-type conformation and upregulate p53 gene expression targets. A phase I trial showed 8/25 (32.0%) evaluable patients with multiple cancer types with *TP53* Y220C mutation treated at higher dose levels of PC14586 had response, and among 6 evaluable pancreatic cancer patients, there was 1 unconfirmed partial response [167]. This trial continues to enroll patients (NCT04585750).

Mutant *TP53* also generates neoantigens that can elicit adaptive immune responses, and HLA-restricted T cells recognizing a range of *TP53* mutations have been identified from multiple patients with a range of epithelial cancers, with a total of 21 reactive unique TILs and a total of 39 TCRs found to date, recognizing multiple mutant TP53s [168, 169]. Reinfusion of ex vivo expanded mutant TP53-targeting autologous TILs resulted in only 2/12 partial responses in *TP53* mutant cancers, but the TILs had high degree of exhaustion. Instead, a strategy to engineer peripherally harvested T cells with appropriate HLA-restricted TCRs may be more effective, and this strategy indeed resulted in a partial response in a patient with metastatic *TP53* R175H mutant breast cancer [169]. Like the potential for *KRAS* mutation-targeting T-cell therapies, study of CAR-T cell receptor therapy targeting mutant *TP53* is ongoing.

MTAP Deletion

Methylthioadenosine phosphorylase (*MTAP*), an enzyme needed in adenine and methionine salvage, is codeleted with the tumor suppressor *CDKN2A* (p16) in 20–25% of pancreatic cancers. As a consequence of *MTAP* loss, its substrate methylthioadenosine (MTA) accumulates and inhibits the activity of protein arginine methyltransferase 5 (PRMT5), and MTAP-deficient cells are then susceptible to further suppression of PRMT5 activity. *MTAP*-deficient cells are thus vulnerable to PRMT5 inhibitors [170, 171] and methionine adenosyltransferase 2a (MAT2A) inhibitors, which further decrease PRMT5 activity and impair PRMT5-mediated critical functions such as mRNA splicing [172, 173]. Clinical trials of the PRMT5-MTA inhibitor MRTX1719 (NCT05245500), MAT2A inhibitor IDE397 (NCT04794699), and selective PRMT5 inhibitor TNG908 (NCT05275478) are ongoing in *MTAP* homozygously deleted cancers.

Claudin 18.2 Targeted and Cellular Therapies

Claudin 18.2 is a tight junction protein that is normally specifically expressed on differentiated gastric epithelial cells, but is aberrantly expressed in several malignancies, including pancreatic cancer [174]. Immunohistochemical staining for claudin 18.2 was 2+ or greater in 54.6% of pancreatic adenocarcinomas and exceeded 60% in lymph node metastases and liver metastases [175]. Given this limited distribution and high frequency of expression in pancreatic cancer, claudin 18.2 is an attractive target for antibody therapy and antibody-drug conjugates and used for immune therapies like CAR-T cell therapies and CD3-bispecific antibody therapies. Preclinical models showed the anti-claudin 18.2 antibody zolbetuximab induced antibody-dependent cellular cytotoxicity and complement-dependent cytotoxicity in claudin 18.2-expressing pancreatic cancer cells [176]. There is an ongoing clinical trial of the claudin 18.2 targeting antibody zolbetuximab combined with gemcitabine and nab-paclitaxel for first-line therapy of claudin 18.2 expressing metastatic pancreatic cancer (NCT03816163). TST001 is another humanized antibody against claudin 18.2 being studied as monotherapy or in combination with nivolumab (NCT04396821). There is also an ongoing phase I trial of BNT141, an mRNA encoding an antibody against claudin 18.2 (NCT04683939). SOT102 is an antibody-drug conjugate with an anti-claudin 18.2 antibody linked with an anthracycline (NCT05525286). Claudin 18.2-targeting cellular therapies are also being studied in claudin 18.2-expressing gastric and pancreatic cancers. A phase I clinical trial of CT041 CAR-CLDN18.2 T cells showed 1/5 pancreatic cancer patients enrolled had a partial response [177, 178], and the study is ongoing (NCT04404595). ASP2138 is a claudin 18.2 x CD3-bispecific antibody that is now in phase I trials (NCT05365581).

Conclusions

Germline mutation profiling, somatic sequencing, and testing for additional potentially predictive biomarkers for targeted therapies are now standard of care for patients with metastatic pancreatic cancer and are critical for identifying potential clinical trial options. Immediately, actionable biomarkers that impact standard of care options include germline *BRCA1/2* testing, microsatellite instability and/or mismatch repair testing, and somatic NGS including identifying the rare patients whose tumors have *BRAF* V600E mutations or actionable fusions, particularly *NTRK1/2/3* or *RET* fusions, which also have tumor-agnostic FDA approvals for targeted agents. The likelihood of finding other actionable aberrations is significantly higher among the 7–10% of patients who have *KRAS* wild-type pancreatic cancer. Among the remaining 90–93% of patients whose cancers harbor a *KRAS* mutation, it is critical to identify the 1% with *KRAS* G12C mutations, as this mutation is now directly targetable with small molecule inhibitors. Ongoing efforts to render previously "undruggable" targets like mutant *KRAS* or *TP53* as druggable are in progress, though knowledge of the specific mutant allele is required to identify potential targeted therapy trial options.

References

1. Siegel RL, Miller KD, Fuchs HE, Jemal A. Cancer statistics, 2022. CA Cancer J Clin. 2022;72(1):7–33.
2. Conroy T, Desseigne F, Ychou M, Bouche O, Guimbaud R, Becouarn Y, et al. FOLFIRINOX versus gemcitabine for metastatic pancreatic cancer. N Engl J Med. 2011;364(19):1817–25.
3. Von Hoff DD, Ervin T, Arena FP, Chiorean EG, Infante J, Moore M, et al. Increased survival in pancreatic cancer with nab-paclitaxel plus gemcitabine. N Engl J Med. 2013;369(18):1691–703.
4. Tempero MA, Malafa MP, Al-Hawary M, Behrman SW, Benson AB, Cardin DB, et al. Pancreatic adenocarcinoma, version 2.2021, NCCN clinical practice guidelines in oncology. J Natl Compr Cancer Netw. 2021;19(4):439–57.
5. Shindo K, Yu J, Suenaga M, Fesharakizadeh S, Cho C, Macgregor-Das A, et al. Deleterious germline mutations in patients with apparently sporadic pancreatic adenocarcinoma. J Clin Oncol. 2017;35(30):3382–90.
6. Hu C, Hart SN, Polley EC, Gnanaolivu R, Shimelis H, Lee KY, et al. Association between inherited germline mutations in cancer predisposition genes and risk of pancreatic cancer. JAMA. 2018;319(23):2401–9.
7. Yurgelun MB, Chittenden AB, Morales-Oyarvide V, Rubinson DA, Dunne RF, Kozak MM, et al. Germline cancer susceptibility gene variants, somatic second hits, and survival outcomes in patients with resected pancreatic cancer. Genet Med. 2019;21(1):213–23.

8. Holter S, Borgida A, Dodd A, Grant R, Semotiuk K, Hedley D, et al. Germline BRCA mutations in a large clinic-based cohort of patients with pancreatic adenocarcinoma. J Clin Oncol. 2015;33(28):3124–9.

9. Grant RC, Selander I, Connor AA, Selvarajah S, Borgida A, Briollais L, et al. Prevalence of germline mutations in cancer predisposition genes in patients with pancreatic cancer. Gastroenterology. 2015;148(3):556–64.

10. Lowery MA, Wong W, Jordan EJ, Lee JW, Kemel Y, Vijai J, et al. Prospective evaluation of germline alterations in patients with exocrine pancreatic neoplasms. J Natl Cancer Inst. 2018;110(10):1067–74.

11. Li S, Silvestri V, Leslie G, Rebbeck TR, Neuhausen SL, Hopper JL, et al. Cancer risks associated with BRCA1 and BRCA2 pathogenic variants. J Clin Oncol. 2022;2022:JCO2102112.

12. O'Reilly EM, Lee JW, Zalupski M, Capanu M, Park J, Golan T, et al. Randomized, multicenter, phase II trial of gemcitabine and cisplatin with or without veliparib in patients with pancreas adenocarcinoma and a germline BRCA/PALB2 mutation. J Clin Oncol. 2020;38(13):1378–88.

13. Park W, Chen J, Chou JF, Varghese AM, Yu KH, Wong W, et al. Genomic methods identify homologous recombination deficiency in pancreas adenocarcinoma and optimize treatment selection. Clin Cancer Res. 2020;26(13):3239–47.

14. Pommier Y, O'Connor MJ, de Bono J. Laying a trap to kill cancer cells: PARP inhibitors and their mechanisms of action. Sci Transl Med. 2016;8:362.

15. Golan T, Hammel P, Reni M, Van Cutsem E, Macarulla T, Hall MJ, et al. Maintenance olaparib for germline BRCA-mutated metastatic pancreatic cancer. N Engl J Med. 2019;381(4):317–27.

16. Hammel P, Kindler HL, Reni M, Van Cutsem E, Macarulla T, Hall MJ, et al. Health-related quality of life in patients with a germline BRCA mutation and metastatic pancreatic cancer receiving maintenance olaparib. Ann Oncol. 2019;30(12):1959–68.

17. Golan T, Hammel P, Reni M, Cutsem EV, Macarulla T, Hall MJ, et al. Overall survival from the phase 3 POLO trial: maintenance olaparib for germline BRCA-mutated metastatic pancreatic cancer. J Clin Oncol. 2021;39:378.

18. Grellety T, Peyraud F, Sevenet N, Tredan O, Dohollou N, Barouk-Simonet E, et al. Dramatic response to PARP inhibition in a PALB2-mutated breast cancer: moving beyond BRCA. Ann Oncol. 2020;31(6):822–3.

19. Horak P, Weischenfeldt J, von Amsberg G, Beyer B, Schutte A, Uhrig S, et al. Response to olaparib in a PALB2 germline mutated prostate cancer and genetic events associated with resistance. Cold Spring Harb Mol Case Stud. 2019;5(2):3657.

20. Tung NM, Robson ME, Ventz S, Santa-Maria CA, Nanda R, Marcom PK, et al. TBCRC 048: phase II study of olaparib for metastatic breast cancer and mutations in homologous recombination-related genes. J Clin Oncol. 2020;38(36):4274–82.

21. Binder KAR, Mick R, O'Hara M, Teitelbaum U, Karasic T, Schneider C, et al. A phase II, single arm study of maintenance rucaparib in patients with platinum-sensitive advanced pancreatic cancer and a pathogenic germline or somatic mutation in BRCA1, BRCA2 or PALB2. Cancer Res. 2019;79:234.

22. Reislander T, Lombardi EP, Groelly FJ, Miar A, Porru M, Di Vito S, et al. BRCA2 abrogation triggers innate immune responses potentiated by treatment with PARP inhibitors. Nat Commun. 2019;10(1):3143.

23. Ding L, Kim HJ, Wang Q, Kearns M, Jiang T, Ohlson CE, et al. PARP inhibition elicits STING-dependent antitumor immunity in Brca1-deficient ovarian cancer. Cell Rep. 2018;25(11):2972–80.

24. Seeber A, Zimmer K, Kocher F, Puccini A, Xiu J, Nabhan C, et al. Molecular characteristics of BRCA1/2 and PALB2 mutations in pancreatic ductal adenocarcinoma. ESMO Open. 2020;5(6):e000942.

25. Reiss KA, Mick R, Teitelbaum UR, O'Hara MH, Schneider CJ, Massa RC, et al. A randomized phase Ib/II study of niraparib (nira) plus nivolumab (nivo) or ipilimumab (ipi) in

patients (pts) with platinum-sensitive advanced pancreatic cancer (aPDAC). J Clin Oncol. 2022;40:4021.

26. Shroff RT, Hendifar A, McWilliams RR, Geva R, Epelbaum R, Rolfe L, et al. Rucaparib monotherapy in patients with pancreatic cancer and a known deleterious BRCA mutation. JCO Precis Oncol. 2018;2018:316.

27. Mohyuddin GR, Aziz M, Britt A, Wade L, Sun W, Baranda J, et al. Similar response rates and survival with PARP inhibitors for patients with solid tumors harboring somatic versus Germline BRCA mutations: a Meta-analysis and systematic review. BMC Cancer. 2020;20(1):507.

28. Brand R, Borazanci E, Speare V, Dudley B, Karloski E, Peters MLB, et al. Prospective study of germline genetic testing in incident cases of pancreatic adenocarcinoma. Cancer. 2018;124(17):3520–7.

29. Gout J, Perkhofer L, Morawe M, Arnold F, Ihle M, Biber S, et al. Synergistic targeting and resistance to PARP inhibition in DNA damage repair-deficient pancreatic cancer. Gut. 2021;70(4):743–60.

30. Hsu FC, Roberts NJ, Childs E, Porter N, Rabe KG, Borgida A, et al. Risk of pancreatic cancer among individuals with pathogenic variants in the ATM gene. JAMA Oncol. 2021;7(11):1664–8.

31. Bailey P, Chang DK, Nones K, Johns AL, Patch AM, Gingras MC, et al. Genomic analyses identify molecular subtypes of pancreatic cancer. Nature. 2016;531(7592):47–52.

32. Perkhofer L, Schmitt A, Romero Carrasco MC, Ihle M, Hampp S, Ruess DA, et al. ATM deficiency generating genomic instability sensitizes pancreatic ductal adenocarcinoma cells to therapy-induced DNA damage. Cancer Res. 2017;77(20):5576–90.

33. Borazanci E, Korn R, Liang WS, Guarnieri C, Haag S, Snyder C, et al. An analysis of patients with DNA repair pathway mutations treated with a PARP inhibitor. Oncologist. 2020;25(1):60–7.

34. Martino C, Pandya D, Lee R, Levy G, Lo T, Lobo S, et al. ATM-mutated pancreatic cancer: clinical and molecular response to gemcitabine/nab-paclitaxel after genome-based therapy resistance. Pancreas. 2020;49(1):143–7.

35. Jette NR, Kumar M, Radhamani S, Arthur G, Goutam S, Yip S, et al. ATM-deficient cancers provide new opportunities for precision oncology. Cancer. 2020;12(3):687.

36. Armstrong SA, Schultz CW, Azimi-Sadjadi A, Brody JR, Pishvaian MJ. ATM dysfunction in pancreatic adenocarcinoma and associated therapeutic implications. Mol Cancer Ther. 2019;18(11):1899–908.

37. Yap TA, Tan DSP, Terbuch A, Caldwell R, Guo C, Goh BC, et al. First-in-human trial of the oral ataxia telangiectasia and RAD3-related (ATR) inhibitor BAY 1895344 in patients with advanced solid tumors. Cancer Discov. 2021;11(1):80–91.

38. Yap TA, Plummer R, Azad NS, Helleday T. The DNA damaging revolution: PARP inhibitors and beyond. Am Soc Clin Oncol Educ Book. 2019;39:185–95.

39. Luchini C, Brosens LAA, Wood LD, Chatterjee D, Shin JI, Sciammarella C, et al. Comprehensive characterisation of pancreatic ductal adenocarcinoma with microsatellite instability: histology, molecular pathology and clinical implications. Gut. 2021;70(1):148–56.

40. Ahmad-Nielsen SA, Bruun Nielsen MF, Mortensen MB, Detlefsen S. Frequency of mismatch repair deficiency in pancreatic ductal adenocarcinoma. Pathol Res Pract. 2020;216(6):152985.

41. Kastrinos F, Mukherjee B, Tayob N, Wang F, Sparr J, Raymond VM, et al. Risk of pancreatic cancer in families with Lynch syndrome. JAMA. 2009;302(16):1790–5.

42. Le DT, Durham JN, Smith KN, Wang H, Bartlett BR, Aulakh LK, et al. Mismatch repair deficiency predicts response of solid tumors to PD-1 blockade. Science. 2017;357(6349):409–13.

43. Marabelle A, Le DT, Ascierto PA, Di Giacomo AM, De Jesus-Acosta A, Delord JP, et al. Efficacy of pembrolizumab in patients with noncolorectal high microsatellite instability/mismatch repair-deficient cancer: results from the phase II KEYNOTE-158 study. J Clin Oncol. 2020;38(1):1–10.

44. Chakrabarti S, Bucheit L, Starr JS, Innis-Shelton R, Shergill A, Dada H, et al. Detection of microsatellite instability-high (MSI-H) by liquid biopsy predicts robust and

durable response to immunotherapy in patients with pancreatic cancer. J Immunother Cancer. 2022;10(6):e004485.

45. Andre T, Berton D, Curigliano G, Jimenez-Rodriguez B, Ellard S, Gravina A, et al. Efficacy and safety of dostarlimab in patients (pts) with mismatch repair deficient (dMMR) solid tumors: analysis of 2 cohorts in the GARNET study. J Clin Oncol. 2022;40:2587.

46. Marabelle A, Fakih M, Lopez J, Shah M, Shapira-Frommer R, Nakagawa K, et al. Association of tumour mutational burden with outcomes in patients with advanced solid tumours treated with pembrolizumab: prospective biomarker analysis of the multicohort, open-label, phase 2 KEYNOTE-158 study. Lancet Oncol. 2020;21(10):1353–65.

47. Lawlor RT, Mattiolo P, Mafficini A, Hong SM, Piredda ML, Taormina SV, et al. Tumor mutational burden as a potential biomarker for immunotherapy in pancreatic cancer: systematic review and still-open questions. Cancer. 2021;13(13):3119.

48. Karamitopoulou E, Andreou A, Wenning AS, Gloor B, Perren A. High tumor mutational burden (TMB) identifies a microsatellite stable pancreatic cancer subset with prolonged survival and strong anti-tumor immunity. Eur J Cancer. 2022;169:64–73.

49. McGrail DJ, Pilie PG, Rashid NU, Voorwerk L, Slagter M, Kok M, et al. High tumor mutation burden fails to predict immune checkpoint blockade response across all cancer types. Ann Oncol. 2021;32(5):661–72.

50. Valero C, Lee M, Hoen D, Zehir A, Berger MF, Seshan VE, et al. Response rates to Anti-PD-1 immunotherapy in microsatellite-stable solid tumors with 10 or more mutations per megabase. JAMA Oncol. 2021;7(5):739–43.

51. Cancer Genome Atlas Research Network. Integrated genomic characterization of pancreatic ductal adenocarcinoma. Cancer Cell. 2017;32(2):185–203.

52. Waddell N, Pajic M, Patch AM, Chang DK, Kassahn KS, Bailey P, et al. Whole genomes redefine the mutational landscape of pancreatic cancer. Nature. 2015;518(7540):495–501.

53. Moore AR, Rosenberg SC, McCormick F, Malek S. RAS-targeted therapies: is the undruggable drugged? Nat Rev Drug Discov. 2020;19(8):533–52.

54. Waters AM, Der CJ. KRAS: the critical driver and therapeutic target for pancreatic cancer. Cold Spring Harb Perspect Med. 2018;8(9):31435.

55. Singhi AD, George B, Greenbowe JR, Chung J, Suh J, Maitra A, et al. Real-time targeted genome profile analysis of pancreatic ductal adenocarcinomas identifies genetic alterations that might be targeted with existing drugs or used as biomarkers. Gastroenterology. 2019;156(8):2242–53.

56. Hofmann MH, Gerlach D, Misale S, Petronczki M, Kraut N. Expanding the reach of precision oncology by drugging All KRAS mutants. Cancer Discov. 2022;12(4):924–37.

57. Canon J, Rex K, Saiki AY, Mohr C, Cooke K, Bagal D, et al. The clinical KRAS(G12C) inhibitor AMG 510 drives anti-tumour immunity. Nature. 2019;575(7781):217–23.

58. Hallin J, Engstrom LD, Hargis L, Calinisan A, Aranda R, Briere DM, et al. The KRAS(G12C) inhibitor MRTX849 provides insight toward therapeutic susceptibility of KRAS-mutant cancers in mouse models and patients. Cancer Discov. 2020;10(1):54–71.

59. Hong DS, Fakih MG, Strickler JH, Desai J, Durm GA, Shapiro GI, et al. KRAS(G12C) inhibition with sotorasib in advanced solid tumors. N Engl J Med. 2020;383(13):1207–17.

60. Strickler JH, Satake H, Hollebecque A, Sunakawa Y, Tomasini P, Bajor DL, et al. First data for sotorasib in patients with pancreatic cancer with KRAS p.G12C mutation: a phase I/II study evaluating efficacy and safety. J Clin Oncol. 2022;40:360490.

61. Jänne PA, Rybkin II, Spira AI, Riely GJ, Papadopoulos KP, Sabari JK, et al. KRYSTAL-1: activity and safety of Adagrasib (MRTX849) in advanced/metastatic non–small-cell lung cancer (NSCLC) harboring KRAS G12C mutation. Eur J Cancer. 2020;138:S1.

62. Bekaii-Saab TS, Spira AI, Yaeger R, Buchschacher GL, McRee AJ, Sabari JK, et al. KRYSTAL-1: updated activity and safety of adagrasib (MRTX849) in patients (Pts) with unresectable or metastatic pancreatic cancer (PDAC) and other gastrointestinal (GI) tumors harboring a KRASG12C mutation. J Clin Oncol. 2022;40:519.

63. Awad MM, Liu S, Rybkin II, Arbour KC, Dilly J, Zhu VW, et al. Acquired resistance to KRAS(G12C) inhibition in cancer. N Engl J Med. 2021;384(25):2382–93.

64. Zhao Y, Murciano-Goroff YR, Xue JY, Ang A, Lucas J, Mai TT, et al. Diverse alterations associated with resistance to KRAS(G12C) inhibition. Nature. 2021;599(7886):679–83.

65. Amodio V, Yaeger R, Arcella P, Cancelliere C, Lamba S, Lorenzato A, et al. EGFR blockade reverts resistance to KRAS(G12C) inhibition in colorectal cancer. Cancer Discov. 2020;10(8):1129–39.

66. Molina-Arcas M, Moore C, Rana S, van Maldegem F, Mugarza E, Romero-Clavijo P, et al. Development of combination therapies to maximize the impact of KRAS-G12C inhibitors in lung cancer. Sci Transl Med. 2019;11:510.

67. Wang X, Allen S, Blake JF, Bowcut V, Briere DM, Calinisan A, et al. Identification of MRTX1133, a noncovalent, potent, and selective KRAS(G12D) inhibitor. J Med Chem. 2022;65(4):3123–33.

68. Hallin J, Bowcut V, Calinisan A, Briere DM, Hargis L, Engstrom LD, et al. Anti-tumor efficacy of a potent and selective non-covalent KRAS(G12D) inhibitor. Nat Med. 2022;28(10):2171–82.

69. Kelsey S, editor Approaches to inhibiting RAS driven tumors beyond KRAS-G12C. In: 2nd annual RAS-targeted drug development conference; 2020 September 14-16, 2020; Virtual Meeting.

70. Gustafson WC, Wildes D, Rice MA, Lee BJ, Jiang J, Wang Z, et al. Direct targeting of RAS in pancreatic ductal adenocarcinoma with RMC-6236, a first-in-class, RAS-selective, orally bioavailable, tri-complex RASMULTI(ON) inhibitor. J Clin Oncol. 2022;40:591.

71. Nichols RJ, Yang YC, Cregg J, Schulze CJ, Wang Z, Dua R, et al. RMC-6291, a next-generation tri-complex KRASG12C(ON) inhibitor, outperforms KRASG12C(OFF) inhibitors in preclinical models of KRASG12C cancers. Cancer Res. 2022;82:3595.

72. Knox JE, Jiang J, Burnett GL, Liu Y, Weller CE, Wang Z, et al. RM-036, a first-in-class, orally-bioavailable, Tri-Complex covalent KRASG12D(ON) inhibitor, drives profound anti-tumor activity in KRASG12D mutant tumor models. Cancer Res. 2022;82:3596.

73. Hillig RC, Sautier B, Schroeder J, Moosmayer D, Hilpmann A, Stegmann CM, et al. Discovery of potent SOS1 inhibitors that block RAS activation via disruption of the RAS-SOS1 interaction. Proc Natl Acad Sci U S A. 2019;116(7):2551–60.

74. Rozakis-Adcock M, van der Geer P, Mbamalu G, Pawson T. MAP kinase phosphorylation of mSos1 promotes dissociation of mSos1-Shc and mSos1-EGF receptor complexes. Oncogene. 1995;11(7):1417–26.

75. Hobbs GA, Baker NM, Miermont AM, Thurman RD, Pierobon M, Tran TH, et al. Atypical KRAS(G12R) mutant is impaired in PI3K signaling and macropinocytosis in pancreatic cancer. Cancer Discov. 2020;10(1):104–23.

76. Hunter JC, Manandhar A, Carrasco MA, Gurbani D, Gondi S, Westover KD. Biochemical and structural analysis of common cancer-associated KRAS mutations. Mol Cancer Res. 2015;13(9):1325–35.

77. Hofmann MH, Gmachl M, Ramharter J, Savarese F, Gerlach D, Marszalek JR, et al. BI-3406, a potent and selective SOS1-KRAS interaction inhibitor, is effective in KRAS-driven cancers through combined MEK inhibition. Cancer Discov. 2020;11(1):142–57.

78. Gerlach D, Gmachl M, Ramharter J, Teh J, Fu S-C, Trapani F, et al. Abstract 1091: BI-3406 and BI 1701963: potent and selective SOS1: KRAS inhibitors induce regressions in combination with MEK inhibitors or irinotecan. Cancer Res. 2020;80:1091.

79. Johnson ML, Gort E, Pant S, Lolkema MP, Sebastian M, Scheffler M, et al. 524P - a phase I, open-label, dose-escalation trial of BI 1701963 in patients (pts) with KRAS mutated solid tumours: a snapshot analysis. Ann Oncol. 2021;32:591–2.

80. Ketcham JM, Haling J, Khare S, Bowcut V, Briere DM, Burns AC, et al. Design and discovery of MRTX0902, a potent, selective, brain-penetrant, and orally bioavailable inhibitor of the SOS1: KRAS protein-protein interaction. J Med Chem. 2022;65(14):9678–90.

81. Nichols RJ, Haderk F, Stahlhut C, Schulze CJ, Hemmati G, Wildes D, et al. RAS nucleotide cycling underlies the SHP2 phosphatase dependence of mutant BRAF-, NF1- and RAS-driven cancers. Nat Cell Biol. 2018;20(9):1064–73.

82. Ruess DA, Heynen GJ, Ciecielski KJ, Ai J, Berninger A, Kabacaoglu D, et al. Mutant KRAS-driven cancers depend on PTPN11/SHP2 phosphatase. Nat Med. 2018;24(7):954–60.

83. Ahmed TA, Adamopoulos C, Karoulia Z, Wu X, Sachidanandam R, Aaronson SA, et al. SHP2 drives adaptive resistance to ERK signaling inhibition in molecularly defined subsets of ERK-dependent tumors. Cell Rep. 2019;26(1):65–78.

84. Lu H, Liu C, Velazquez R, Wang H, Dunkl LM, Kazic-Legueux M, et al. SHP2 inhibition overcomes RTK-mediated pathway reactivation in KRAS-mutant tumors treated with MEK inhibitors. Mol Cancer Ther. 2019;18(7):1323–34.

85. Liu C, Lu H, Wang H, Loo A, Zhang X, Yang G, et al. Combinations with allosteric SHP2 inhibitor TNO155 to block receptor tyrosine kinase signaling. Clin Cancer Res. 2021;27(1):342–54.

86. Fedele C, Li S, Teng KW, Foster CJR, Peng D, Ran H, et al. SHP2 inhibition diminishes KRASG12C cycling and promotes tumor microenvironment remodeling. J Exp Med. 2021;218(1):e20201414.

87. Brana I, Shapiro G, Johnson ML, Yu HA, Robbrecht D, Tan DS-W, et al. Initial results from a dose finding study of TNO155, a SHP2 inhibitor, in adults with advanced solid tumors. J Clin Oncol. 2021;39:3005.

88. Wang QJ, Yu Z, Griffith K, Hanada K, Restifo NP, Yang JC. Identification of T-cell receptors targeting KRAS-mutated human tumors. Cancer Immunol Res. 2016;4(3):204–14.

89. Cafri G, Yossef R, Pasetto A, Deniger DC, Lu YC, Parkhurst M, et al. Memory T cells targeting oncogenic mutations detected in peripheral blood of epithelial cancer patients. Nat Commun. 2019;10(1):449.

90. Poole A, Karuppiah V, Hartt A, Haidar JN, Moureau S, Dobrzycki T, et al. Therapeutic high affinity T cell receptor targeting a KRAS(G12D) cancer neoantigen. Nat Commun. 2022;13(1):5333.

91. Tran E, Robbins PF, Lu YC, Prickett TD, Gartner JJ, Jia L, et al. T-Cell transfer therapy targeting mutant KRAS in cancer. N Engl J Med. 2016;375(23):2255–62.

92. Sim MJW, Lu J, Spencer M, Hopkins F, Tran E, Rosenberg SA, et al. High-affinity oligoclonal TCRs define effective adoptive T cell therapy targeting mutant KRAS-G12D. Proc Natl Acad Sci U S A. 2020;117(23):12826–35.

93. Leidner R, Sanjuan Silva N, Huang H, Sprott D, Zheng C, Shih YP, et al. Neoantigen T-cell receptor gene therapy in pancreatic cancer. N Engl J Med. 2022;386(22):2112–9.

94. Bear AS, Blanchard T, Cesare J, Ford MJ, Richman LP, Xu C, et al. Biochemical and functional characterization of mutant KRAS epitopes validates this oncoprotein for immunological targeting. Nat Commun. 2021;12(1):4365.

95. Mullard A. Cracking KRAS. Nat Rev Drug Discov. 2019;18(12):887–91.

96. Steinbuck M, DeMuth P, Seenappa L. Lymph node-targeted AMP-vaccine enables tumor-directed mKRAS-specific immune responses with potent polyfunctional and cytolytic activity. J Immunother Cancer. 2020;8:723.

97. Roberts TC, Langer R, Wood MJA. Advances in oligonucleotide drug delivery. Nat Rev Drug Discov. 2020;19(10):673–94.

98. Zorde Khvalevsky E, Gabai R, Rachmut IH, Horwitz E, Brunschwig Z, Orbach A, et al. Mutant KRAS is a druggable target for pancreatic cancer. Proc Natl Acad Sci U S A. 2013;110(51):20723–8.

99. Golan T, Khvalevsky EZ, Hubert A, Gabai RM, Hen N, Segal A, et al. RNAi therapy targeting KRAS in combination with chemotherapy for locally advanced pancreatic cancer patients. Oncotarget. 2015;6(27):24560–70.

100. Kamerkar S, LeBleu VS, Sugimoto H, Yang S, Ruivo CF, Melo SA, et al. Exosomes facilitate therapeutic targeting of oncogenic KRAS in pancreatic cancer. Nature. 2017;546(7659):498–503.

101. Pecot CV, Wu SY, Bellister S, Filant J, Rupaimoole R, Hisamatsu T, et al. Therapeutic silencing of KRAS using systemically delivered siRNAs. Mol Cancer Ther. 2014;13(12):2876–85.

102. Papke B, Azam SH, Feng AY, Gutierrez-Ford C, Huggins H, Pallan PS, et al. Silencing of oncogenic KRAS by mutant-selective small interfering RNA. ACS Pharmacol Transl Sci. 2021;4(2):703–12.
103. Mendt M, Kamerkar S, Sugimoto H, McAndrews KM, Wu CC, Gagea M, et al. Generation and testing of clinical-grade exosomes for pancreatic cancer. JCI Insight. 2018;3(8):e99263.
104. Infante JR, Somer BG, Park JO, Li CP, Scheulen ME, Kasubhai SM, et al. A randomised, double-blind, placebo-controlled trial of trametinib, an oral MEK inhibitor, in combination with gemcitabine for patients with untreated metastatic adenocarcinoma of the pancreas. Eur J Cancer. 2014;50(12):2072–81.
105. Ko AH, Bekaii-Saab T, Van Ziffle J, Mirzoeva OM, Joseph NM, Talasaz A, et al. A multicenter, open-label phase II clinical trial of combined MEK plus EGFR inhibition for chemotherapy-refractory advanced pancreatic adenocarcinoma. Clin Cancer Res. 2016;22(1):61–8.
106. Bodoky G, Timcheva C, Spigel DR, La Stella PJ, Ciuleanu TE, Pover G, et al. A phase II open-label randomized study to assess the efficacy and safety of selumetinib (AZD6244 [ARRY-142886]) versus capecitabine in patients with advanced or metastatic pancreatic cancer who have failed first-line gemcitabine therapy. Investig New Drugs. 2012;30(3):1216–23.
107. Kenney C, Kunst T, Webb S, Christina D Jr, Arrowood C, Steinberg SM, et al. Phase II study of selumetinib, an orally active inhibitor of MEK1 and MEK2 kinases, in KRAS(G12R)-mutant pancreatic ductal adenocarcinoma. Investig New Drugs. 2021;39(3):821–8.
108. Ardalan B, Cotta JA, Gombosh M, Azqueta JI. Cobimetinib plus gemcitabine is an active combination in KRAS G12R-mutated in previously chemotherapy-treated and failed pancreatic patients. J Clin Oncol. 2020;38:4642.
109. Bryant KL, Stalnecker CA, Zeitouni D, Klomp JE, Peng S, Tikunov AP, et al. Combination of ERK and autophagy inhibition as a treatment approach for pancreatic cancer. Nat Med. 2019;25(4):628–40.
110. Kinsey CG, Camolotto SA, Boespflug AM, Guillen KP, Foth M, Truong A, et al. Protective autophagy elicited by RAF→MEK→ERK inhibition suggests a treatment strategy for RAS-driven cancers. Nat Med. 2019;25(4):620–7.
111. Rahib L, Chen K, Ocean AJ, Xie C, Duffy A, Manji GA, et al. Use of a real-world data approach to rapidly generate outcomes data following a case study of a novel treatment combination in pancreatic adenocarcinoma. J Clin Oncol. 2020;38:e16735.
112. Heining C, Horak P, Uhrig S, Codo PL, Klink B, Hutter B, et al. NRG1 fusions in KRAS wild-type pancreatic cancer. Cancer Discov. 2018;8(9):1087–95.
113. Zhang X, Mao T, Zhang B, Xu H, Cui J, Jiao F, et al. Characterization of the genomic landscape in large-scale Chinese patients with pancreatic cancer. EBioMedicine. 2022;77:103897.
114. Windon AL, Loaiza-Bonilla A, Jensen CE, Randall M, Morrissette JJD, Shroff SG. A KRAS wild type mutational status confers a survival advantage in pancreatic ductal adenocarcinoma. J Gastrointest Oncol. 2018;9(1):1–10.
115. Topham JT, Tsang ES, Karasinska JM, Metcalfe A, Ali H, Kalloger SE, et al. Integrative analysis of KRAS wildtype metastatic pancreatic ductal adenocarcinoma reveals mutation and expression-based similarities to cholangiocarcinoma. Nat Commun. 2022;13(1):5941.
116. Jones MR, Williamson LM, Topham JT, Lee MKC, Goytain A, Ho J, et al. NRG1 gene fusions are recurrent, clinically actionable gene rearrangements in KRAS wild-type pancreatic ductal adenocarcinoma. Clin Cancer Res. 2019;25(15):4674–81.
117. Philip PA, Azar I, Xiu J, Hall MJ, Hendifar AE, Lou E, et al. Molecular characterization of KRAS wild-type tumors in patients with pancreatic adenocarcinoma. Clin Cancer Res. 2022;28(12):2704–14.
118. Schultheis B, Reuter D, Ebert MP, Siveke J, Kerkhoff A, Berdel WE, et al. Gemcitabine combined with the monoclonal antibody nimotuzumab is an active first-line regimen in KRAS wildtype patients with locally advanced or metastatic pancreatic cancer: a multicenter, randomized phase IIb study. Ann Oncol. 2017;28(10):2429–35.
119. Qin S, Bai Y, Wang Z, Chen Z, Xu R, Xu J, et al. Nimotuzumab combined with gemcitabine versus gemcitabine in K-RAS wild-type locally advanced or metastatic pancreatic cancer: a

prospective, randomized-controlled, double-blinded, multicenter, and phase III clinical trial. J Clin Oncol. 2022;40:LBA4011.

120. Drilon A, Somwar R, Mangatt BP, Edgren H, Desmeules P, Ruusulehto A, et al. Response to ERBB3-directed targeted therapy in NRG1-rearranged cancers. Cancer Discov. 2018;8(6):686–95.

121. Cadranel J, Liu SV, Duruisseaux M, Branden E, Goto Y, Weinberg BA, et al. Therapeutic potential of afatinib in NRG1 fusion-driven solid tumors: a case series. Oncologist. 2021;26(1):7–16.

122. Laskin J, Liu SV, Tolba K, Heining C, Schlenk RF, Cheema P, et al. NRG1 fusion-driven tumors: biology, detection, and the therapeutic role of afatinib and other ErbB-targeting agents. Ann Oncol. 2020;31(12):1693–703.

123. Schram AM, Odintsov I, Espinosa-Cotton M, Khodos I, Sisso WJ, Mattar MS, et al. Zenocutuzumab, a HER2xHER3 bispecific antibody, is effective therapy for tumors driven by NRG1 gene rearrangements. Cancer Discov. 2022;12(5):1233–47.

124. Schram AM, Goto K, Kim D-W, Martin-Romano P, Ou S-HI, O'Kane GM, et al. Efficacy and safety of zenocutuzumab, a HER2 x HER3 bispecific antibody, across advanced NRG1 fusion (NRG1+) cancers. J Clin Oncol. 2022;40:105.

125. Seghers AK, Cuyle PJ, Van Cutsem E. Molecular targeting of a BRAF mutation in pancreatic ductal adenocarcinoma: case report and literature review. Target Oncol. 2020;15(3):407–10.

126. Hyman DM, Puzanov I, Subbiah V, Faris JE, Chau I, Blay JY, et al. Vemurafenib in multiple nonmelanoma cancers with BRAF V600 mutations. N Engl J Med. 2015;373(8):726–36.

127. Grinshpun A, Zarbiv Y, Roszik J, Subbiah V, Hubert A. Beyond KRAS: practical molecular targets in pancreatic adenocarcinoma. Case Rep Oncol. 2019;12(1):7–13.

128. Li HS, Yang K, Wang Y. Remarkable response of BRAF (V600E)-mutated metastatic pancreatic cancer to BRAF/MEK inhibition: a case report. Gastroenterol Rep. 2022;10:31.

129. Hendifar A, Blais EM, Wolpin B, Subbiah V, Collisson E, Singh I, et al. Retrospective case series analysis of RAF family alterations in pancreatic cancer: real-world outcomes from targeted and standard therapies. JCO Precis Oncol. 2021;5:494.

130. Yao Z, Torres NM, Tao A, Gao Y, Luo L, Li Q, et al. BRAF mutants evade erk-dependent feedback by different mechanisms that determine their sensitivity to pharmacologic inhibition. Cancer Cell. 2015;28(3):370–83.

131. Dankner M, Rose AAN, Rajkumar S, Siegel PM, Watson IR. Classifying BRAF alterations in cancer: new rational therapeutic strategies for actionable mutations. Oncogene. 2018;37(24):3183–99.

132. Yao Z, Yaeger R, Rodrik-Outmezguine VS, Tao A, Torres NM, Chang MT, et al. Tumours with class 3 BRAF mutants are sensitive to the inhibition of activated RAS. Nature. 2017;548(7666):234–8.

133. Johnson DB, Zhao F, Noel M, Riely GJ, Mitchell EP, Wright JJ, et al. Trametinib activity in patients with solid tumors and lymphomas harboring BRAF non-V600 mutations or fusions: results from NCI-MATCH (EAY131). Clin Cancer Res. 2020;26(8):1812–9.

134. Foster SA, Whalen DM, Ozen A, Wongchenko MJ, Yin J, Yen I, et al. Activation mechanism of oncogenic deletion mutations in BRAF, EGFR, and HER2. Cancer Cell. 2016;29(4):477–93.

135. Chen SH, Zhang Y, Van Horn RD, Yin T, Buchanan S, Yadav V, et al. Oncogenic BRAF deletions that function as homodimers and are sensitive to inhibition by RAF dimer inhibitor LY3009120. Cancer Discov. 2016;6(3):300–15.

136. Wrzeszczynski KO, Rahman S, Frank MO, Arora K, Shah M, Geiger H, et al. Identification of targetable BRAF DeltaN486_P490 variant by whole-genome sequencing leading to dabrafenib-induced remission of a BRAF-mutant pancreatic adenocarcinoma. Cold Spring Harb Mol Case Stud. 2019;5(6):4424.

137. Chmielecki J, Hutchinson KE, Frampton GM, Chalmers ZR, Johnson A, Shi C, et al. Comprehensive genomic profiling of pancreatic acinar cell carcinomas identifies recurrent RAF fusions and frequent inactivation of DNA repair genes. Cancer Discov. 2014;4(12):1398–405.

138. Botton T, Talevich E, Mishra VK, Zhang T, Shain AH, Berquet C, et al. Genetic heterogeneity of BRAF fusion kinases in melanoma affects drug responses. Cell Rep. 2019;29(3):573–88.

139. Hainsworth JD, Meric-Bernstam F, Swanton C, Hurwitz H, Spigel DR, Sweeney C, et al. Targeted therapy for advanced solid tumors on the basis of molecular profiles: results from MyPathway, an open-label, phase IIa multiple basket study. J Clin Oncol. 2018;36(6):536–42.

140. Li J, Lu H, Ng PK, Pantazi A, Ip CKM, Jeong KJ, et al. A functional genomic approach to actionable gene fusions for precision oncology. Sci Adv. 2022;8(6):2382.

141. Yang WW, Yang L, Lu HZ, Sun YK. Long-term survival of a patient with pancreatic cancer and lung metastasis: a case report and review of literature. World J Clin Cases. 2021;9(30):9134–43.

142. Allen MJ, Zhang A, Bavi P, Kim JC, Jang GH, Kelly D, et al. Molecular characterisation of pancreatic ductal adenocarcinoma with NTRK fusions and review of the literature. J Clin Pathol. 2021;76(3):158–65.

143. Westphalen CB, Krebs MG, Le Tourneau C, Sokol ES, Maund SL, Wilson TR, et al. Genomic context of NTRK1/2/3 fusion-positive tumours from a large real-world population. NPJ Precis Oncol. 2021;5(1):69.

144. Doebele RC, Drilon A, Paz-Ares L, Siena S, Shaw AT, Farago AF, et al. Entrectinib in patients with advanced or metastatic NTRK fusion-positive solid tumours: integrated analysis of three phase 1-2 trials. Lancet Oncol. 2020;21(2):271–82.

145. Demetri GD, De Braud F, Drilon A, Siena S, Patel MR, Cho BC, et al. Updated integrated analysis of the efficacy and safety of entrectinib in patients with NTRK fusion-positive solid tumors. Clin Cancer Res. 2022;28(7):1302–12.

146. Hyman D, Tan DSW, Tilburg CV, Albert C, Geoerger B, Farago A, et al. Durability of response with larotrectinib in adult and pediatric patients with TRK fusion cancer. Ann Oncol. 2019;30:ix123.

147. Drilon A, Laetsch TW, Kummar S, DuBois SG, Lassen UN, Demetri GD, et al. Efficacy of larotrectinib in TRK fusion-positive cancers in adults and children. N Engl J Med. 2018;378(8):731–9.

148. Drilon AE, Hong DS, Tilburg CM, Doz F, Tan DS, Kummar S, et al. Long-term efficacy and safety of larotrectinib in a pooled analysis of patients with tropomyosin receptor kinase (TRK) fusion cancer. J Clin Oncol. 2022;40:3100.

149. O'Reilly EM, Hechtman JF. Tumour response to TRK inhibition in a patient with pancreatic adenocarcinoma harbouring an NTRK gene fusion. Ann Oncol. 2019;30(8):36–40.

150. Pishvaian MJ, Garrido-Laguna I, Liu SV, Multani PS, Chow-Maneval E, Rolfo C. Entrectinib in TRK and ROS1 fusion-positive metastatic pancreatic cancer. JCO Precis Oncol. 2018;2:1–7.

151. Drilon AE, Subbiah V, Oxnard GR, Bauer TM, Velcheti V, Lakhani NJ, et al. A phase 1 study of LOXO-292, a potent and highly selective RET inhibitor, in patients with RET-altered cancers. J Clin Oncol. 2018;36:102.

152. Subbiah V, Wolf J, Konda B, Kang H, Spira A, Weiss J, et al. Tumour-agnostic efficacy and safety of selpercatinib in patients with RET fusion-positive solid tumours other than lung or thyroid tumours (LIBRETTO-001): a phase 1/2, open-label, basket trial. Lancet Oncol. 2022;23(10):1261–73.

153. Subbiah V, Hu MI-N, Gainor JF, Mansfield AS, Alonso G, Taylor MH, et al. Clinical activity of the RET inhibitor pralsetinib (BLU-667) in patients with RET fusion+ solid tumors. J Clin Oncol. 2020;38:109.

154. Subbiah V, Cassier PA, Siena S, Garralda E, Paz-Ares L, Garrido P, et al. Pan-cancer efficacy of pralsetinib in patients with RET fusion-positive solid tumors from the phase 1/2 ARROW trial. Nat Med. 2022;28(8):1640–5.

155. Subbiah V, Iannotti NO, Gutierrez M, Smith DC, Feliz L, Lihou CF, et al. FIGHT-101, a first-in-human study of potent and selective FGFR 1-3 inhibitor pemigatinib in pan-cancer patients with FGF/FGFR alterations and advanced malignancies. Ann Oncol. 2022;33(5):522–33.

156. Fusco MJ, Saeed-Vafa D, Carballido EM, Boyle TA, Malafa M, Blue KL, et al. Identification of targetable gene fusions and structural rearrangements to foster precision medicine in KRAS wild-type pancreatic cancer. JCO Precis Oncol. 2021;5:65–74.

157. Ng CF, Glaspy J, Placencio-Hickok VR, Thomassian S, Gong J, Osipov A, et al. Exceptional response to erdafitinib in FGFR2-mutated metastatic pancreatic ductal adenocarcinoma. J Natl Compr Cancer Netw. 2022;20(10):1076–9.
158. Poon D, Tan MH, Khor D. Stage 4 pancreatic adenocarcinoma harbouring an FGFR2-TACC2 fusion mutation with complete response to erdafitinib a pan-fibroblastic growth factor receptor inhibitor. BMJ Case Rep. 2021;14(9):e244271.
159. Singhi AD, Ali SM, Lacy J, Hendifar A, Nguyen K, Koo J, et al. Identification of targetable ALK rearrangements in pancreatic ductal adenocarcinoma. J Natl Compr Cancer Netw. 2017;15(5):555–62.
160. Gower A, Golestany B, Gong J, Singhi AD, Hendifar AE. Novel ALK fusion, PPFIBP1-ALK, in pancreatic ductal adenocarcinoma responsive to Alectinib and Lorlatinib. JCO Precis Oncol. 2020;4:865.
161. Ou K, Liu X, Li W, Yang Y, Ying J, Yang L. ALK rearrangement-positive pancreatic cancer with brain metastasis has remarkable response to ALK inhibitors: a case report. Front Oncol. 2021;11:724815.
162. Meric-Bernstam F, Hainsworth J, Bose R III, Friedman CF, Kurzrock R, et al. MyPathway HER2 basket study: pertuzumab (P) + trastuzumab (H) treatment of a large, tissue-agnostic cohort of patients with HER2-positive advanced solid tumors. J Clin Oncol. 2021;39(15):3004.
163. Tsurutani J, Iwata H, Krop I, Janne PA, Doi T, Takahashi S, et al. Targeting HER2 with trastuzumab deruxtecan: a dose-expansion, phase I study in multiple advanced solid tumors. Cancer Discov. 2020;10(5):688–701.
164. Levine AJ. Targeting the P53 protein for cancer therapies: the translational impact of P53 research. Cancer Res. 2022;82(3):362–4.
165. Weissmueller S, Manchado E, Saborowski M, Morris JP, Wagenblast E, Davis CA, et al. Mutant p53 drives pancreatic cancer metastasis through cell-autonomous PDGF receptor beta signaling. Cell. 2014;157(2):382–94.
166. Kim MP, Li X, Deng J, Zhang Y, Dai B, Allton KL, et al. Oncogenic KRAS recruits an expansive transcriptional network through mutant p53 to drive pancreatic cancer metastasis. Cancer Discov. 2021;11(8):2094–111.
167. Dumbrava EE, Johnson ML, Tolcher AW, Shapiro G, Thompson JA, El-Khoueiry AB, et al. First-in-human study of PC14586, a small molecule structural corrector of Y220C mutant p53, in patients with advanced solid tumors harboring a TP53 Y220C mutation. J Clin Oncol. 2022;40:3003.
168. Malekzadeh P, Pasetto A, Robbins PF, Parkhurst MR, Paria BC, Jia L, et al. Neoantigen screening identifies broad TP53 mutant immunogenicity in patients with epithelial cancers. J Clin Invest. 2019;129(3):1109–14.
169. Kim SP, Vale NR, Zacharakis N, Krishna S, Yu Z, Gasmi B, et al. Adoptive cellular therapy with autologous tumor-infiltrating lymphocytes and T-cell receptor-engineered T cells targeting common p53 neoantigens in human solid tumors. Cancer Immunol Res. 2022;10(8):932–46.
170. Kryukov GV, Wilson FH, Ruth JR, Paulk J, Tsherniak A, Marlow SE, et al. MTAP deletion confers enhanced dependency on the PRMT5 arginine methyltransferase in cancer cells. Science. 2016;351(6278):1214–8.
171. Mavrakis KJ, McDonald ER 3rd, Schlabach MR, Billy E, Hoffman GR, deWeck A, et al. Disordered methionine metabolism in MTAP/CDKN2A-deleted cancers leads to dependence on PRMT5. Science. 2016;351(6278):1208–13.
172. Kalev P, Hyer ML, Gross S, Konteatis Z, Chen CC, Fletcher M, et al. MAT2A inhibition blocks the growth of MTAP-deleted cancer cells by reducing PRMT5-dependent mRNA splicing and inducing DNA damage. Cancer Cell. 2021;39(2):209–24.
173. Marjon K, Cameron MJ, Quang P, Clasquin MF, Mandley E, Kunii K, et al. MTAP deletions in cancer create vulnerability to targeting of the MAT2A/PRMT5/RIOK1 axis. Cell Rep. 2016;15(3):574–87.
174. Sahin U, Koslowski M, Dhaene K, Usener D, Brandenburg G, Seitz G, et al. Claudin-18 splice variant 2 is a pan-cancer target suitable for therapeutic antibody development. Clin Cancer Res. 2008;14(23):7624–34.

175. Woll S, Schlitter AM, Dhaene K, Roller M, Esposito I, Sahin U, et al. Claudin 18.2 is a target for IMAB362 antibody in pancreatic neoplasms. Int J Cancer. 2014;134(3):731–9.
176. Tureci M-KR, Woll S, Yamada T, Sahin U. Characterization of zolbetuximab in pancreatic cancer models. Onco Targets Ther. 2019;8(1):e1523096.
177. Zhan X, Wang B, Li Z, Li J, Wang H, Chen L, et al. Phase I trial of Claudin 18.2-specific chimeric antigen receptor T cells for advanced gastric and pancreatic adenocarcinoma. J Clin Oncol. 2019;37:2509.
178. Qi C, Gong J, Li J, Liu D, Qin Y, Ge S, et al. Claudin18.2-specific CAR T cells in gastrointestinal cancers: phase 1 trial interim results. Nat Med. 2022;28(6):1189–98.

Immunotherapy in Pancreatic Cancer

6

Zachary P. Yeung and Madappa N. Kundranda

Introduction

Pancreatic ductal adenocarcinoma (PDAC) carries a dismal prognosis and is predicted to be the number two cause of cancer-related mortality in the United States by 2040 [1]. While advances in the management of pancreatic cancer have incrementally improved 5-year OS, the proportion of patients alive at this 5-year landmark remains a disappointing 11% in all-stage SEER analysis [2]. Even in the curative setting, greater than 75% of the patients develop recurrence or metastatic disease within 2 years [3]. Current standard of care approaches with pancreatic ductal adenocarcinoma have relied on multidisciplinary combinations of the traditional pillars of cancer therapy including surgery, radiation, and intensive cytotoxic chemotherapies. More recent data have incorporated biomarker-driven approaches including targeting *BRAFV600E* and *KRASG12C*. Given growing recognition that pancreatic cancer is a disease with early metastatic potential that requires systemic treatment [4], interest has turned to immunotherapy given its promise in achieving durable responses in multiple tumor types in the metastatic setting. However, outside of the tumor agnostic indication for microsatellite instability high (MSI-H) and deficient mismatch repair (dMMR) tumors, immunotherapy has not emerged as a major therapeutic option for pancreatic cancer and has failed to improve overall survival. In this chapter, we will review the current understanding of immunobiology of pancreatic cancer with a particular focus on the tumor microenvironment implicated in the immunosuppressive phenotype of this malignancy. We summarize available insights on biomarkers for immunotherapy in selected populations and recapitulate prior trial findings while describing the landscape of investigational immunotherapies.

Z. P. Yeung · M. N. Kundranda (✉)
Gastrointestinal Cancer Program, Division of Cancer Medicine, Banner MD Anderson Cancer Center, Gilbert, AZ, USA
e-mail: madappa.kundranda@bannerhealth.com

S. Pant (ed.), *Pancreatic Cancer*, https://doi.org/10.1007/978-3-031-38623-7_6

Pancreatic Tumor Microenvironment (TME)

The "cold" pancreatic TME arises from a histopathologic milieu defined by a lack of effector T cells and multiple mechanisms whereby cancer cells avoid host immune responses. We briefly review the immune landscape of PDAC tumor stroma with a focus on intratumoral heterogeneity and complex interactions of effector cells. We contextualize how cancer-associated fibroblasts coordinate via paracrine signaling with immunosuppressive actors to promote PDAC evasion of host immunity that leads to tumor growth and invasion.

Stroma

Both primary pancreatic tumors and metastases are characterized by a desmoplastic stroma comprising 80–90% of tumor volume [5, 6]. This dense fibrotic tissue is generated by cancer-associated fibroblasts (CAFs), myofibroblasts, pancreatic stellate cells (PSC), and cancer cells with overabundance of extracellular matrix (ECM) components that act as a barrier to immune surveillance and compress blood vessels blocking drug delivery [7]. ECM components such as hyaluronan, collagen, and tenascin C have been implicated in inhibitory signaling pathways that suppress neoplasia-directed immune responses [8]. Other hallmarks include distortion of tumor vasculature, hypoxia, high interstitial pressures, and low pH. In combination, these features hinder trafficking and effector function of immune cells to promote tumor growth through a balance of immunotolerance and immunosuppression.

Effector T cells and Tumor Heterogeneity

A preponderance of the literature has correlated effector cell population signatures with overall survival—grossly enriched CD3+ and CD8+ subsets are associated with prolonged survival and regulatory FoxP3+ infiltration prognostically unfavorable for OS [9]. Past understandings of stroma have described its role as physical barrier that limits accumulation of effector cells of which T cells are the dominant component found in primary tumors [10]. However, more recent spatial analysis of multiple cellular types within PDAC tissue has elucidated that the spatial distribution and proximity of T cells to cancer cells correlates with survival. Carstens et al. found that desmoplastic elements such as alpha-SMA$^+$ fibroblasts were not associated with decreased cytotoxic T-cell infiltration suggesting that desmoplasia may not be in itself a physical barrier [11]. These findings of CD8+ infiltration as a survival correlate were validated in another cohort that further refined this prognostic association with specifically higher CD8+ cell density in the tumor center but not in the tumor margin [12].

Additional pathologic characterization of the distribution of immune infiltration reveals distinct fibroblastic stroma phenotypes or "sub-tumor microenvironments:" (1) "deserted" regions with thin fibroblasts, ECM deposition, and CD20+ immune cells associated with chemoresistance, (2) immune hot "reactive" regions rich in inflammatory CD8+ T cell infiltrates in direct contact with tumor cells with high neoantigen counts and SNVs associated with progression, and (3) regions with intermediate levels of these features. Tumor heterogeneity with co-occurrence of multiple phenotypes within the same tumor was associated with worse survival [13].

Cancer-Associated Fibroblasts

Cancer-associated fibroblasts deposit the ECM and produce tumor growth factors. They are the predominant non-neoplastic cell type in the TME. They modulate tumor progression via production of TGF-β, VEGF, IL-6, and CXCL12 [14–16]. CAFs also immunosuppress by acting on CD8+ T cells, T regs, and macrophages via IL-6, CXCL9, and TGFβ [17]. They have been implicated as integral to resistance to immunotherapy [18]. Sequencing has revealed that subpopulations of these fibroblasts are responsible for the heterogeneity of tumors [13]. Smooth muscle actin has been used to differentiate different fibroblasts populations that appear to have opposing functions. SMA-high CAFs are driven by TGFβ of which LRRC15+ subsets predominate in PDAC and are associated with poor response to anti-PD-L1 therapy [19]. Another unique CAF population is the antigen-presenting CAF that expresses MHC class II molecules and induces expansion of regulatory T cells [20].

Inhibitory Paracrine Signaling and Cell Populations

CAF-secreted VEGF mediates angiogenic remodeling of the TME and inhibition of cytotoxic T-cell trafficking and function and antigen presentation [21]. VEGF expression favors CAF/PSC-directed cytokine-mediated (e.g., TGFβ, IDO, IL6, 8, 10, CSF) enrichment and recruitment of adenosine-secreting PD-L1+ M2-polarized tumor-associated macrophages (TAMs), immunosuppressive myeloid-derived suppressor cells (MDSCs), and FOXP3+ regulatory T cells (Tregs) [22]. In contrast, the TME has a relative lack of pro-inflammatory M1 macrophages, dendritic cells, natural killer cells, and effector CD4+ and CD8+ T lymphocytes (fivefold fewer compared to "hot tumors") [23].

TME host factors include obesity, a known risk factor for development of PDAC [24]. Elevated levels of lipocalin-2 (LCN2), an adipokine elevated in the serum and in adipose tissue of obese individuals, have been implicated in adversely modulating the TME via activation of PSCs, stromal remodeling, and upregulation of tumor-associated macrophages (TAMs) precipitating ductal metaplasia and predisposing to PDAC development [25].

TAMs

TAMs serve as major nodes of paracrine activity within the intricate network of interactions within the TME receiving signals and releasing growth factors and cytokines. They promote tumor cell invasion, induce angiogenesis, and facilitate metastasis [26]. Researchers have primarily focused on M2-polarized anti-inflammatory TAMs that secrete immunosuppressive cytokines including TGFβ and IL-10. They interfere with effector T-cell metabolism and recruit T regs. Simultaneously, they suppress activation of CD8+ cytotoxic T-cell activation while upregulating PSCs further promoting evasion of immune surveillance [27, 28]. These M2-polarized TAMs were found to be associated with more advanced nodal disease in resected patients and worse overall survival [29]. Long-term survivors have lower densities of these M2 macrophages [30]. One proposed therapeutic strategy involves immunotherapy in combination with inhibition of colony-stimulating factor-1 receptor (CSF1R), which recruits TAMs to the TME. CSF1R blockade has been demonstrated to upregulate PDL1 and CTLA4 to synergize with checkpoint immunotherapy [31, 32].

MDSCs

Enriched by IL-6 [33], MDSCs suppress effector T cells via reactive oxygen species and adenosine. Through their production of Interferon-γ and IL-10, MDSCs mediate maturation of de novo Tregs [34, 35]. MDSCs modulate CD8+ T-cell activity, promote proliferation of CD4+ Tregs, stimulate angiogenesis via secretion of VEGF, and upregulate PD-L1 and LAG3 to further immunosuppression [36–38]. Elevated levels of the chemokine CXCL5 linked to MDSC recruitment have been correlated with infiltration of granulocytic types of MDSCs associated with inferior median overall survival (38.5 months in high vs. 64 months in low) [39]. Transgenic mouse models where myeloid cells were depleted demonstrated prevented KRAS-driven tumorigenesis. In tumors, myeloid depletion arrested tumor growth and led to some instances of regression associated with CD8+ T-cell infiltration [40]. MDSCs inhibit CD8+ T-cell activity by inducing PD-L1 expression via EGFR/MAPK pathways.

Tregs

Regulatory T cells (Tregs) are forkhead box protein 3 (FOXP3) expressing cells that represent a major obstacle to tumor immunotherapy by binding to dendritic cells and preventing them from activating CD8+ T-cell responses. Patient with tumors harboring high prevalence of Tregs often had poorly differentiated tumors with poor prognosis [41–43]. Competitive binding of Treg CTLA-4 to B7 downregulates the number of B7 receptors on dendritic cells preventing antigen presentation [44]. However, their exact role in tumor dynamics requires further study, as experimental depletion of CD4+Foxp3+Tregs yielded rapid growth of tumors in a transgenic mouse model via interactions with fibroblasts [45].

TANs

Tumor-associated neutrophils (TANs) are increasingly recognized to promote tumor progression, mediate resistance to therapy, and regulate immunosuppression. Systemic elevation of CXCR2$^+$ neutrophils in the peripheral blood and bone marrow correlates with overall survival in patients with PDAC [46]. TANs accumulate in tumors in a CXCR2-dependent fashion to establish an immunosuppressive niche [47]. The complex interactions of TANs are illustrated by the finding that depletion of CXCR2+ neutrophils suppress metastasis, but this leads to compensatory upregulation of CR2+ TAMs [48]. TANs also induce apoptosis of CD8+ cytotoxic lymphocytes [49]. They uniquely produce neutrophil extracellular traps (NETs) induced by IL-17 in a tumor-cell-dependent fashion that foster resistance to checkpoint blockade [50].

TH17

In the setting of chronic pancreatitis, T-Helper-17 (TH17) cells contribute to tumorigenesis by secreting IL-17. Binding of this ligand to a KRAS-dependent receptor induces downstream expression of genes related to embryonic stemness and secretion of chemokines that attract MDSCs and neutrophils to the TME [51]. Secreted granulocyte-macrophage colony-stimulating factor (GM-CSF) recruits suppressive myeloid cells that interfere with CD8+ T-cell infiltration and cytotoxicity [52].

Conventional Immunotherapy Biomarkers in PDAC

Anti-programmed death receptor-1/programmed death receptor-ligand 1 (anti-PD-1/PD-L1) and anticytotoxic T-lymphocyte-associated protein 4 (anti-CTLA-4) checkpoint blockade in unselected patients with PDAC has failed to confer any meaningful clinical benefit. Attempts to select patients using available biomarkers such as TMB and PD-L1 have failed to predict activity, while dramatic responses seen with MSI-H/DMMR tumors are less common in PDAC

Tumor Mutational Burden and Neoantigens

Despite tumor-agnostic FDA regulatory approval for pembrolizumab based on 29% ORR from KEYNOTE-158 suggesting survival benefits with IO in elevated TMB, notably, no patients with PDAC were included in this basket trial. Biomarker analysis of Keynote-028 to correlate outcomes to TMB and PD-L1 excluded PDAC cases because there were no responders [53]. Critics have noted that responders in these trials often were *POLE* mutated or were MSI-H [54].

High TMB comprises only 1.1% of PDAC cancers and is usually associated with MSI-H/dMMR [55]. The low tumor mutational burden of PDAC (~3.5 mut/Mb in the MSK IMPACT cohort; median 1.8 mut/Mb in Foundation) [56] has been one explanation for why PDAC is unresponsive to immunotherapy. Analysis at Memorial Sloan Kettering Cancer Center demonstrated only two patients with elevated TMB of 10; none responded to anti-PD-1 therapy [57]. The authors suggested that cancer-type-specific TMB cutoffs may be appropriate for determining likely responses to immune checkpoint blockade, illustrating the lack of harmonized thresholds described in the literature [58]. McGrail and colleagues demonstrated that TMB-H classification varies by tumor type and analyzed responses based on CD8+ T-cell infiltration and neoantigen load. Pancreatic cancer was classified in a subset where TMB did not predict response to ICB. Their survival analysis suggested that TMB-H tumors in this category II exhibited worse OS compared to TMB-L tumors. They questioned TMB as a tissue agnostic marker [59]. While long term survivors often have elevated TMB in some cohorts [60], more recent evidence has shown that quality of neoepitopes matters, not just quantity. Long-term survivors of pancreatic cancers showed no correlation between neoantigen load and survival and developed tumors with fewer neoantigens. Neoantigens that resembled bacterial epitopes were observed in these long-term survivors [61, 62].

DMMR/MSI-H

Only 1–2% of pancreatic cancer patients have MSI-H or dMMR tumors, representing a unique genomic subset. A large proportion of these patients harbor alteration of a gene implicated in autosomal dominant Lynch syndrome. MSI-H PDAC is strongly associated with medullary and mucinous/colloid histology and genomically *KRAS-TP53* wild type enriched with co-occurring JAK and KMT2 mutations [63].

Trial data from KEYNOTE-158 studying pembrolizumab in patients with non-colorectal solid tumors that were MSI-high showed a lower response in patients with PDAC (18.2%) versus the ORR of 34.3% in the entire cohort of MSI-H solid tumors [64]. An analysis of MSI-H/dMMR GI cancers by Chida and colleagues found that low TMB and alteration of PTEN predicted negative responses to PD-1 blockade; both pancreatic cancer patients in this cohort harbored PTEN mutations [65]. Given that overlap between MSI-H and TMB high PDACs is not 100% [66], work by Salem et al. demonstrated that individual variants in mismatch repair genes *MLH1*, *PMS2*, *MSH2*, and *MSH6* produce different levels of tumor mutational burden that displayed variability by histology, which may explain why dMMR PDAC responds differently to immunotherapy as compared to dMMR colon adenocarcinoma [67].

PD-L1

PD-L1 expression is low in the stroma in PDAC as compared to expression in other tumor types.

Upregulation of PD-L1 via glucocorticoid signaling has been associated with poor survival and promotes immune tolerance by inhibiting T-cell activity [68–70]. As a biomarker, there are no clinically useful cut points to inform clinical utility of immune checkpoint inhibition. While not a predictive tool, PD-L1 expression in certain cell populations within the TME is prognostic. Analysis of TCGA data has demonstrated that PD-L1 expression was associated with poor overall survival. Patients with tumors found to be enriched in subsets that were PD-L1^{negative}/CD8+^{high} had a positive prognosis [71], suggesting that those patients with T-cell infiltration without concomitant adaptive immune evasion are a unique subset with prolonged survival. Similar findings of an inverse relationship between PD-L1 expression and disease-specific survival have been described in a resected cohort [70].

Immunotherapeutic Approaches in Unselected PDAC

Earlier attempts at harnessing immunotherapy to treat pancreatic cancer have largely been in an all comers unresectable or metastatic population. To date, various studies have trialed monotherapy and combinations of checkpoint inhibitors targeting PD-1/PD-L1 and/or CTLA4 with or without standard of care chemotherapy backbones. The results have been less than impressive. We review past approaches based on mechanism of action and review the rationale for therapy before summarizing findings. Our review will also describe efforts at formulating viruses, oncolytic viruses, adoptive cell therapies, and cancer vaccines.

Immune Checkpoint Inhibitors: Anti-CTLA-4 Monotherapy

On T cells, the CTLA-4 receptor competes with higher affinity against CD28 for the CD80 and CD86 ligands on antigen-presenting cells [72]. Lower CTLA-4 and higher CD80 expression in PDAC have been correlated with improved survival [73]. Binding of CTLA-4 limits priming of naïve T cells and impedes antitumor effector T-cell activity. While favorable responses were observed in melanoma, such success have not been observed in pancreatic cancer. Royal et al. carried out a phase II trial of single agent Ipilimumab for locally advanced or metastatic PDAC [74]. Of 27 subjects, there were no responders by RECIST criteria, but a subject experienced a delayed response after initial progressive disease. Select clinical trial data is displayed in Table 6.1.

Table 6.1 Checkpoint inhibition in PDAC

Trial ID	Phase	Therapy arms	Mechanism of action	# patients ($n=$)	Response rate (%)	Median overall survival (months)
Royal et al.	II	Ipililumab 3 mg/kg q3wks × 4 × 2	Anti-CTLA4	27	0; 1 patient with delayed tumor shrinkage at 12 weeks but PD at 33 weeks	~4
Brahmer et al. NCT00729664	I	Pembrolizumab	Anti-PD-L1	207, 14 pancreatic	0	
Marabelle et al. KEYNOTE-158, NCT02628067	II	Pembrolizumab	Anti-PD-L1 in DMMR/MSI-H	N = 223, 22 pancreatic	18.2%; 1 CR, 3 PR	4
O'Reilly et al. NCT02558894	II	Durvalumab ± tremelimumab	Anti-PD-1 vs. Anti-PD-1 + anti-CLTA4	64 (32 D + T; 33 D)	3.1%	3.1 (D + T); 3.6 (D)
Aglietta et al. NCT00556023	Ib	Tremelimumab + gemcitabine	Anti-CTLA4 + chemo	34	10.5%	7.4
Kamath et al. NCT01473940	Ib	Ipililumab + gemcitabine	Anti-CTLA4 + chemo	21	14%	6.9
Weiss et al. NCT02331251	Ib/II	pembrolizumab + gemcitabine/ nab-paclitaxel	Anti-PD-L1 + chemo	15	17.6%, 27% in chemo-naive	15 for chemo-naive
Renouf et al. PA.7 trial. NCT02879318		Gemcitabine/nab-paclitaxel + D ± T vs. Gemcitabine abraxane	Anti-PD-1 + anti-CLTA4 + Chemo	180	30.3% (G + N + D + T) vs. 23% (G + N)	9.8 (G + N + D + T) vs. 8.8 (G + N)

Immune Checkpoint Inhibitors: Anti-PD-1/ Anti-PD-L1 Monotherapy

PD-1 ligand binding promotes self-tolerance by inhibiting T-cell activation and proliferation. Simultaneously, this signaling axis interferes with downstream signaling from the TCR complex and CD28 to promote apoptosis of T-cell effectors [75, 76]. As previously stated, PD-L1 is uncommonly overexpressed in PDAC and inversely correlates with CD8+ T-cell infiltration and clinical prognosis [77, 78]. The results with monotherapy have been disappointing. The original basket trials demonstrated lack of response in MSS patients and lower response rate in MSI-H and dMMR PDAC patients (18%) compared to other cancer types [79, 80].

Immune Checkpoint Inhibitors: Combination Anti-PD-1 and Anti-CTLA4 Blockade

Given the synergy observed in other tumor types, dual anti-PD-1 and anti-CTLA4 combination was trialed in a multicenter phase 2 randomized control trial [81]. Patients received durvalumab plus tremelimumab combination therapy for 4 cycles followed by durvalumab therapy (or durvalumab monotherapy for up to 12 months or until onset of progression or unacceptable toxicity). Objective response rate for combination therapy was a mere 3.1%. No responders were seen in the single agent durvalumab arm. Adding anti-CTLA-4 to anti-PD-L1 in pretreated mPDAC patients (n = 65) did not improve survival compared to anti-PD-L1 monotherapy (mOS 3.1 months vs. 3.6 months; mPFS 1.5 months vs. 1.5 months).

Immune Checkpoint Inhibitors with Chemotherapy

Given the lack of efficacy in the checkpoint blockade only studies, investigators in the field turned to see if addition of these agents to standard cytotoxic chemotherapy regimens would enhance efficacy and improve outcomes. This is in context of expanding recognition that cytotoxic drugs can synergize with immunotherapy by stimulating immunogenic tumor cell death, reduce tumor-induced immune suppression, and increase effector T-cell function and infiltration.

The first published trial to explore the combination of chemotherapy and checkpoint blockade in PDAC explored addition of tremelimumab with gemcitabine [82]. Median OS was 7.4 months with two patients achieving partial response, both of which were in the 15 mg/kg dose escalation phase, which was comparable to historical outcomes with single-agent gemcitabine of 6.8 months [83, 84]. Addition of CTLA-4 blockade to gemcitabine was trialed in a phase Ib study in an advanced PDAC patient population. Median OS of 6.9 months and mPFS 2.5 months were similar to single-agent gemcitabine historical outcomes [85–87].

More promising results were noted by the PembroPlus phase Ib/II trial that added pembrolizumab to gemcitabine/nab-paclitaxel backbone [88, 89]. In this cohort of

17 patients, 11 were chemotherapy naïve. This chemotherapy naïve group exhibited median PFS of 9.1 months and median OS of 15.1 months, which is over 6 months longer than median trial outcomes for gemcitabine/nab-paclitaxel alone. The study was also notable for utilization of tumor cell-free DNA copy number instability, which correlated with longer PFS and improved OS.

The Canadian phase II PA.7 trial looked at gemcitabine/nab-paclitaxel with or without durvalumab and tremelimumab in the first line. The trial was negative and showed no significant improvement in OS, PFS, or ORR at a median follow-up of 28.5 months in this cohort of 180 patients [90].

Taken together, these trials have shown that combining checkpoint inhibition of PD-1/PD-L1 and CTLA-4 with chemotherapy has not changed practice away from conventional cytotoxic regimens. However, it is unclear what the optimal chemo regimen to combine with immunotherapy. The results of two larger trials are eagerly awaited (NCT04674956 and NCT03983057; camrelizumab with gemcitabine/nab-paclitaxel and camrelizumab with FOLFIRINOX).

Novel Checkpoint Inhibitors

Increasing understanding of T-cell immunity has revealed novel checkpoints that involved in T-cell exhaustion. Balli et al. found that cytolytic high tumors had higher expression of several immune checkpoints, except for PD-L1 which was uniformly low. They also proposed categorizing PDAC based on co-expression of CTLA-4, TIGIT, TIM-3, and VISTA for clinical targeting purposes [91].

The TIGIT receptor, expressed on NK cells and activated CD4+ and C8+ T cells, has been described in directly inhibiting NK cytotoxicity and T-cell activity [92, 93]. TIGIT-ligand interactions with CD155 and C112 on tumor and myeloid cells promote NK and T-cell tolerance [94, 95]. Expression of CD155 in tumor tissue has been found to inversely correlate with TIL frequency and survival [96]. TIGIT competes for ligands against CD226 that promotes NK and T-cell activation. Blockade of TIGIT in the preclinical setting selectively affects CD226hiCD8+ T cells, which also increase in the setting of FOLRIFIRNOX therapy, suggesting possible synergy [97]. Modified FOLFIRINOX treatment in mPDAC patients increased the proportion of CD226hiCD8+ T cells, implying that this chemotherapeutic combination may increase tumor sensitivity to anti-TIGIT treatment. A phase 1b/2 randomized trial is currently assessing anti-TIGIT combined with gemcitabine/nab-paclitaxel in the metastatic setting under the MORPHEUS platform trials (NCT03193190).

TIM-3 is overexpressed on exhausted T cells as well as tumoral DCs [98, 99]. Additional staining studies show moderate to high expression in 29% of pancreatic patients [100]. TIM-3 putatively leads to invasion, metastatic spread, and recurrence [101]. TIM-3 binds Gal-9, phosphatidylserine carcinoembryonic antigen-related cell adhesion molecule 1 (CEACAM1) and high mobility group protein B1 (HMGB1) to downregulate immunity [102–104]. Gal-9 binding with TIM-3 on T cells and NK cells leads to diminished activation and inhibition. This is particularly salient, since Gal-9 is increased in the tumor tissue and blood of PDAC patients

[105]. While anti-TIM-3 therapy is being pursued in other tumor types, no active therapeutic trials are enrolling pancreatic cancer patients.

Recent work reported overexpression of VISTA (V-domain Ig suppressor of T-cell activation), an inhibitory checkpoint molecule, in PDAC in comparison to melanoma, and postulated that VISTA represents a more dominant inhibitory pathway and may represent a more efficacious target for immunotherapy in PDAC [106]. Other validation studies have demonstrated that VISTA is moderately or highly expressed on the protein level of 63% pancreatic cancer patient samples [100]. Development of a novel antibody HMBD-002 has allowed for preclinical work to show that blockade of this axis to reduce myeloid-derived suppression of T-cell activity and prevent neutrophil migration in mouse models of multiple cancer types [107]. HMBD-002 significantly inhibited tumor growth while decreasing infiltration of suppressive myeloid cells and increasing T-cell activity with TH1/TH17 immune signature. Accordingly, NCT05082610 is recruiting patients for evaluation of HMBD-002 with or without pembrolizumab in advanced solid tumors including pancreatic cancer.

LAG-3 represents another inhibitory molecule present on PDAC tumor-infiltrating lymphocytes (TILs) which works by binding MHCII molecules on tumor cells. LAG-3 has been found upregulated on infiltrating lymphocytes in PDAC [108]. However, recent correlative work has demonstrated moderate or high expression of LAG3 in only 6.8% of PDAC tissue samples, which calls into question its usefulness as a target. A LAG3 bispecific XmAb22841 is undergoing active trials in NCT03849469, but it is not actively recruiting. It is unclear if pancreatic cancer has been included.

Targeting TME + Immunotherapy

Given that the tumor microenvironment strongly attenuates the immune regulation of pancreatic environment, rational therapeutic approaches at targeting the TME have been the most recent landscape of trials. The CCL2/CCR2 and chemokine receptor type 4 (CXCR4) receptor pathways involved in the recruitment of immunosuppressive monocytes to the TME are currently under evaluation as drug targets in combination with chemotherapy and immunotherapy [109]. Small molecule inhibition of the CXCR2 receptor expressed on tumor-associated neutrophils and MDSCs has been shown to induce antitumor immunity against PDAC in mouse models when combined with chemotherapy [110]. Combined CCR2 and CXCR2 blockade, along with FOLFIIRINOX chemotherapy, increases overall survival in a KPC mouse model. Based on this work, an early phase trial was carried out with CCR2 inhibition with FOLFIRINOX, which demonstrated response rate of 49% with disease control rate of 97% [111]. Unfortunately, the drug maker has decided not to pursue further development of PF-04136309. Currently, SX-682, an allosteric inhibitor to CXCR1 and CXCR2, is under investigation in combination with nivolumab as maintenance therapy in PDAC (NCT04477343). BMS-813160 is a

CCR2/CCR5 dual antagonist which is being studied in combination with SBRT, nivolumab, and GVAX (NCT03767582).

Although a trial of combining the anti-CXCR4 drug mogamulizumab with durvalumab or tremelimumab yielded a paltry ORR of 5.3%, the phase 2a COMBAT trial suggested that chemotherapy concurrent with anti-PD-1 and C-X-C motif chemokine receptor (CXCR)4 antagonist motixafortide may augment chemotherapeutic effects. Patients in this cohort of 22 patients achieved a mOS of 7.8 months from the start of pembrolizumab in the second-line pretreated setting with an ORR of 32% and 77% DCR [112]. Biomarker analysis following this trial demonstrated that high CXCR expression is associated with improved survival and a pro-inflammatory phenotype that may identify a subset of tumors with greater responsiveness to immunotherapy [113]. An additional phase II trial called Chemo4MetPanc will study motixafortide with gemcitabine/nab-paclitaxel and cemiplimab in the 1L mPDAC setting (NCT04543071) [114]. A trial combining plerixafor for CXCR4 blockade with cemiplimab check point inhibition is recruiting (NCT04177810). Unfortunately, other trials attempting to deplete immunosuppressive cells, including a study combining ibrutinib with PD-L1 inhibition, showed lack of efficacy (mOS 4.2 months, mPFS 1.7 months) [115].

Despite initial signals of promise in phase I data [116], an attempt to target M2 TAM inhibition in a phase II clinical study evaluating the colony-stimulating factor-1 receptor (CSF1R) inhibitor cabiralizumab with nivolumab and chemotherapy in advanced PDAC patients did not improve progression-free survival compared with chemotherapy alone (NCT03336216) [117]. A multicenter phase Ib/II trial evaluated a fully human IgG2 monoclonal anti-CSF1R antibody, AMG 820, in combination with pembrolizumab, and enrolled 116 patients including 31 patients with metastatic PDAC (NCT02713529). Despite showing target-specific immune changes, this trial did not meet its primary efficacy endpoint. In another phase Ib/II trial that included patients with metastatic PDAC, limited activity was observed with the anti-CSF1 antibody, lacnotuzumab, given in combination with anti-PD1 spartalizumab (NCT02807844). In a phase I study, pexidartinib (PLX3397), a CSF1R kinase inhibitor, was studied in combination with anti-PD-L1 durvalumab in patients with PDAC, resulting in a modest 21% clinical benefit rate (4/19 stable disease, including two patients with microsatellite instability-high colorectal cancers; NCT02777710) [118].

Another target of interest is activation of CD40 expressed on dendritic cells and B cells. Based on translational work in murine models, studies sought to recapitulate immune-priming and reversal of T-cell exhaustion through the upregulation of cytokines, antigen-presenting molecules, costimulatory molecules, and adhesion molecules [119]. Chemotherapy incorporating gemcitabine and nab-paclitaxel with concomitant CD40 activation induced T-cell-dependent immunity and memory in mouse models that correlated with tumor regression and survival. The phase Ib/II PRINCE trial evaluated combining sotigalimab, a CD40 agonist, with gemcitabine and nab-paclitaxel with or without nivolumab. Initial phase Ib results showed a response in 14 of 24 evaluable patients (58%) [120]. However, phase II results showed that while the nivolumab + chemo in the first-line treatment of PDAC resulted in a 57.7% 12-month overall survival rate, sotigalimab + chemo resulted in 58.1% 1-year survival ratel while sotigalimab + nivolumab + chemo yielded a rate of 41.3%. Median OS in the nivolumab + chemo arm was 16.7 months. No patient subset benefitted from the triplet of sotigalimab, nivolumab, and chemo. While negative, the PRINCE trial biomarker analyses correlated survival after nivolumab/ chemo with a less suppressive tumor microenvironment and higher numbers of activated antigen-experienced circulating T cells at baseline suggesting potential treatment-specific correlates of efficacy with the potential for biomarker-selected patient populations. Another CD40 agonist selicrelumab also demonstrated limited efficacy in conjunction with atezolizumab and chemotherapy in an unselected population within the MORPHEUS trial [121]. In the neoadjuvant setting, it yielded an OS of 23.4 months [122].

CD73, which enzymatically generates extracellular adenosine, is upregulated in PDA and exerts an immunosuppressive effect on T cells [123]. MEDI9447 or oleclumab is a monoclonal antibody directed to CD73 to prevent adenosine generation. It was combined with durvalumab therapy in a phase I trial that produced a partial response in 2 of 20 PDAC patients and disease control rate of 25%. Current trials are underway with Oleclumab in the neoadjuvant setting with durvalumab and gemcitabine/nab-paclitaxel in resectable/borderline resectable PDAC (NCT04940286) [124]. A small molecule inhibitor of CD73 (AB 680) is also under active investigation in combination with gemcitabine/nab-paclitaxel chemotherapy and PD-1 inhibition with zimberelimab (AB122; NCT04104672) [125]. Targeting the adenosine receptors A2aR and A2bR with AB928 is also being investigated in the MORPHEUS phase 1b/2 platform with atezolizumab and gemcitabine/nab-paclitaxel (NCT03193190).

Targeting IL-6, which is implicated in the inflammation of the TME, has been attempted. Combination of nivolumab, ipilimumab, and tocilizumab in conjunction with SBRT did not meet the primary endpoint in the TRIPPLE-R trial (NCT04258150). Tocilizumab is being studied in combination with atezolizumab and chemo in the MORPHEUS platform trial (NCT03193190).

Given the prominence of the unique stroma in PDAC, a target that gained prominence is high interstitial fluid pressures (IFP) seen in the PDAC microenvironment. KPC mice models suggested IPF was associated with hyaluronic acid (HA) deposition in the pancreatic tumor ECM; administration of pegylated recombinant human hyaluronidase (PEGPH20) obliterated patent vascularization in the TME and normalized IFP in these mice. Accordingly, the investigators proceeded to combine PEGPH20 with gemcitabine, which prolonged overall survival compared with gemcitabine alone [126]. Based on these findings, investigators carried out a phase Ib/II trial of PEGPH20 in combination with gemcitabine/nab-paclitaxel versus gemcitabine/nab-paclitaxel alone; PFS was not improved, but subgroup analysis stratified by HA content showed a significant improvement in overall response rate (52% vs. 24%, $p = 0.038$) in patients with tumors of high-HA vs. low-HA [127]. The SWOG 1313 phase IB/II randomized trial of FOLFIRINOX plus human hyaluronidase PEGPH20 versus FOLFIRINOX alone was performed in patients with metastatic PDAC. The trial was closed early because interim analysis found a signal of increased incidence of thrombotic events and GI bleeding in addition to an inferior worse OS of 7.7 months vs. the 14.4 months in the chemo-only control arm [128]. A phase III trial of combination of PEGPH20 and gemcitabine/nab-paclitaxel versus gemcitabine/nab-paclitaxel in high HA-expression in metastatic PDAC demonstrated no OS benefit (11.2 months compared to 11.5 months, HR = 1.00, p = 0.97) [129]. No further development of PEGPH20 for metastatic PDAC is planned.

Another putative strategy focusing on the stroma that has been outlined is targeting the vitamin D receptor (VDR) theorized to participate in stromal reprogramming and conversion of quiescent to activated pancreatic stellate cells (PSCs). Therapy with calcipotriol, which agonistically engages VDR, decreases inflammation and fibrosis in a pancreatitis murine model while shifting CAFs toward a more quiescent phenotype, reduced tumor growth, and improved chemotherapy penetration [130]. Based on this finding, paricalcitol plus gemcitabine/nab-paclitaxel is being studied in NCT 03520790 in the metastatic setting. NCT 04524702 is investigating hydroxychloroquine and paricalcitol combination with gemcitabine/nab-paclitaxel in advanced PDAC. NCT02754726 is investigating nivolumab + gemcitabine/nab-paclitaxel/cisplatin.

Hedgehog (Hh) pathway is upregulated in pancreatic cancer stem cells (CSCs), which interact with stromal fibroblasts via paracrine signaling resulting in PTEN-related promotion of a fibrotic and immune suppressive stroma leading to tumorigenesis [131]. Further preclinical research suggested Shh inhibition resulted in major improvement in outcomes by facilitating entry of chemotherapy into pancreatic tumors [132]. Unfortunately, a phase II trial that assessed gemcitabine/nab-paclitaxel plus vismodegib (a hedgehog inhibitor) in patients with metastatic PDAC produced no clinical benefit [133].

Focal adhesion kinase 1 (FAK1) is a nonreceptor tyrosine kinase implicated in activating pro-inflammatory cytokines and upregulating pathologic fibrosis. FAK1 is upregulated in PDAC, and tumors with high FAK1 expression had higher levels of total stromal collagen and collagen I deposition. The combination of a FAK-inhibitor, gemcitabine, and anti-PD1 immunotherapy in a KPC mouse model reduced tumor burden and improved overall survival with immune correlates showing significantly increased CD8+ tumor-infiltrating lymphocytes compared with mice treated with gemcitabine and anti-PD1 immunotherapy alone [134]. NCT03727880 is investigating pembrolizumab with or without the FAK inhibitor defactinib following chemotherapy as a neoadjuvant/adjuvant treatment for resectable PDAC.

Desmoplasia is a product of connective tissue growth factor (CTGF). CTGF overexpression is associated with aberrant fibrous tissue in mouse models, which was successfully abrogated with the anti-CTGF antibody pamrevlumab. Clinical trials initiated in the neoadjuvant setting for LAPC demonstrated that addition of pamrevlumab to standard neoadjuvant gemcitabine/nab-paclitaxel increased chemotherapy completion, increased radiographic response by PET, and increased eligibility for surgery and resection rate. ORR was 30%. Among those eligible for surgery, the antibody arm demonstrated improvement in OS (27.73 months vs.

18.40 months) [135]. The phase III LAPIs trial will follow up these findings in a larger patient population (NCT03941093).

Overcoming the drug delivery issue in the PDAC stroma is being trialed. NCT05042128 is examining CEND-1, a novel cyclic tumor-penetrating peptide iRGD (internalizing arginylglycylaspartic acid) in combination with gemcitabine/nab-paclitaxel.

Harnessing mesothelin as a biomarker is currently underway with anetumab ravtansine—a fully human IgG1 antibody-drug conjugate targeted to mesothelin to deliver DM4 chemotherapy payload—with either nivolumab, nivolumab + ipilimumab, or gemcitabine + nivolumab (NCT03816358). Stable disease was observed in pancreatic cancer patients in the phase I portion [136].

Claudin 18.2 aberrant expression in PDAC is well described. A 1L Ph II gem/nab-P ± zolbetuximab (IgG1 mAb targeting Claudin 18.2) in metastatic PDAC is active (NCT03816163). Histologically confirmed high CLDN18.2 expression ($\geq 75\%$ of tumor cells demonstrate moderate-to-strong IHC staining) is required for enrollment [137].

Targeting the communication between PSCs and PDAC tumor cells has implicated leukemia inhibitory factor (LIF) as a key paracrine mediator in stromal crosstalk. LIF blockade slows tumor progression and augments the effects of chemo in prolonging OS in mouse models [138]. NCT04999969 is a phase II trial examining an inhibitor of LIF (AZD0171) in combination with gemcitabine/nab-paclitaxel chemo and durvalumab checkpoint inhibition.

Vaccines

One of the most durable efforts at immunotherapy in pancreatic cancer has been the development of vaccines. Table 6.2 summarizes select vaccine trials in PDAC.

The first vaccine developed was GVAX (granulocyte-macrophage colony-stimulating factor gene transfected tumor cells vaccine) containing irradiated allogeneic pancreatic cancer cells virally transduced with GM-CSF and administered intradermally. GVAX demonstrated the ability to recruit antigen-presenting cells (APCs), predominantly dendritic cells (DCs), to the inoculation site resulting in CD8+ T cells cross-priming [139].

A second vaccine, CRS-207, consists of deactivated Listeria expressing mesothelin, a tumor-associated antigen highly expressed in PDAC [140]. Mesothelin is often co-expressed with CA-125 (MUC-16). Binding of CA-125 with secreted mesothelin enhances tumor cell motility and invasion [141]. Translational murine studies have suggested efficacy of mixing vaccines with checkpoint inhibition [142]. A trial with GVAX/cyclophosphamide followed by CRS-207 with or without nivolumab was completed, and though the primary endpoint of improving OS was not met, an increase of CD8+T cells and decrease in TAMS and MDSCs were observed in the TME of biopsied tumors in patient with better OS [143]. GVAX in combination with ipilimumab in a cohort of 15 patients was also disappointing with a median OS of a mere 5.7 months [144]. Among patients with an OS >4.3 months,

Table 6.2 Selected vaccine trials in PDAC

Trial ID	Phase	Therapy arms (metastatic unless otherwise indicated)	Mechanism of action	# patients ($n=$)	Response rate (%)	Median overall survival (months)
Laheru et al.	II	CG8020/CG2505 alone (A) ± cyclophosphamide (B)	GM-CSF secreting allogeneic PDAC tumor cells (GVAX)	50 (30 in A, 20 in B)	0%	2.3 (A) and 4.3 (B)
Le et al. NCT01417000	II	Cy/GVAX × 2 + CRS-207 × 4 (arm A) vs. Cy/GVAX × 6 (arm B)	GVAX ± Listeria expressing mesothelin	90 (arm A, $n = 61$; arm B, $n = 29$)	N/A	6.1 m (A) vs. 3.9 m (B); patients who received ≥3 doses, 9.7 (A) vs. 4.6 (B)
Tsujikawa et al. NCT02243371	II	GVAX + CRS-207 ± nivolumab (A vs. B)	GVAX ± Listeria expressing mesothelin ± anti-PD-1	93 (A 51; B 42)	4% (A); 2% (B)	5.9 (A) vs. 6.1 (B)
Le et al. NCT00836407	Ib	Ipilimumab 10 mg/kg (arm 1) vs. ipilimumab 10 mg/kg + GVAX (arm 2)	Anti-CTLA 4 ± GVAX	30	0%	3.6 vs. 5.7
Wu et al.	II	Induction FOLFIRINOX then (A) GVAX + ipilimumab vs. (B) FOLFIRINOX continuation	GVAX + anti-CTLA4	82 (40; 42)	6%	9.4 vs. 14.7
Kaida et al.	I	WT1 peptide vaccine + gemcitabine	WT-1 + chemo	9 pancreas	DCR at 2 months 89%	8.6
Nishida et al.	I	WT1 peptide vaccine + gemcitabine	WT-1 peptide + chemo	32	20%	8.1
Koido et al.	I	MHC I restricted + gemcitabine vs. MHC II restricted + gemcitabine vs. MHCI/II restricted	DC WT-1 + chemo	10 Pancreas	0%	>20 w/ strong DTH reaction
Tsukinaga et al.	I	WT-1 MHI/II vaccine + gemcitabine	DC WT-1 + chemo	7	0%	10.8
Mayanagi et al.	I	WT-1 peptide-pulsed DC vaccine + gemcitabine	DC WT-1 + chemo	10	0%	8
Yanagisawa et al.	I	WT1 DC vaccine + gemcitabine/S1 after resection	DC WT-1 vaccine + chemo	9	N/A	2 years OS 62.5%
Nishida et al.	II	GEM ± WT1 DC vaccine gemcitabine in advanced	chemo ± DC WT-1 vaccine	91	14% vs. 12%	9.6 vs. 8.9
Hanada et al.	I	WT-1 DC + chemo ± radiation ± surgery	DC WT-1 vaccine	6	ND	59

Nagai et al.	I/IIa	WT-1/MUC1 DC after resection	DC WT-1 and MUC-1 peptide-pulsed vaccine	10	N/A	77.8% 3 years survival
Rong et al.	I	MUC1 vaccine	MUC1-peptide-pulsed DC	7	0%	ND
Asahara et al.	I/II	Vaccine in gemcitabine refractory advanced patients	KIF20A peptide vaccine	29	0%	4.75
Miyazawa et al.	II	OCV-C01 vaccine combined with gemcitabine as adjuvant therapy after resection	KIF20A, VEGFR1, and VEGFR2 epitope peptide vaccine + chemo	30	N/A	69% OS at 18 months; median NR
Yamaue et al.	II/III	Elpamotide + gemcitabine vs. gemcitabine + placebo	VEGFR2 peptide vaccine + chemo vs. chemo	153 (100 vs. 53 placebo)	ND	8.36 vs. 8.54
Shima et al.	II	(1) Survivin 2B peptide (SVN-2B) + interferon-β (IFNβ); (2) SVN-2B only; or (3) placebo	Survivin 2B peptide vaccine	44	0%	3.4 months vs. 3.2 months vs. 3.7 months
Middleton et al. TeloVac, ISRCTN4382138	III	Gemcitabine + Capecitabine alone vs. + sequential GV1001 vs. + concurrent GV1001 LA/Metastatic	hTERT, class II 16mer peptide vaccine	1062	14%	7.9 vs. 6.9 vs. 8.4
Weden et al.	II	CTN-95002 or CTN-98010 after resection	KRAS peptide vaccine	23	N/A	27.5 months
Palmer et al. NCT02261714	I/II	TG01/GM-CSF + gemcitabine after resection	KRAS peptide vaccine + GMCSF	33	N/A	33.1
Yanagimoto et al.	II	Personalized peptide vaccine + gemcitabine	Personalized peptide vaccine + chemo	21	33%	9
Qiu et al.	I	Vaccine following gemcitabine/oxaliplatin + radiation	Alpha-Gal DC and NK cell vaccine	14	14%	24.7
Mehrotra et al. NCT01410968	I	Poly(IC:LC) and peptide autologous DC	Peptide-pulsed hTERT DC vaccine, carcinoembryonic antigen (CEA) and survivin with an intramuscular TLR-3 agonist	8	0%	7.7
Hewitt et al. NCT01836432.	III	Neoadjuvant chemo and chemoXRT ± Algenpantucel-L (Hyper-acute-pancreas) BR/LA	Allogeneic PDAC cells expressing murine α(1,3)GT gene	282	ND	14.3 vs. 14.9

a mesothelin-specific T-cell signature was enhanced with significant augmentation of the T-cell repertoire, suggesting at least a partial induction of a T-cell-mediated immune response. Another RCT examined GVAX + anti-CTLA-4 in a maintenance setting following 4–6 cycles of FOLFIRINOX. Unfortunately, this GVAX + anti-CTLA combination produced significantly inferior survival compared to FOLFIRINOX (mOS 9.4 months vs. 14.7 months, ORR 6% vs. 14%, $p = 0.019$) [145].

Wilm's tumor gene WT-1 has been implicated in tumor growth, invasion, angiogenesis, and metastatic processes and is overexpressed in approximately 75% of PDAC tumors [146]. WT-1 peptide vaccines and WT-1-peptide-pulsed DCs have been utilized in combination with chemo [147–155]. Nishida et al. described the largest cohort of 85 patients with recurrent, LAPC, or mPDAC randomized to receive an intradermal WT-1 peptide vaccine plus gemcitabine ($n = 42$) or gemcitabine monotherapy ($n = 43$). Treatment in the vaccine plus chemo arm produced no significant difference in overall survival compared to the chemo-only arm (mOS 9.6 months vs. 8.9 months ($p = 0.4$)). A subset of patient with a delayed-type hypersensitivity (DTH) had a substantially improved PFS ($p > 0.001$).

MUC-1 is differentially expressed in >60% of PDAC patients and correlates with tumor size and dysplasia, suggesting a pivotal role in tumor progression [156]. A WT-1/MUC-1 peptide-pulsed DC vaccine combined with gemcitabine as adjuvant therapy in resected PDAC patients produced a measurable WT-1-specific CD8+ T-cell response in 40% of patients. Survival outcomes of mPFS and mOS of 17.7 and 46.4 months from the first vaccination were encouraging.

Earlier efforts with a MUC-1-pulsed DC vaccine in seven advanced PDAC patients with aberrant MUC-1 expression previously treated with chemotherapy and surgery showed no clinical responses [157], which suggests possible benefit with targeting multiple antigens.

KIF20A is a motor protein highly expressed in pancreatic cancer implicated in tumor growth and is highly expressed in >90% of PDAC patients [158, 159] Asahara et al. assessed an injected KIF20A66 protein vaccine in gemcitabine refractory, unresectable, or recurrent metastatic PDAC patients ($n = 29$), resulting in a peptide-specific CD8+ effector T-cell response and an mOS of 4.2 months, compared to 2.2 months with best supportive care ($p = 0.047$) [160].

A peptide-cocktail vaccine OCV-C01 containing epitope peptides derived from KIF20A and VEGF1/2 in combination with gemcitabine was trialed in the adjuvant setting after resection. Median DFS was 15.8 months and OS at 18 months was 69%. DFS was significantly longer in patients demonstrating KIF20A T-cell responses with no recurrences in patients with this immune correlate who underwent R0 resection [161]. VEGFR-directed vaccines from this same group were tested in a phase 2/3 RCT that allocated VEGFR2 peptide vaccine combined with gemcitabine ($n = 100$) or a placebo with gemcitabine ($n = 53$) to a chemoradiation naïve LAPC and mPDAC patients. Survival outcomes were similar between the two treatment groups (8.4 months and 8.5 months, $p = 0.9$, respectively) [162].

Survivin is typically only expressed during embryonic and fetal development where it participates in cell cycle regulation and apoptosis. In PDAC, it is pathologically expressed in about 80% of patients, with elevated expression associated with worse prognosis and treatment resistance [163, 164]. Utility of a survivin 2B-vaccine (SVN2B) was investigated in the phase 2 setting that included 83 pretreated advanced PDAC patients. Arms demonstrated no difference in median OS despite survivin-specific CD8+ T-cell signature enrichment when allocated to receive SVN-2B + IFN-α ($n = 30$), SVN-2B only ($n = 34$), or a placebo ($n = 19$) [165].

Pancreatic cancer cells achieve immortalization via activation of telomerase to avoid senescence [166]. Middleton and colleagues tested an intradermal telomerase peptide vaccine GV1001 (TeloVac) on LAPC and mPDAC patients [167]. Arms compared gemcitabine/capecitabine doublet chemotherapy versus sequential chemotherapy/vaccine or concurrent chemo with vaccine. The trial was negative, and GV1001 did not improve survival. Immune correlates stratified by sequential or concurrent chemo + vaccine did not relate to overall survival.

KRAS is classic alteration in 90% of PDAC patients associated with overall worse prognosis and treatment insensitivity [168]. Two major varieties of KRAS-directed vaccines have been tested in clinical trials: (1) Epstein Barr Virus-transformed lymphoblastoid cell line (CLC) [169] or (2) combined with adjuvant GM-CSF in PDAC patients with a confirmed KRAS mutation [170, 171]. Combination with gemcitabine as adjuvant therapy after resection has yielded initial favorable results. Palmer et al. trialed their vaccine on 32 PDAC patients who underwent primary resection. These patients received an intradermal injection of a seven-peptide vaccine covering most known mutations of KRAS (TG01), co-administered with recombinant GM-CSF (TG01/GM-CSF), and combined with gemcitabine. Median OS (33.1–34.3 months) and mPFS (13.9–19.5 months) were favorable when compared to historical outcomes (mOS 17–27 months) [172]. Peptide-specific-T-cell activation was detected in >74% of patients.

Preclinical work has more recently investigated a combinatorial strategy of neoantigen vaccine and STING adjuvant that produced transient tumor regression in a mouse model [173]. Addition of anti-PD-1 and an OX40 agonist augmented responses [174]. Building on sparse proof of concept work [175], multiple clinical trials are currently testing neoantigen vaccine treatments: NCT03558945, NCT03953235 (vaccine + nivolumab/ipilimumab), and NCT03956056.

Tumor-based vaccines and multi-antigen vaccines, with or without DCs as delivery vector, have been utilized clinically for PDAC more recently. A small trial combined personalized peptide vaccine with gemcitabine in 21 LAPC and mPDAC patients, resulting in an mOS of 9 months and mPFS of 7 months, comparable to gemcitabine/nabpaclitaxel alone (8.5 months) [176]. Alpha-galactosyl (α-Gal)-expressing tumor lysate-pulsed DCs were combined with cytokine-induced killer cells (CIK) in pretreated LAPC and mPDAC patients ($n = 14$) that achieved an mOS of 24.7 months. Immune correlates of CD8+ T cells, CD45+RO+ T cells, and CD56+ NK cell levels were increased. DTH was positive in 86% of patients and significantly correlated with prognosis [177]. Another immunotherapy consisting of a peptide-pulsed hTERT DC vaccine, carcinoembryonic antigen (CEA), and survivin with an intramuscular TLR-3 agonist (poly-ICLC) in pretreated LAPC and mPDAC patients resulted in an mOS and mPFS of 7.7 and 3 months with measurable tumor-specific T-cell populations [178]. Overall, studies have indicated that vaccines can illicit immune responses, but clinically relevant survival outcomes indicate the need for further research.

Recent publication described a phase III trial assessing algenpantucel-L [HyperAcute-Pancreas algenpantucel-L (HAPa)] consisting of allogeneic pancreatic cancer cells engineered to express the murine $\alpha(1,3)GT$ gene in a vaccine formulation. They compared HAPa in combination with SOC chemo/chemoradiation vs. standard of care chemo in locally advanced and borderline resectable disease. PFS and OS unfortunately were lower in the treatment group [179].

Immune Stimulators

Immune stimulation has been another mechanism that has been proposed as an adjunct to improve the effectiveness of immunotherapy. The most commonly altered signal transduction pathway in pancreatic cancer is the TGF-beta axis [180]. Inhibitors of TGF-β signaling have been explored in preclinical models and showed enhanced antitumor activity in combination with gemcitabine [181]. In combination with gemcitabine, galunisertib demonstrated low toxicity and 1.8 months increase in median overall survival compared to single-agent gemcitabine [182]. When combined with durvalumab PD-1 blockade in a phase Ib study, clinical activity was limited [183]. Currently, NIS793, a fully human IgG2 mAb blockinf TGFβ, is under investigation in two trials: 1L Ph III daNIS-2: Gem/nab-P $\pm$ NIS793 TGFβ/placebo (NCT04935359) and 1L Ph II daNIS-1 Gem/nab-P $\pm$ NIS793 $\pm$ Spartalizumab in 1L Metastatic disease (NCT04390763).

A phase I trial was attempted with eftilagimod alpha (IMP321) in combination with gemcitabine chemotherapy based on preclinical data that MHC class II agonist triggers maturation of APCs followed by activation of CD8+ T cells. This trial recruited treatment-naïve advanced PDAC patients. While safe ad well tolerated, doses administered in the trial demonstrated did not elicit correlative immunological response [184].

OX40 receptor activation signals downstream enhancement of effector functions, memory formation, and survival of CD4+ and CD8+ T cells [185]. Combination of an OX40 agonist with PD-1 blockade induced tumor cell rejection, depleted regulatory/exhausted T-cell complement, and stimulated T-cell immune memory in a mouse model [186]. While data from human trials is yet available, a phase 1b/2 trial combining an OX40 agonist with a toll-like receptor (TLR)-9 ligand is currently recruiting cancer patients including those with mPDAC (NCT04387071).

RO6874281 is a novel monomeric bispecific IL-2v immunocytokine that shows binding affinity to tumor-associated fibroblasts in the TME via FAP. Binding initiates CD8+ T-cell and NK effectors [187]. The drug will be combined with atezolizumab in the MORPHEUS platform trial (NCT03193190).

Adjuvants

In immunotherapy, adjuvants are usually added to vaccines in order to modulate or increase an immune response against the antigens contained within them [188]. They target the priming phase or the effector phase but can also be utilized as immune modulators to condition the microenvironment of both tumors and their draining lymph nodes in order to support both phases. Adjuvants bind onto pattern recognition receptors (PRRs), including toll-like receptors (TLRs), stimulator of IFN genes (STING), and NOD-like receptors (NLRs) to initiate immune responses and trigger release of chemokines/cytokines that can attract T cells [189]. Peritumoral administration has demonstrated superior antitumor efficacy in terms of DC and tumor-specific CD8+ T-cell activation and long-lasting tumor protection in mice when compared to systemic administration [190].

Binding of ligand to the toll-like receptors has been studied in the context of increasing inflammation via IL-12, INF-alpha, and TNF-alpha. Activation leads to dendritic cell maturation and T-cell and NK effector function. Some TLR expression has been associated with better prognosis in pancreatic cancer patients [191–193]. However, there is conflicting data that implicates activation of TLRs with tumorigenesis and angiogenesis [194, 195]. Preclinical work with orthotopic models of pancreatic cancer demonstrates activity in combination with other modalities such as chemo, radiotherapy, and checkpoint blockade [196–200] phase 2 data in human subjects comparing combination of gemcitabine, and IMM-101, a TLR2/1 agonist, with chemo alone demonstrated a modest overall survival benefit in favor of IMM-101 (7 months vs. 4.4 months) [201]. The results of the PANFIRE-III trial (NCT04612530) combining irreversible electroporation and nivolumab with administration of intratumoral TLR ligand are eagerly awaited [202]. Data from NCT04050085 that combined nivolumab with radiation and a TLR9 agonist SD-101 has yet to be presented.

The cyclic GMP-AMP synthase (cGAS)-STING pathway in innate immune cells detects cytosolic double-stranded DNA fragments and initiates inflammatory responses, resulting in DC maturation and infiltration of NK and T-cell effectors into PDAC [203, 204]. Mouse models have shown the efficacy of targeting STING in combination with vaccines, checkpoint inhibitors, and radiation to prolong survival and shrink tumors [173, 174, 205]. While efforts with STING agonists in NCT03010176 and NCT03172936 failed to induce tumor regression, NCT04144140 is ongoing.

Oncolytic Viruses

Oncolytic viral therapy harnesses the lytic therapy of viruses that can differentially target cancer cells that harbor upregulated oncogenic signaling and defective interferon-mediated immunity. The newly produced oncolytic viruses, virus-derived PAMPs, DAMPs, and tumor antigens are released into the TME, infecting other tumor cells; they also serve to activate DCs and prime T cells in the draining lymph nodes. CXCL9 and CXCL10 act as chemoattractants for immune effector trafficking [206]. Genetic modifications of these viruses allow for arming with immune modulator transgenes, so that immune-activating products are released by infected tumor cells upon lysis, decreasing immune suppression in the TME and/or increasing immune activation [207].

In mouse models of pancreatic cancer, oncolytic viruses caused tumor shrinkage and prolonged survival via downregulation of TAMs and increasing infiltration and function of Th1 cell responses [208, 209]. Clinical use of these viruses was first described in the unresectable setting [210, 211]. Other efforts have sought to augment therapy in resectable patients [212]. In one RCT, patients received IV pelareorep (an oncolytic reovirus) combined with carboplatin/paclitaxel ($n = 36$) or carboplatin/paclitaxel alone ($n = 37$). The primary outcome, mPFS, did not significantly differ between the treatment groups (4.9 months vs. 5.2 months, $p = 0.6$), but the oncolytic virus arm produced measurable increases in systemic Th1 CD4+ and CD8+ T cells [213]. Addition of that same viral construct to anti-PD-1 and chemotherapy yielded novel T-cell clones and transcriptional evidence of systemic immune activation associated with clinical benefit [214]. Another trial utilized intratumoral HF-10, a natural oncolytic HSV-1 virus, in combination with erlotinib (anti-EGFR) and gemcitabine in ten LAPC patients, achieving an mOS of 15.5 months [215]. A German trial of an oncolytic parvovirus H-1PB. (ParvOryx) in seven patients refractory to 1L therapy in the metastatic setting showed responses in two patients with no dose-limiting toxicities and survival of 326 and 555 days [216]. All patients showed T-cell responses to viral proteins. Patient who exhibited a partial response was found to have a distinct immunologic pattern in both tumor tissues and in blood suggestive of immune activation after administration of ParvOryx.

NCT03252808 is a Japanese study of the oncolytic herpes simplex virus canerpaturev (C-REV, formerly HF10) in combination with gemcitabine/nab-paclitaxel. Best overall response rate at 16 weeks was 66% with a DCR of 100% in the cohort of six patients. Further data from this study has not been released since 2019 [217].

Musher et al. recently presented promising results from NCT02705196 that investigated LOAd703, an oncolytic adenovirus with transgenes encoding TMZ-CD40L and 4-1BBL, in conjunction with gemcitabine/nab-paclitaxel standard of care chemo in patients with unresectable or metastatic PDAC. Of the 21 patients treated, 57% had already been exposed to chemo. Objective response was observed in 5/11 patients (55%) in the highest dose level. Of all evaluable patients, ORR was 44% with a DCR of 94%. Median OS in the patients who received at least one injection was 8.7 months. Post-injection immune correlates showed the proportion of T effector memory cells increase while T regs and MDSCs decreased. A follow-up trial adding atezolizumab to this promising combination is underway [218].

NCT02045589 is a phase I multicenter, open-label study of IV VCN-01, an oncolytic adenovirus that was trialed with or without gemcitabine/nab-paclitaxel. ORR in patient with PDAC was 50% [219]. Of 22 patients in the pancreatic cancer arms that were evaluable, eight patients experienced disease stabilization lasting more than 1 year with median OS 11–13.5 months. Subgroup analysis of patients at the RP2D demonstrated impressive outcomes; ORR was 83% with PFS of

6.3 months and OS of 20.8 months. Other trials are recruiting: NCT04637698 is seeking to evaluate OH2, a type 2 herpes simplex virus expressing GM-CSF.

Adoptive Cellular Therapy

Adoptive cell therapy involves infusion autologous or allogeneic effector cells (usually T or NK cells) to eradicate cancer. Cells are harvested, selected, and modified. Modifications in the processing may include expression of a chimeric antigen receptor that targets a specific protein moiety or a TCR to specifically recognize a peptide/MHC complex. Successes have been observed in hematologic malignancies, but responses in solid tumors have been limited. Selected cellular therapies are detailed in Table 6.3.

As described by Watanabe and colleagues, preclinical mouse models showed promise with a mesothelin-directed CAR-T construct combined with armed oncolytic viruses expressing IL-2 and TNF-alpha. Clinical development still requires optimization and remains in early stages.

Trials of a mesothelin CAR-T in humans showed limited activity [220, 221]. In NCT01897415, autologous T cells were engineered using mRNA electroporation, inducing transient expression of a second-generation anti-MSLN CAR construct coupled to 4-1BB and CD3ζ. The best response observed was stabilization of disease in two individuals for 3.8 and 5.4 months.

In NCT02159716, lentiviral transduced anti-MSLN CAR-T cells were also investigated. No patients responded, but 11 of 15 individuals did achieve stable disease. Later analysis demonstrated that only 3 of 15 patient samples displayed greater than 75% MSLN expression, suggesting that upfront patient selection by biomarkers would be a necessary future optimization. This trial (NCT03054298) is currently recruiting. NCT03638193 is a Chinese study of autologous T cells lentivirally transduced to express anti-mesothelin scFv fused to TCRζ and 4-1BB costimulatory domains in patients with metastatic pancreatic cancer. Patients will undergo lymphodepletion with cyclophosphamide. No results have been released.

Efforts to use Vγ9Vδ2 T cells in the adjuvant setting failed to prolong survival [222].

More promising results have been described by Kumai et al. [223] αβ T-cell therapy ± chemotherapy resulted in mOS of 11.3 months from start of immunotherapy and 18.7 months from diagnosis, which is longer than historical references for cytotoxic regimens.

NCT02541370 was a phase 1 clinical trial where T cells were engineered using lentiviral vectors to target CD133. Of the 23 patients treated, seven had PDAC that was advanced. Patient tumor samples demonstrated CD133 expression greater than 50%. The conditioning regimen involved cyclophosphamide and nab-paclitaxel. Three patient achieved stable disease, two achieved partial response, and two patients progressed. Repeated cell infusions provided a greater period of disease control within the pancreatic cohort. Post-treatment biopsies showed that tumor tissue no longer expressed CD133 [224].

Table 6.3 Selected adoptive cellular therapy studies incorporating PDAC patients

Trial ID	Phase	Therapy arms	Target	# patients ($n=$)	Response rate (%)	Median overall survival (months)
Haas et al. NCT02159716	I	3 + 3 (CART-meso ± cyclophosphamide)	anti-MSLN CAR construct coupled to 4-1BB and CD3ζ	5 PDAC	0	NR
Beatty et al. NCT01897415	I	CART-meso	lentiviral transduced anti-MSLN CAR-T cells	6	0	NR
Aoki et al.	I	Gemcitabine γδ T cells in resected PDAC	Vγ9Vδ2 T cells	28	N/A	NR
Kumai et al.	II	αβ T cells ± chemotherapy or chemoradiation	αβ T cell therapy ± chemotherapy	67	NR	18.7
Wang et al. NCT02541370	I	Cyclophosphamide + nab-paclitaxel + anti-CD133 CAR-T	Anti-CD 133 lentiviral transduced T cells	23 (7 PDAC)	28.6% (2/7 PDAC)	ND
Liu et al. NCT01869166	I	Cyclophosphamide/nab-paclitaxel and CAR-T in patients with >50% EGFR expression	EGFR-directed CART	16	25%	4.9
Feng et al. NCT01935843	I	CART with nab-paclitaxel and cyclophosphamide conditioning in patients >50% HER-2+ tumor cells	ERBB2-directed CART	11 (2 PDAC)	0%	ND
Katz et al. HTM-SURE NCT02850536	Ib	Anti-CEA CAR-T using hepatic artery infusion with IL-2	Second generation anti-CEA CAR-T	1 PDAC	1 CR as best response for 13 months	23.2 months
Leidner et al.	I	TCR, high dose IL2, tocilizumab, and cyclophosphamide	HLA-restricted T cell receptor targeting two separate KRASG12D peptides	1 PDAC	PR	Ongoing response

Another group targeted EGFR given its presence in 90% of PDAC tumors. NCT01869166 used EGFR-directed CAR-T cells in 16 patients with >50% EGFR expression [225]. Preconditioning was performed with cyclophosphamide and nab-paclitaxel. Patients were allowed to undergo palliative radiotherapy for tumor-associated pain. Of the 16 patients, eight achieved stable disease for 2–4 months, four were partial responders for 2–4 months, and two had disease progression. Two patients were lost to follow up.

One of the earliest attempts to design CAR-Ts involved targeting ERBB2. Unfortunately, within 15 min of infusion on NCI-09-C-0041, a patient experience severe on-target/off-tumor response resulting in death. Despite this, NCT01935843 enrolled two PDAC patients with >50% HER-2+ tumor cells. Preconditioning utilized cyclophosphamide and nab-paclitaxel. At final assessment, both individuals with pancreatic cancer achieved stable disease for 5.3 and 8.3 months [226]. NCT03740256 is investigating combination of a binary oncolytic adenovirus (CAdVEC) in combination with a HER2-specific autologous VAR VST in advanced HER2 positive solid tumors including PDAC and is actively recruiting.

CAR-T therapy targeting CEA given to a patient via hepatic artery infusion (NCT02850536) demonstrated a complete metabolic response in the liver that was durable and sustained for 13 months with normalization in tumor markers in one instance. Post-treatment tumor specimens demonstrated abundance of CAR+ cells [227]. Unfortunately, other attempts at targeting CEA have not made it off the launching pad. NCT04037241 was originally designed to study an anti-CEA CAR-T + chemotherapy vs. chemotherapy alone in patient with CEA+ pancreatic cancer and liver metastases. The trial was withdrawn under sponsor termination. NCT03818165 and NCT03682744 targeting the same moiety was terminated for limited enrollment. Other targets for CAR include CD70 (NCT02830724), Claudin 18.2 with CT041 (NCT04404595), PSCA with BPX-601 in NCT02744287, and HER2-Targeted Dual Switch CAR-T Cells (BPX-603) in NCT04650451.

Continued development of CAR-T cells will require further investigation in how best to increase tumor infiltration, to select proper antigens for targeting, to modulate the immunosuppressive TME, and to ensure fitness and survival of the infused cells [228–231]. Target engagement between CAR-T and PDAC cells occurs slowly, creating an additional challenge, as T cells, once activated and exposed to consistent antigen, begin a process of terminal differentiation towards an exhausted and hypo-functional state [232]. Third-generation CARs engineered to secrete checkpoint inhibitors to target PD-1, which enhanced antitumor activity and prolonged functional persistence [233, 234]. Newer fourth-generation CARs (also termed armored CARs or TRUCKS) have engineered CAR-T cells to express receptors for chemokines to aid in recruitment of immune cells to tumors [235–237]. Significant interest has also combining oncolytic viruses with CAR-T cells [238].

Allogeneic CAR-T cells have been suggested as a more available standardized off-the-shelf alternative to manufactured autologous CARs [239]. However, the allogeneic nature introduces the risk of graft versus host disease (GvHD) via HLA mismatch, which may also threaten the CAR persistence via immune elimination.

There is a fine balance: both life-threatening risks and donor availability decrease with higher-resolution HLA typing.

NK cells have been identified as an alternative to CAR-T cells. NK cells are innate immune effects that target foreign or damaged cells but recognize targets in a non-antigen-specific manner without the need for prior sensitization [240]. Froelich has described NK cells isolated from umbilical cord blood modified to express an anti-PSCA CAR construct with soluble IL-15 [241]. These PSCA-directed CAR NK cells were tested in a metastatic humanized pancreatic cancer mouse model. An increase in cytotoxic function, suppressed tumor growth, and prolonged survival were observed. On Day 48, pancreatic biopsies revealed minimal tumor cells and a high number of NK cells, indicating persistence of the immune cells within the TME. A number of trials are examining allogeneic NK cell infusions in PDAC but have not recently published any updates on results (NCT02839954, NCT03941457, NCT03634501; NCT03093688). There is initial data to suggest that allogeneic NK cell infusions targeting ROBO1 in PDAC are feasible [242]. Other recent proposals have included generating CAR NK cells from induced pluripotent stem cells derived from triple homozygous HLA donors so that immune suppression genes can be removed to prolong NK persistence and efficacy while minimizing rejection [243].

TILs are mononuclear immune cells that infiltrate tumor tissue during the initial immune response [244]. TIL therapy is limited by IL-2 AEs because high-dose IL-2 is required after infusion [245]. TIL therapy in PDAC is currently being tested in phase I and phase II clinical trials (NCT05098197, NCT03935893, NCT03610490, NCT04426669). TILs with gene encoding checkpoint inhibition of CISH through CIRSPR genetic engineering in NCT04426669 will make the results particularly interesting.

CAR macrophages have also been described targeting HER2 [246]. Phase I trial with CT-0508 (NCT04660929) is recruiting.

Great attention returned to TCR-based therapy with recent publication of a dramatic response.

Following a single infusion of autologous T cells genetically engineered to clonally express two allogeneic HLA-C*08:02-restricted T-cell receptors (TCRs) targeting mutant KRAS G12D expressed by the tumors, a patient with progressive pancreatic cancer had regression of visceral metastases (overall partial response of 72% by RECIST 1.1). The response was ongoing at 6 months. The engineered T cells constituted more than 2% of all the circulating peripheral-blood T cells 6 months after the cell transfer demonstrating persistence. This case report demonstrates proof of concept for TCR gene therapy targeting the KRAS driver mutations in mediating the objective regression of metastatic pancreatic cancer [247].

Multimodality Therapy with Local Ablation and Immunotherapy

Another approach that has gained interest is harnessing radiotherapy and/or radiofrequency ablation in conjunction with immunotherapy to circumvent the suppressive TME. From the theoretical perspective, investigators have posited that radiation can generate neoantigens in an "abscopal effect" that would act as systemic immune stimulant to act on distant metastatic sites.

Phase II data has demonstrated in microsatellite stable PDAC, addition of radiation to nivolumab and ipilimumab yielded a disease control rate of 29% (5/17 patients) with immune correlates enriched in NK cells in those that responded [248]. This proof of principle has been extended to more ablative techniques. Irreversible electroporation (IRE) is a nonthermal ablative technique in which high-voltage electrical pulses are applied directly to the tumor. It has been shown to transiently alleviate immune suppression and create a window for antitumor T-cell activation [249, 250]. Combining other therapeutics with IRE has coined terms such as electrochemotherapy and electroimmunotherapy [251]. Based on survival outcomes and tumor regression in mouse models [252, 253], O'Neill and colleagues initiated a phase 1 trial of concurrent checkpoint inhibition with IRE in LAPC following stable disease after chemotherapy [254]. Median OS was 18 months with mPFS of 6.3 months. This was further explored in the phase 2 PANFIRE trial in the locally advanced or recurrent PDAC setting in conjunction with cytotoxic chemotherapy. The target median OS was surpassed, and a phase 3 trial in conjunction with immunotherapy is ongoing (NCT04612530) [255]. PANFIRE-III will evaluate IRE + systemic anti-PD-1 with or without an intratumoral TLR-9 agonist in mPDAC patient with stable or responsive disease following eight cycles of FOLFIRINOX [202].

Percutaneous IRE has also been combined with NK cell therapy [256]. Compared to IRE alone, IRE + NK cells resulted in a modest improvement of mOS in patients with LAPC (12.2 months vs. 13.6 months, $p = 0.033$, $n = 35$) and mPDAC (9.1 months vs. 10.2 months, $p = 0.037$, $n = 32$), as well as improved mPFS in LAPC (9.1 months vs. 7.9 months, $p = 0.043$). Systemic measures of CD8+ T cells, NK cells, and pro-inflammatory cytokines increased to suggest positive immune correlates of survival.

Another trial compared IRE + allogeneic Vγ9Vδ2 T cells ($n = 30$) versus IRE alone ($n = 32$) in 62 LAPC patients, of whom 49 had previously received chemotherapy. Median OS for IRE + Vγ9Vδ2 T cells was significantly prolonged compared to IRE alone (mOS 14.5 months vs. 11 months, $p = 0.01$; mPFS 11 months vs. 8 months, $p = 0.03$). Patients receiving multiple T-cell infusions survived significantly longer compared to patients receiving a single infusion (mOS 17 months vs. 13.5 months, $p > 0.05$) [257].

Combination of SABR and immunomodulation with anti-CD40 or IL-12 microspheres have been promising in preclinical models of pancreatic cancer [258, 259]. Trials in a cohort of 59 pretreated mPDAC patients showed that in the 39 evaluable patients, SABR+ durvalumab produced better survival outcomes compared to SABR + durvalumab + tremelimumab dual blockade. Cohorts that received higher doses of radiation over five fractions had better survival. Overall response rate was a disappointing 5.1% [260].

Another trial interrogated the combination of neoadjuvant oregovomab with chemoimmunotherapy followed by stereotactic body radiotherapy and nelfinavir for radiosensitization in the locally advanced setting. Reported mOS and mPFS were an unimpressive 13 months and 8.6 months, respectively [261]. Multiple trials are ongoing that combine SABR with various immunotherapies in PDAC: Losartan + Nivolumab in combination with FOLFIRINOX and XBRT in localized PDAC (NCT03563248); chemotherapy versus chemotherapy + aldoxorubicin HCl, L-15 cytokine fusion protein N-803, and PD-L1 t-high affinity NK cell (NCT04390399); Nivolumab + SBRT (NCT04098432). NCT04327986 was terminated because of toxicity with bintrafusp alfa.

Microbiome

PDAC-associated microbes have been associated with immunosuppression, and their ablation is linked to improved responses to therapies. Mouse models have demonstrated differential evolution of the gut microbiome throughout the pancreatic tumorigenesis process vs. control mice. The microbiome promotes oncogenesis by induction of innate and adaptive immune suppression [262, 263]. Bacterial eradication in PDAC mouse models led to a reduction in immune-suppressive M2 TAMs, an increased intratumoral CD8:CD4 T cell ratio, and upregulation in PD-1 expression. Combination therapy of anti-PD1 antibodies and antibiotics displayed synergistic activity when compared to anti-PD1 alone. These findings were validated in another study that antibiotics could slow cancer growth and decrease the number of metastases [264].

Decreased diversity of the microbiome in PDAC patients has also piqued interest [265]. A unique pancreatic intratumoral microbiome has been implicated in resistance to gemcitabine via enzymatic conversion of the drug to its inactive form by gammaproteobacteria [266]. Long-term survivors have been shown to have higher tumor microbial diversity correlated with higher cytotoxic T-cell infiltration [267]. Mouse models for fecal microbial transplants (FMT) demonstrate that tumor microbiome diversity and composition influence pancreatic cancer outcomes in a CD8+ T-cell-dependent manner and that tumor progression can be altered by FMT [268]. Trials in humans for FMT have demonstrated success in reversing immunotherapy resistance in melanoma [269, 270]. Trials are underway in other tumor types including pancreatic cancer.

Immunotherapy in Selected Populations: Biomarker-Driven Combinations

Immunotherapy in Homologous Repair-Deficient PDAC

Given that immunotherapy has ineffective in unselected PDAC patients, much interest has turned to investigating subsets harboring subsets of alterations that could indicate benefit. Key findings in these clinical efforts have been summarized in Table 6.4.

While multiple gene and scoring systems comprise heterogeneous definitions of homologous recombination deficiency (HRD), germline pathogenic alteration of

Table 6.4 Select immunotherapy findings targeting DNA repair response

Trial ID	Phase	Therapy arms	Target	# patients ($n=$)	Response rate (%)	Median overall survival (months)
Renouf et al. CCTG PA.7, NCT02879318	II	GEM, Nab-P, D, +T (arm A) vs. GEM + Nab-P (arm B)	Germline *ATM*: 12 in arm A and 4 in arm B.	180	ND	ATM mutation 13.9 vs. WT 4.9
Terrero et al.	Retrospective	Nivolumab/ipilimumab in chemorefractory patients	Germline pathogenic variants in HRD genes	12 (10 PDAC)	40% in PDAC	ND
Riess et al. NCT03404960	Ib/II	Niraparib + nivolumab or Niraparib + ipilimumab in platinum-sensitive patients	Platinum sensitivity	84	N/A	Niraparib + Ipi 59.6% 6-month PFS

BRCA1/BRCA2 1 has been extensively recognized as a biomarker in 3–10% of patients and somatic alterations in 15–17% of tumors. Biallelic alterations of BRCA1/BRCA2 are associated with higher median tumor mutational burden and overall increased incidence of loss of heterozygosity when compared to wild-type tumors [271–273]. BRCA1/2-altered tumors are more susceptible to platinum-based cytotoxic regimens, and when platinum sensitive, HRD tumors are candidates for PARP inhibitors as illustrated by the POLO trial [274]. The benefit of PARP inhibitors as maintenance in these patients has been underwhelming with final overall survival analysis showing no difference with the addition of Olaparib.

The molecular underpinnings of this susceptibilityare thought to be synthetic lethality with production of mutations and neoantigens that signal for catastrophic cell death. Based on findings that PD-L1, tumor-infiltrating lymphocytes, and neoantigens are enriched in other BRCA1/2 malignancies [275], it has been theorized that these patients would be more susceptible to immunotherapy possibly in combination with other modalities such as poly(ADP-ribose) polymerase (PARP) inhibitors or radiation that generates mutations. Analysis of the CARIS database has demonstrated that BRCA-mutated PDAC samples had a mean TMB of 8.7 Mut/Mb with higher rate of PD-L1 expression (22%) as compared to WT (6.5% and 11.1%, respectively) [276].

Biomarker analysis of the negative CCTG PA.7 trial presented by Renouf and colleagues suggested that while plasma TMB did not predict the usefulness of combining PD-L1 and CTLA-4 inhibition with a gemcitabine/nab-paclitaxel backbone in all comers, a subset of patients with germline *ATM* alteration garnered an overall survival benefit. In the 12 patients with germline *ATM* mutation treated in the chemotherapy/immunotherapy arm, median survival was 13.9 months versus 4.9 months in the chemotherapy-only arm (four patients) with hazard ratio of 0.1. This difference was not observed in ATM wildtype. Germline ATM mutation status was independent of plasma TMB levels [277].

Preclinical work by Zhang et al. showed that DNA repair inhibition by pharmacologic blockade or siRNA silencing of ataxia telangiectasia mutated (ATM) results in induction of type I IFN-mediated innate immune response in PDAC that is increased by radiation, which potentiates increased sensitivity to PD-L1 blockade

[278]. Building on these findings, a recent single-center retrospective analysis by Terrero and colleagues suggests that some germline mutations in DNA repair genes may signal a potential therapeutic niche for immunotherapy. They analyzed ten pancreatic cancer patients, one cholangiocarcinoma patient, and one ampullary cancer patient with pathogenic genetic variants (PGVs) in HRD genes with chemotherapy-resistant disease that was microsatellite stable treated with ipilimumab 1 mg/kg and nivolumab 3 mg/kg every 21 days for 4 doses, followed by nivolumab 480 mg every 28 days [279]. Of the ten pancreatic cancer patients treated, two complete responses (20%) were achieved with one partial response (10%), and stable disease in two patients (20%) were observed as best response. Five had progressive disease (50%). For pancreatic patients, response rate was 30% with disease control rate of 50%. All patients with complete or partial responses had biallelic alteration on somatic testing. PD-L1 CPS score was not available in their published analysis for these responders. The two complete responders had germline alterations in BRCA 1 and RAD51C with tumor mutational burdens of 4 and 8 mutations per Mb; their durations of response were 41.6 months and 26.4 months, respectively. Analysis of biopsies in responders indicated increased densities of tumor-infiltrating lymphocytes and increased of inflammatory cytokines CCL4 and CXCL10.

Another case report noted exceptional response to olaparib and pembrolizumab following platinum therapy in a patient harboring a germline BRCA1 pathogenic variant with PDAC that demonstrated high mutational burden. Interestingly in this case, the exceptionally high tumor burden was not correlated with a detected *POLE* mutation, and addition of olaparib when oligoprogression in the liver was observed on scans resulted in radiographic complete response [280].

Several trials are underway to further investigate HRD PDAC and immunotherapy.

A randomized phase II study evaluating maintenance pembrolizumab plus olaparib versus olaparib monotherapy in platinum-sensitive, PDAC *gBRCA1/2*-mutated metastatic PDAC is open to accrual (NCT04548752). A phase II study is evaluating the role of dostarlimab and niraparib in patients with metastatic PDAC harboring either somatic or germline mutation in one of six HR genes (*BRCA1/2, PALB2, BARD1, RAD51c, RAD51d*) following platinum-based chemotherapy (NCT04493060). In a similar vein, the phase II POLAR study is evaluating pembrolizumab plus olaparib in the postplatinum, maintenance setting in patients with PDAC with a HR gene mutation or in participants with an exceptional response to platinum-based chemotherapy with no HR gene mutations (NCT04666740).

Platinum Sensitivity

Besides upfront treatment regimens, there is an unmet need for maintenance strategies in pancreatic cancer given the neuropathy and cytopenias associated with extended lifelong therapy traditional cytotoxic agents. Recent work by Riess and colleagues has examined maintenance with PARP inhibition with checkpoint block-ade in patients sensitive to platinum-containing chemotherapy [281]. Patients were randomized to niraparib 200 mg daily plus either nivolumab ($n = 44$) or ipilimumab ($n = 40$). Of the 84 evaluable patients, 6-month progression-free survival was 20.6% in the niraparib plus nivolumab group and 59.6% niraparib plus ipilimumab arm. Ten (22%) of 46 patients in the niraparib plus nivolumab group and 23 (50%) of 45 patients in the niraparib plus ipilimumab group had a grade 3 or worse treatment-related adverse event. The primary endpoint of 6-month progression-free survival was met in the niraparib plus ipilimumab maintenance group, whereas niraparib plus nivolumab yielded inferior progression-free survival. Biomarker analysis has not been published but is eagerly awaited to further refine which sets of patients may benefit from this maintenance strategy.

SWI/SNF Complex

SWItch/Sucrose Nonfermentable (SWI/SNF) complex is a subfamily of adenosine triphosphate-dependent (ATP-dependent) chromatin remodeling proteins that alter nucleosome topology and DNA access, ultimately regulating gene transcription. In some malignancies, they have been associated with responsiveness to immune checkpoint inhibitors via CD8+ T-cell cytotoxicity. Retrospective work by Botta et al. demonstrated that of patients with SWI/SNF-alterations treated with immuno-therapy, 8 of 9, 89% responded. When the three patients with MSI-H/dMMR tumors were removed (three patients), five of nine responded (55.5%). The PFS in the patients attaining PR ranged from 3 to 33+ months with at least three durable responses. The TMB in these patients ranged from 0 to 11 mut/Mb. These patients had alterations in *ARID1A*, *PBRM1*, *ARID1B*, and *SMARCA4.*

Conclusion

Pancreatic cancer has been resistant to immunotherapy in unselected patients who have received checkpoint inhibition owing to significant immunosuppressive tumor biology. Rational combinatorial approaches to therapy based on targets within the TME have so far shown no survival benefit but remain under investigation. Additional refinement of those subsets of patients who have benefited from therapy in setting of altered DNA repair mechanisms has indicated that biomarker-driven approaches may be more promising; immune signatures of T-cell responses have often correlated with better outcomes. Vaccines, oncogenic viruses, and cellular therapy continue be areas of active research to generalize the dramatic responses that have been recently reported to a larger patient population.

References

1. Rahib L, Wehner MR, Matrisian LM, Nead KT. Estimated projection of US cancer incidence and death to 2040. JAMA Netw Open. 2021;4(4):e214708. https://doi.org/10.1001/jamanetworkopen.2021.4708. PMID: 33825840; PMCID: PMC8027914.
2. American Cancer Society. Cancer facts & figures 2022. Atlanta, GA: American Cancer Society; 2022. https://www.cancer.org/content/dam/cancer-org/research/cancer-facts-and-statistics/annual-cancer-facts-and-figures/2022/2022-cancer-facts-and-figures.pdf.
3. Groot VP, Rezaee N, Wu W, Cameron JL, Fishman EK, Hruban RH, Weiss MJ, Zheng L, Wolfgang CL, He J. Patterns, timing, and predictors of recurrence following pancreatectomy for pancreatic ductal adenocarcinoma. Ann Surg. 2018;267(5):936–45. https://doi.org/10.1097/SLA.0000000000002234. PMID: 28338509.
4. Sohal DPS, Walsh RM, Ramanathan RK, Khorana AA. Pancreatic adenocarcinoma: treating a systemic disease with systemic therapy. J Natl Cancer Inst. 2014;106(3):dju011. https://doi.org/10.1093/jnci/dju011.
5. Mahadevan D, Von Hoff DD. Tumor-stroma interactions in pancreatic ductal adenocarcinoma. Mol Cancer Ther. 2007;6(4):1186–97. https://doi.org/10.1158/1535-7163.MCT-06-0686. Epub 2007 Apr 3. PMID: 17406031.
6. Whatcott CJ, Diep CH, Jiang P, Watanabe A, LoBello J, Sima C, Hostetter G, Shepard HM, Von Hoff DD, Han H. Desmoplasia in primary tumors and metastatic lesions of pancreatic cancer. Clin Cancer Res. 2015;21:3561–8. https://doi.org/10.1158/1078-0432.CCR-14-1051.
7. Ebelt ND, Zamloot V, Manuel ER. Targeting desmoplasia in pancreatic cancer as an essential first step to effective therapy. Oncotarget. 2020;11(38):3486–8. https://doi.org/10.18632/oncotarget.27745. PMID: 33014284; PMCID: PMC7517960.
8. Chandana S, Babiker HM, Mahadevan D. Therapeutic trends in pancreatic ductal adenocarcinoma (PDAC). Expert Opin Investig Drugs. 2019;28:161–77. https://doi.org/10.1080/13543784.2019.1557145.
9. Orhan A, Vogelsang RP, Andersen MB, Madsen MT, Hölmich ER, Raskov H, Gögenur I. The prognostic value of tumour-infiltrating lymphocytes in pancreatic cancer: a systematic review and meta-analysis. Eur J Cancer. 2020;132:71–84. https://doi.org/10.1016/j.ejca.2020.03.013. Epub 2020 Apr 22. PMID: 32334338.
10. Shibuya KC, et al. Pancreatic ductal adenocarcinoma contains an effector and regulatory immune cell infiltrate that is altered by multimodal neoadjuvant treatment. PLoS One. 2014;9:e96565.
11. Carstens J, Correa de Sampaio P, Yang D, et al. Spatial computation of intratumoral T cells correlates with survival of patients with pancreatic cancer. Nat Commun. 2017;8:15095. https://doi.org/10.1038/ncomms15095.
12. Masugi YAT, Ueno A, et al. Characterization of spatial distribution of tumor-infiltrating CD8+ T cells refines their prognostic utility for pancreatic cancer survival. Mod Pathol. 2019;32:1495–507.
13. Grünwald BT, Devisme A, Andrieux G, Vyas F, Aliar K, McCloskey CW, Macklin A, Jang GH, Denroche R, Romero JM, Bavi P, Bronsert P, Notta F, O'Kane G, Wilson J, Knox J, Tamblyn L, Udaskin M, Radulovich N, Fischer SE, Boerries M, Gallinger S, Kislinger T, Khokha R. Spatially confined sub-tumor microenvironments in pancreatic cancer. Cell. 2021;184(22):5577–5592.e18. https://doi.org/10.1016/j.cell.2021.09.022. Epub 2021 Oct 12. PMID: 34644529.
14. Ahmadzadeh M, Rosenberg SA. TGF-beta 1 attenuates the acquisition and expression of effector function by tumor antigen-specific human memory CD8 T cells. J Immunol. 2005;174:5215–23. https://doi.org/10.4049/jimmunol.174.9.5215.
15. Feig C, Jones JO, Kraman M, Wells RJ, Deonarine A, Chan DS, Connell CM, Roberts EW, Zhao Q, Caballero OL, et al. Targeting CXCL12 from FAP-expressing carcinoma-associated

fibroblasts synergizes with anti-PD-L1 immunotherapy in pancreatic cancer. Proc Natl Acad Sci U S A. 2013;110:20212–7. https://doi.org/10.1073/pnas.1320318110.

16. Shi Y, Gao W, Lytle NK, Huang P, Yuan X, Dann AM, Ridinger-Saison M, DelGiorno KE, Antal CE, Liang G, et al. Targeting LIF-mediated paracrine interaction for pancreatic cancer therapy and monitoring. Nature. 2019;569:131–5. https://doi.org/10.1038/s41586-019-1130-6.

17. Monteran L, Erez N. The dark side of fibroblasts: cancer-associated fibroblasts as mediators of immunosuppression in the tumor microenvironment. Front Immunol. 2019;10:1835. https://doi.org/10.3389/fimmu.2019.01835.

18. Chakravarthy A, Khan L, Bensler NP, Bose P, De Carvalho DD. TGF-beta-associated extracellular matrix genes link cancer-associated fibroblasts to immune evasion and immunotherapy failure. Nat Commun. 2018;9:4692. https://doi.org/10.1038/s41467-018-06654-8.

19. Dominguez CX, Müller S, Keerthivasan S, Koeppen H, Hung J, Gierke S, Breart B, Foreman O, Bainbridge TW, Castiglioni A, Senbabaoglu Y, Modrusan Z, Liang Y, Junttila MR, Klijn C, Bourgon R, Turley SJ. Single-cell RNA sequencing reveals stromal evolution into LRRC15⁺ myofibroblasts as a determinant of patient response to cancer immunotherapy. Cancer Discov. 2020;10(2):232–53. https://doi.org/10.1158/2159-8290.CD-19-0644. Epub 2019 Nov 7. PMID: 31699795.

20. Huang H, Wang Z, Zhang Y, Pradhan RN, Ganguly D, Chandra R, Murimwa G, Wright S, Gu X, Maddipati R, Müller S, Turley SJ, Brekken RA. Mesothelial cell-derived antigen-presenting cancer-associated fibroblasts induce expansion of regulatory T cells in pancreatic cancer. Cancer Cell. 2022;40(6):656–673.e7. https://doi.org/10.1016/j.ccell.2022.04.011. Epub 2022 May 5. PMID: 35523176; PMCID: PMC9197998.

21. Fukumura D, Kloepper J, Amoozgar Z, Duda DG, Jain RK. Enhancing cancer immunotherapy using antiangiogenics: opportunities and challenges. Nat Rev Clin Oncol. 2018;15(5):325–40. PubMed: 29508855.

22. Lindau D, Gielen P, Kroesen M, Wesseling P, Adema GJ. The immunosuppressive tumour network: myeloid-derived suppressor cells, regulatory T cells and natural killer T cells. Immunology. 2013;138:105–15.

23. Padoan A, Plebani M, Basso D. Inflammation and pancreatic cancer: focus on metabolism, cytokines, and immunity. Int J Mol Sci. 2019;20:676. https://doi.org/10.3390/ijms20030676.

24. Eibl G, Cruz-Monserrate Z, Korc M, Petrov MS, Goodarzi MO, Fisher WE, et al. Diabetes mellitus and obesity as risk factors for pancreatic cancer. J Acad Nutr Diet. 2018;118(4):555–67. PubMed: 28919082.

25. Gomez-Chou SS-SA, Badi N, et al. Lipocalin-2 promotes pancreatic ductal adenocarcinoma by regulating inflammation in the tumor microenvironment. Cancer Res. 2017;77:2647–60. PubMed: 28249896.

26. Helm O, Held-Feindt J, Grage-Griebenow E, Reiling N, Ungefroren H, Vogel I, Krüger U, Becker T, Ebsen M, Röcken C, et al. Tumor-associated macrophages exhibit pro- and anti-inflammatory properties by which they impact on pancreatic tumorigenesis: role of macrophages in pancreatic cancer. Int J Cancer. 2014;135:843–61.

27. Noy R, Pollard JW. Tumor-associated macrophages: from mechanisms to therapy. Immunity. 2014;41(1):49–61. PubMed: 25035953.

28. Ren B, Cui M, Yang G, Wang H, Feng M, You L, et al. Tumor microenvironment participates in metastasis of pancreatic cancer. Mol Cancer. 2018;17(1):108. PubMed: 30060755.

29. Kurahara H, Shinchi H, Mataki Y, Maemura K, Noma H, Kubo F, Sakoda M, Ueno S, Natsugoe S, Takao S. Significance of M2-polarized tumor-associated macrophage in pancreatic cancer. J Surg Res. 2011;167:e211–9.

30. Sadozai H, Acharjee A, Eppenberger-Castori S, Gloor B, Gruber T, Schenk M, Karamitopoulou E. Distinct stromal and immune features collectively contribute to long-term survival in pancreatic cancer. Front Immunol. 2021;12:643529.

31. Zhu Y, Knolhoff BL, Meyer MA, Nywening TM, West BL, Luo J, Wang-Gillam A, Goedegebuure SP, Linehan DC, DeNardo DG. CSF1/CSF1R blockade reprograms tumor-infiltrating macrophages and improves response to T-cell checkpoint immunotherapy in

pancreatic cancer models. Cancer Res. 2014;74(18):5057–69. https://doi.org/10.1158/0008-5472.CAN-13-3723. Epub 2014 Jul 31. PMID: 25082815; PMCID: PMC4182950.

32. Young KHD, Cunningham D, Starling N. Immunotherapy and pancreatic cancer: unique challenges and potential opportunities. Ther Adv Med Oncol. 2018;10:1–20.

33. Weber R, Groth C, Lasser S, Arkhypov I, Petrova V, Altevogt P, Utikal J, Umansky V. IL-6 as a major regulator of MDSC activity and possible target for cancer immunotherapy. Cell Immunol. 2021;359:104254.

34. Marigo I, Dolcetti L, Serafini P, Zanovello P, Bronte V. Tumor-induced tolerance and immune suppression by myeloid derived suppressor cells. Immunol Rev. 2008;222:162–79.

35. Groth C, Hu X, Weber R, Fleming V, Altevogt P, Utikal J, et al. Immunosuppression mediated by myeloid-derived suppressor cells (MDSCs) during tumour progression. Br J Cancer. 2019;120(1):16–25. PubMed: 30413826.

36. Stromnes IM, Brockenbrough JS, Izeradjene K, Carlson MA, Cuevas C, Simmons RM, Greenberg PD, Hingorani SR. Targeted depletion of an MDSC subset unmasks pancreatic ductal adenocarcinoma to adaptive immunity. Gut. 2014;63(11):1769–81. https://doi.org/10.1136/gutjnl-2013-306271. Epub 2014 Feb 20. PMID: 24555999; PMCID: PMC4340484.

37. Huang B, Pan PY, Li Q, Sato AI, Levy DE, Bromberg J, Divino CM, Chen SH. Gr-1+CD115+ immature myeloid suppressor cells mediate the development of tumor-induced T regulatory cells and T-cell anergy in tumor-bearing host. Cancer Res. 2006;66(2):1123–31. https://doi.org/10.1158/0008-5472.CAN-05-1299. PMID: 16424049.

38. Pinton L, Solito S, Damuzzo V, Francescato S, Pozzuoli A, Berizzi A, Mocellin S, Rossi CR, Bronte V, Mandruzzato S. Activated T cells sustain myeloid-derived suppressor cell-mediated immune suppression. Oncotarget. 2016;7(2):1168–84. https://doi.org/10.18632/oncotarget.6662. PMID: 26700461; PMCID: PMC4811451.

39. Li A, King J, Moro A, Sugi MD, Dawson DW, Kaplan J, Li G, Lu X, Strieter RM, Burdick M, et al. Overexpression of CXCL5 is associated with poor survival in patients with pancreatic cancer. Am J Pathol. 2011;178:1340–9.

40. Zhang Y, Velez-Delgado A, Mathew E, Li D, Mendez FM, Flannagan K, et al. Myeloid cells are required for PD-1/PD-L1 checkpoint activation and the establishment of an immunosuppressive environment in pancreatic cancer. Gut. 2017;66(1):124–36. PubMed: 27402485.

41. Tang Y, Xu X, Guo S, Zhang C, Tang Y, Tian Y, Ni B, Lu B, Wang H. An increased abundance of tumor-infiltrating regulatory T cells is correlated with the progression and prognosis of pancreatic ductal adenocarcinoma. PLoS One. 2014;9:e91551.

42. Wartenberg M, Zlobec I, Perren A, Koelzer VH, Gloor B, Lugli A, Karamitopoulou E. Accumulation of FOXP3+T-cells in the tumor microenvironment is associated with an epithelial-mesenchymal-transition-type tumor budding phenotype and is an independent prognostic factor in surgically resected pancreatic ductal adenocarcinoma. Oncotarget. 2015;6:4190–201.

43. Ino Y, Yamazaki-Itoh R, Shimada K, Iwasaki M, Kosuge T, Kanai Y, Hiraoka N. Immune cell infiltration as an indicator of the immune microenvironment of pancreatic cancer. Br J Cancer. 2013;108:914–23.

44. Jang J-E, et al. Crosstalk between regulatory T cells and tumor-associated dendritic cells negates anti-tumor immunity in pancreatic cancer. Cell Rep. 2017;20(3):558–71.

45. Zhang Y, Lazarus J, Steele NG, Yan W, Lee H-J, Nwosu ZC, Halbrook CJ, Menjivar RE, Kemp SB, Sirihorachai V, et al. Regulatory T-cell depletion alters the tumor microenvironment and accelerates pancreatic carcinogenesis. Cancer Discov. 2020;10:422–39. https://doi.org/10.1158/2159-8290.CD-19-0958.

46. Nywening TM, Belt BA, Cullinan DR, Panni RZ, Han BJ, Sanford DE, Jacobs RC, Ye J, Patel AA, Gillanders WE, Fields RC, DeNardo DG, Hawkins WG, Goedegebuure P, Linehan DC. Targeting both tumour-associated CXCR2⁺ neutrophils and CCR2⁺ macrophages disrupts myeloid recruitment and improves chemotherapeutic responses in pancreatic ductal adenocarcinoma. Gut. 2018;67(6):1112–23. https://doi.org/10.1136/gutjnl-2017-313738. Epub 2017 Dec 1. PMID: 29196437; PMCID: PMC5969359.

47. Chao T, Furth EE, Vonderheide RH. CXCR2-dependent accumulation of tumor-associated neutrophils regulates T-cell immunity in pancreatic ductal adenocarcinoma. Cancer Immunol Res. 2016;4(11):968–82. https://doi.org/10.1158/2326-6066.CIR-16-0188. Epub 2016 Oct 13. PMID: 27737879; PMCID: PMC5110270.

48. Steele CW, Karim SA, Leach JDG, Bailey P, Upstill-Goddard R, Rishi L, Foth M, Bryson S, McDaid K, Wilson Z, Eberlein C, Candido JB, Clarke M, Nixon C, Connelly J, Jamieson N, Carter CR, Balkwill F, Chang DK, Evans TRJ, Strathdee D, Biankin AV, Nibbs RJB, Barry ST, Sansom OJ, Morton JP. CXCR2 inhibition profoundly suppresses metastases and augments immunotherapy in pancreatic ductal adenocarcinoma. Cancer Cell. 2016;29(6):832–45. https://doi.org/10.1016/j.ccell.2016.04.014. Epub 2016 Jun 2. PMID: 27265504; PMCID: PMC4912354.

49. Michaeli J, Shaul ME, Mishalian I, Hovav AH, Levy L, Zolotriov L, et al. Tumor-associated neutrophils induce apoptosis of non-activated CD8 T-cells in a TNFalpha and NO-dependent mechanism, promoting a tumor-supportive environment. Oncoimmunology. 2017;6(11):e1356965. PubMed: 29147615.

50. Zhang Y, Chandra V, Riquelme Sanchez E, Dutta P, Quesada PR, Rakoski A, et al. Interleukin-17-induced neutrophil extracellular traps mediate resistance to checkpoint blockade in pancreatic cancer. J Exp Med. 2020;217(12):e20190354.

51. McAllister F, Bailey JM, Alsina J, Nirschl CJ, Sharma R, Fan H, et al. Oncogenic Kras activates a hematopoietic-to-epithelial IL-17 signaling axis in preinvasive pancreatic neoplasia. Cancer Cell. 2014;25(5):621–37. PubMed: 24823639.

52. Bayne LJ, Beatty GL, Jhala N, Clark CE, Rhim AD, Stanger BZ, et al. Tumor-derived granulocyte-macrophage colony-stimulating factor regulates myeloid inflammation and T cell immunity in pancreatic cancer. Cancer Cell. 2012;21(6):822–35. PubMed: 22698406.

53. Ott PA, Bang YJ, Piha-Paul SA, Razak ARA, Bennouna J, Soria JC, Rugo HS, Cohen RB, O'Neil BH, Mehnert JM, Lopez J, Doi T, van Brummelen EMJ, Cristescu R, Yang P, Emancipator K, Stein K, Ayers M, Joe AK, Lunceford JK. T-cell-inflamed gene-expression profile, programmed death ligand 1 expression, and tumor mutational burden predict efficacy in patients treated with pembrolizumab across 20 cancers: KEYNOTE-028. J Clin Oncol. 2019;37(4):318–27. https://doi.org/10.1200/JCO.2018.78.2276. Epub 2018 Dec 13. PMID: 30557521.

54. Rousseau B, Foote MB, Maron SB, Diplas BH, Lu S, Argilés G, Cercek A, Diaz LA Jr. The spectrum of benefit from checkpoint blockade in hypermutated tumors. N Engl J Med. 2021;384(12):1168–70. https://doi.org/10.1056/NEJMc2031965. PMID: 33761214; PMCID: PMC8403269.

55. Lawlor RT, Mattiolo P, Mafficini A, Hong SM, Piredda ML, Taormina SV, Malleo G, Marchegiani G, Pea A, Salvia R, Kryklyva V, Shin JI, Brosens LA, Milella M, Scarpa A, Luchini C. Tumor mutational burden as a potential biomarker for immunotherapy in pancreatic cancer: systematic review and still-open questions. Cancers. 2021;13(13):3119. https://doi.org/10.3390/cancers13133119. PMID: 34206554; PMCID: PMC8269341.

56. Chalmers ZR, Connelly CF, Fabrizio D, et al. Analysis of 100,000 human cancer genomes reveals the landscape of tumor mutational burden. Genome Med. 2017;9:34. https://doi.org/10.1186/s13073-017-0424-2.

57. Valero C, Lee M, Hoen D, et al. Response rates to anti–PD-1 immunotherapy in microsatellite-stable solid tumors with 10 or more mutations per megabase. JAMA Oncol. 2021;7:739–43.

58. Luchini C, Bibeau F, Ligtenberg MJL, Singh N, Nottegar A, Bosse T, Miller R, Riaz N, Douillard J-Y, Andre F, et al. ESMO recommendations on microsatellite instability testing for immunotherapy in cancer, and its relationship with PD-1/PD-L1 expression and tumour mutational burden: a systematic review-based approach. Ann Oncol. 2019;30:1232–43. https://doi.org/10.1093/annonc/mdz116.

59. McGrail DJ, Pilié PG, Rashid NU, Voorwerk L, Slagter M, Kok M, Jonasch E, Khasraw M, Heimberger AB, Lim B, Ueno NT, Litton JK, Ferrarotto R, Chang JT, Moulder SL, Lin SY. High tumor mutation burden fails to predict immune checkpoint blockade

response across all cancer types. Ann Oncol. 2021;32(5):661–72. https://doi.org/10.1016/j. annonc.2021.02.006. Epub 2021 Mar 15. PMID: 33736924; PMCID: PMC8053682.

60. Karamitopoulou E, Andreou A, Wenning AS, Gloor B, Perren A. High tumor mutational burden (TMB) identifies a microsatellite stable pancreatic cancer subset with prolonged survival and strong anti-tumor immunity. Eur J Cancer. 2022;169:64–73. https://doi.org/10.1016/j. ejca.2022.03.033. Epub 2022 May 2. PMID: 35512587.

61. Balachandran VP, et al. Identification of unique neoantigen qualities in long-term survivors of pancreatic cancer. Nature. 2017;551:512–6.

62. Łuksza M, Sethna ZM, Rojas LA, et al. Neoantigen quality predicts immunoediting in survivors of pancreatic cancer. Nature. 2022;606:389–95. https://doi.org/10.1038/ s41586-022-04735-9.

63. Luchini C, Brosens LAA, Wood LD, Chatterjee D, Shin JI, Sciammarella C, Fiadone G, Malleo G, Salvia R, Kryklyva V, Piredda ML, Cheng L, Lawlor RT, Adsay V, Scarpa A. Comprehensive characterisation of pancreatic ductal adenocarcinoma with microsatellite instability: histology, molecular pathology and clinical implications. Gut. 2021;70(1):148–56. https://doi.org/10.1136/gutjnl-2020-320726. Epub 2020 Apr 29. PMID: 32350089; PMCID: PMC7211065.

64. Marabelle A, Le DT, Ascierto PA, Di Giacomo AM, De Jesus-Acosta A, Delord JP, et al. Efficacy of pembrolizumab in patients with noncolorectal high microsatellite instability/mismatch repair-deficient cancer: results from the phase II KEYNOTE-158 study. J Clin Oncol. 2020;38(1):1–10. PubMed: 31682550.

65. Chida K, Kawazoe A, Kawazu M, Suzuki T, Nakamura Y, Nakatsura T, Kuwata T, Ueno T, Kuboki Y, Kotani D, Kojima T, Taniguchi H, Mano H, Ikeda M, Shitara K, Endo I, Yoshino T. A low tumor mutational burden and PTEN mutations are predictors of a negative response to PD-1 blockade in MSI-H/dMMR gastrointestinal tumors. Clin Cancer Res. 2021;27(13):3714–24. https://doi.org/10.1158/1078-0432.CCR-21-0401. Epub 2021 Apr 29. PMID: 33926917.

66. Salem ME, Puccini A, Grothey A, Raghavan D, Goldberg RM, Xiu J, Korn WM, Weinberg BA, Hwang JJ, Shields AF, Marshall JL, Philip PA, Lenz HJ. Landscape of tumor mutation load, mismatch repair deficiency, and PD-L1 expression in a large patient cohort of gastrointestinal cancers. Mol Cancer Res. 2018;16(5):805–12. https://doi.org/10.1158/1541-7786. MCR-17-0735. Epub 2018 Mar 9. PMID: 29523759; PMCID: PMC6833953.

67. Salem ME, Bodor JN, Puccini A, Xiu J, Goldberg RM, Grothey A, Korn WM, Shields AF, Worrilow WM, Kim ES, Lenz HJ, Marshall JL, Hall MJ. Relationship between MLH1, PMS2, MSH2 and MSH6 gene-specific alterations and tumor mutational burden in 1057 microsatellite instability-high solid tumors. Int J Cancer. 2020;147(10):2948–56. https://doi. org/10.1002/ijc.33115. Epub 2020 Jun 18. PMID: 32449172; PMCID: PMC7530095.

68. Pandey V, Storz P. Targeting the tumor microenvironment in pancreatic ductal adenocarcinoma. Expert Rev Anticancer Ther. 2019;19:473–82. https://doi.org/10.1080/14737140.201 9.1622417.

69. Deng Y, Xia X, Zhao Y, Zhao Z, Martinez C, Yin W, Yao J, Hang Q, Wu W, Zhang J, Yu Y, Xia W, Yao F, Zhao D, Sun Y, Ying H, Hung MC, Ma L. Glucocorticoid receptor regulates PD-L1 and MHC-I in pancreatic cancer cells to promote immune evasion and immunotherapy resistance. Nat Commun. 2021;12(1):7041. https://doi.org/10.1038/s41467-021-27349-7. PMID: 34873175; PMCID: PMC8649069.

70. Tessier-Cloutier B, Kalloger SE, Al-Kandari M, Milne K, Gao D, Nelson BH, Renouf DJ, Sheffield BS, Schaeffer DF. Programmed cell death ligand 1 cut-point is associated with reduced disease specific survival in resected pancreatic ductal adenocarcinoma. BMC Cancer. 2017;17(1):618. https://doi.org/10.1186/s12885-017-3634-5. PMID: 28870260; PMCID: PMC5584324.

71. Danilova L, Ho WJ, Zhu Q, Vithayathil T, De Jesus-Acosta A, Azad NS, Laheru DA, Fertig EJ, Anders R, Jaffee EM, Yarchoan M. Programmed cell death ligand-1 (PD-L1) and CD8 expression profiling identify an immunologic subtype of pancreatic ductal adenocarcinomas with favorable survival. Cancer Immunol Res. 2019;7(6):886–95. https://

doi.org/10.1158/2326-6066.CIR-18-0822. Epub 2019 May 1. PMID: 31043417; PMCID: PMC6548624.

72. Wei SC, Duffy CR, Allison JP. Fundamental mechanisms of immune checkpoint blockade therapy. Cancer Discov. 2018;8:1069–86. https://doi.org/10.1158/2159-8290.CD-18-0367.

73. Farren M, Mace TA, Geyer S, Mikhail S, Wu C, Ciombor KK, Tahiri S, Ahn D, Noonan A, Villalonacalero M, et al. Systemic immune activity predicts overall survival in treatment-naïve patients with metastatic pancreatic cancer. Clin Cancer Res. 2015;22:2565–74. https://doi.org/10.1158/1078-0432.CCR-15-1732.

74. Royal RE, Levy C, Turner K, Mathur A, Hughes M, Kammula US, Sherry RM, Topalian SL, Yang JC, Lowy I, et al. Phase 2 trial of single agent ipilimumab (anti-CTLA-4) for locally advanced or metastatic pancreatic adenocarcinoma. J Immunother. 2010;33:828–33. https://doi.org/10.1097/CJI.0b013e3181eec14c.

75. Kamphorst AO, Wieland A, Nasti T, Yang S, Zhang R, Barber DL, Konieczny BT, Daugherty CZ, Koenig L, Yu K, et al. Rescue of exhausted CD8 T cells by PD-1–targeted therapies is CD28-dependent. Science. 2017;355:1423–7. https://doi.org/10.1126/science.aaf0683.

76. Hui E, Cheung J, Zhu J, Su X, Taylor MJ, Wallweber HA, Sasmal DK, Huang J, Kim JM, Mellman I, et al. T cell costimulatory receptor CD28 is a primary target for PD-1–mediated inhibition. Science. 2017;355:1428–33. https://doi.org/10.1126/science.aaf1292.

77. Yarchoan M, Albacker LA, Hopkins AC, Montesion M, Murugesan K, Vithayathil TT, Zaidi N, Azad NS, Laheru DA, Frampton GM, et al. PD-L1 expression and tumor mutational burden are independent biomarkers in most cancers. JCI Insight. 2019;4:e126908. https://doi.org/10.1172/jci.insight.126908.

78. Gao H-L, Liu L, Qi Z-H, Xu H-X, Wang W-Q, Wu C-T, Zhang S-R, Xu J-Z, Ni Q-X, Yu X-J. The clinicopathological and prognostic significance of PD-L1 expression in pancreatic cancer: a meta-analysis. Hepatobil Pancreat Dis Int. 2018;17:95–100. https://doi.org/10.1016/j.hbpd.2018.03.007.

79. Brahmer JR, Tykodi SS, Chow LQ, Hwu W-J, Topalian SL, Hwu P, Drake CG, Camacho LH, Kauh J, Odunsi K, et al. Safety and activity of anti–PD-L1 antibody in patients with advanced cancer. N Engl J Med. 2012;366:2455–65. https://doi.org/10.1056/NEJMoa1200694.

80. Marabelle A, Le DT, Ascierto PA, Di Giacomo AM, De Jesus-Acosta A, Delord J-P, Geva R, Gottfried M, Penel N, Hansen A, et al. Efficacy of pembrolizumab in patients with non-colorectal high microsatellite instability/mismatch repair–deficient cancer: results from the phase II KEYNOTE-158 study. J Clin Oncol. 2020;38:1–10. https://doi.org/10.1200/JCO.19.02105.

81. O'Reilly EM, Oh D-Y, Dhani N, Renouf DJ, Lee MA, Sun W, Fisher G, Hezel A, Chang S-C, Vlahovic G, et al. Durvalumab with or without tremelimumab for patients with metastatic pancreatic ductal adenocarcinoma. JAMA Oncol. 2019;5:1431–8. https://doi.org/10.1001/jamaoncol.2019.1588.

82. Aglietta M, Barone C, Sawyer MB, Moore MJ, Miller WH, Bagalà C, Colombi F, Cagnazzo C, Gioeni L, Wang E, et al. A phase I dose escalation trial of tremelimumab (CP-675,206) in combination with gemcitabine in chemotherapy-naive patients with metastatic pancreatic cancer. Ann Oncol. 2014;25:1750–5. https://doi.org/10.1093/annonc/mdu205.

83. Conroy T, Desseigne F, Ychou M, Bouché O, Guimbaud R, Bécouarn Y, Adenis A, Raoul JL, Gourgou-Bourgade S, de la Fouchardière C, Bennouna J, Bachet JB, Khemissa-Akouz F, Péré-Vergé D, Delbaldo C, Assenat E, Chauffert B, Michel P, Montoto-Grillot C, Ducreux M, Groupe Tumeurs Digestives of Unicancer; PRODIGE Intergroup. FOLFIRINOX versus gemcitabine for metastatic pancreatic cancer. N Engl J Med. 2011;364(19):1817–25. https://doi.org/10.1056/NEJMoa1011923. PMID: 21561347.

84. Von Hoff DD, Ervin T, Arena FP, Chiorean EG, Infante J, Moore M, Seay T, Tjulandin SA, Ma WW, Saleh MN, Harris M, Reni M, Dowden S, Laheru D, Bahary N, Ramanathan RK, Tabernero J, Hidalgo M, Goldstein D, Van Cutsem E, Wei X, Iglesias J, Renschler MF. Increased survival in pancreatic cancer with nab-paclitaxel plus gemcitabine. N Engl J Med. 2013;369(18):1691–703. https://doi.org/10.1056/NEJMoa1304369. Epub 2013 Oct 16. PMID: 24131140; PMCID: PMC4631139.

85. Mohindra NA, Kircher SM, Nimeiri HS, Benson AB, Rademaker A, Alonso E, Blatner N, Khazaie K, Mulcahy MF. Results of the phase Ib study of ipilimumab and gemcitabine for advanced pancreas cancer. J Clin Oncol. 2015;33:e15281. https://doi.org/10.1200/jco.2015.33.15_suppl.e15281.

86. Kalyan A, Kircher SM, Mohindra NA, Nimeiri HS, Maurer V, Rademaker A, Benson AB, Mulcahy MF. Ipilimumab and gemcitabine for advanced pancreas cancer: a phase Ib study. J Clin Oncol. 2016;34:e15747. https://doi.org/10.1200/JCO.2016.34.15_suppl.e15747.

87. Kamath SD, Kalyan A, Kircher S, Nimeiri H, Fought AJ, Benson A, Mulcahy M. Ipilimumab and gemcitabine for advanced pancreatic cancer: a phase Ib study. Oncology. 2019;25:e808–15. https://doi.org/10.1634/theoncologist.2019-0473.

88. Weiss GJ, Waypa J, Blaydorn L, Coats J, McGahey K, Sangal A, Niu J, Lynch C, Farley JH, Khemka V. A phase Ib study of pembrolizumab plus chemotherapy in patients with advanced cancer (PembroPlus). Br J Cancer. 2017;117:33–40. https://doi.org/10.1038/bjc.2017.145.

89. Weiss GJ, Blaydorn L, Beck J, Bornemann-Kolatzki K, Urnovitz H, Schütz E, Khemka V. Phase Ib/II study of gemcitabine, nab-paclitaxel, and pembrolizumab in metastatic pancreatic adenocarcinoma. Investig New Drugs. 2017;36:96–102. https://doi.org/10.1007/s10637-017-0525-1.

90. Renouf DJ, Knox JJ, Kavan P, Jonker D, Welch S, Couture F, Lemay F, Tehfe M, Harb M, Aucoin N, et al. LBA65—The Canadian Cancer Trials Group PA.7 trial: results of a randomized phase II study of gemcitabine (GEM) and nab-paclitaxel (Nab-P) vs GEM, Nab-P, Durvalumab (D) and Tremelimumab (T) as first line therapy in metastatic pancreatic ductal adenocarcinoma (MPDAC). Ann Oncol. 2020;31:S1195.

91. Balli D, Rech AJ, Stanger BZ, Vonderheide RH. Immune cytolytic activity stratifies molecular subsets of human pancreatic cancer. Clin Cancer Res. 2017;23(12):3129–38. PubMed: 28007776.

92. Stanietsky N, Simic H, Arapovic J, Toporik A, Levy O, Novik A, et al. The interaction of TIGIT with PVR and PVRL2 inhibits human NK cell cytotoxicity. Proc Natl Acad Sci U S A. 2009;106(42):17858–63. PubMed: 19815499.

93. Yu X, Harden K, Gonzalez LC, Francesco M, Chiang E, Irving B, et al. The surface protein TIGIT suppresses T cell activation by promoting the generation of mature immunoregulatory dendritic cells. Nat Immunol. 2009;10(1):48–57. PubMed: 19011627.

94. Pauken KE, Wherry EJ. TIGIT and CD226: tipping the balance between costimulatory and coinhibitory molecules to augment the cancer immunotherapy toolkit. Cancer Cell. 2014;26:785–7.

95. Johnston RJ, Comps-Agrar L, Hackney J, Yu X, Huseni M, Yang Y, Park S, Javinal V, Chiu H, Irving B, et al. The immunoreceptor TIGIT regulates antitumor and antiviral CD8 + T cell effector function. Cancer Cell. 2014;26:923–37.

96. Nishiwada S, Sho M, Yasuda S, Shimada K, Yamato I, Akahori T, Kinoshita S, Nagai M, Konishi N, Nakajima Y. Clinical significance of CD155 expression in human pancreatic cancer. Anticancer Res. 2015;35:2287–97.

97. Jin H-S, Ko M, Choi D-S, Kim JH, Lee D-H, Kang S-H, Kim I, Lee HJ, Choi EK, Kim K-P, et al. CD226hiCD8+ T cells are a prerequisite for anti-TIGIT immunotherapy. Cancer Immunol Res. 2020;8:912–25.

98. Acharya N, Sabatos-Peyton C, Anderson AC. Tim-3 finds its place in the cancer immunotherapy landscape. J Immunother Cancer. 2020;8:e000911.

99. Du W, Yang M, Turner A, Xu C, Ferris RL, Huang J, Kane LP, Lu B. TIM-3 as a target for cancer immunotherapy and mechanisms of action. Int J Mol Sci. 2017;18:645.

100. Lenzo FL, Kato S, Pabla S, DePietro P, Nesline MK, Conroy JM, Burgher B, Glenn ST, Kuvshinoff B, Kurzrock R, Morrison C. Immune profiling and immunotherapeutic targets in pancreatic cancer. Ann Transl Med. 2021;9(2):119. https://doi.org/10.21037/atm-20-1076. PMID: 33569421; PMCID: PMC7867882.

101. Peng P-J, Li Y, Sun S. On the significance of Tim-3 expression in pancreatic cancer. Saudi J Biol Sci. 2017;24:1754–7.

102. Wolf Y, Anderson AC, Kuchroo VK. TIM3 comes of age as an inhibitory receptor. Nat Rev Immunol. 2019;20:173–85.
103. Cebrián MJG, Bauden M, Andersson R, Holdenrieder S, Ansari D. Paradoxical role of HMGB1 in pancreatic cancer: tumor suppressor or tumor promoter? Anticancer Res. 2016;36:4381–90.
104. Gebauer F, Wicklein D, Horst J, Sundermann P, Maar H, Streichert T, Tachezy M, Izbicki JR, Bockhorn M, Schumacher U. Carcinoembryonic antigen-related cell adhesion molecules (CEACAM) 1, 5 and 6 as biomarkers in pancreatic cancer. PLoS One. 2014;9:e113023.
105. Seifert AM, Reiche C, Heiduk M, Tannert A, Meinecke A-C, Baier S, von Renesse J, Kahlert C, Distler M, Welsch T, et al. Detection of pancreatic ductal adenocarcinoma with galectin-9 serum levels. Oncogene. 2020;39:3102–13.
106. Blando JSA, Higa MG, et al. Comparison of immune infiltrates in melanome and pancreatic cancer highlights VISTA as a potential target in pancreatic cancer. Proc Natl Acad Sci. 2019;116(5):1692–7.
107. Thakkar D, Paliwal S, Dharmadhikari B, Guan S, Liu L, Kar S, Tulsian NK, Gruber JJ, DiMascio L, Paszkiewicz KH, Ingram PJ, Boyd-Kirkup DJ. Rationally targeted anti-VISTA antibody that blockades the C-C′ loop region can reverse VISTA immune suppression and remodel the immune microenvironment to potently inhibit tumor growth in an Fc independent manner. J Immunother Cancer. 2022;10(2):e003382. https://doi.org/10.1136/jitc-2021-003382. Erratum in: J Immunother Cancer. 2022;10(2): PMID: 35131861; PMCID: PMC8823246.
108. Meng Q, Liu Z, Rangelova E, Poiret T, Ambati A, Rane L, et al. Expansion of tumor-reactive T cells from patients with pancreatic cancer. J Immunother. 2016;39(2):81–9. PubMed: 26849077.
109. Rosenberg AMD. Immunotherapy in pancreatic adenocarcinoma -- overcoming barriers to response. J Gastrointest Oncol. 2018;9(1):143–59. PubMed: 29564181.
110. Nywening TM, Belt BA, Cullinan DR, Panni RZ, Han BJ, Sanford DE, et al. Targeting both tumour-associated CXCR2(+) neutrophils and CCR2(+) macrophages disrupts myeloid recruitment and improves chemotherapeutic responses in pancreatic ductal adenocarcinoma. Gut. 2018;67(6):1112–23. PubMed: 29196437.
111. Nywening TMM, Wang-Gillam A, Sanford DEE, et al. Targeting tumour-associated macrophages with CCR2 inhibition in combination with FOLFIRINOX in patients with borderline resectable and locally advanced pancreatic cancer: a single-centre, open-label, dose-finding, non-randomised, phase 1b trial. Lancet Oncol. 2016;17:651–62. https://doi.org/10.1016/S1470-2045(16)00078-4.
112. Bockorny B, Semenisty V, Macarulla T, Borazanci E, Wolpin BM, Stemmer SM, Golan T, Geva R, Borad MJ, Pedersen KS, et al. BL-8040, a CXCR4 antagonist, in combination with pembrolizumab and chemotherapy for pancreatic cancer: the COMBAT trial. Nat Med. 2020;26:878–85. https://doi.org/10.1038/s41591-020-0880-x.
113. Seeber A, et al. J Clin Oncol. 2021;39(15_suppl):4021. https://doi.org/10.1200/JCO.2021.39.15_suppl.4021.
114. Pellicciotta I, et al. J Clin Oncol. 2021;39(3_suppl):TPS454. https://doi.org/10.1200/JCO.2021.39.3_suppl.TPS454.
115. Hong D, Rasco D, Veeder M, Luke JJ, Chandler J, Balmanoukian A, George T, Munster P, Berlin JD, Gutierrez M, et al. A phase 1b/2 study of the Bruton tyrosine kinase inhibitor ibrutinib and the PD-L1 inhibitor durvalumab in patients with pretreated solid tumors. Oncology. 2019;97:102–11. https://doi.org/10.1159/000500571.
116. Wainberg ZA, Piha-Paul SA, Luke JJ, et al. First-in-human phase 1 dose escalation and expansion of a novel combination, anti—CSF-1 receptor (cabiralizumab) plus ant-PD-1 (nivolumab), in patients with advanced solid tumors. Presented at: 32nd SITC Annual Meeting; November 8–12, 2017; National Harbor, MD. Abstract O4. https://go.aws/3c8iEjG.
117. PipelineReview.com. Five prime therapeutics provides update on phase 2 trial of cabiralizumab combined with Opdivo® in pancreatic cancer. 2020. https://pipelinereview.com/index.php/2020021973818/Antibodies/

Five-Prime-Therapeutics-Provides-Update-on-Phase-2-Trial-of-Cabiralizumab-Combined-with-Opdivo-in-Pancreatic-Cancer.html.

118. Ho WJ, Jaffee EM. Macrophage-targeting by CSF1/1R blockade in pancreatic cancers. Cancer Res. 2021;81(24):6071–3. https://doi.org/10.1158/0008-5472.CAN-21-3603. PMID: 34911778; PMCID: PMC9164148.

119. Vonderheide R. The immune revolution: a case for priming, not checkpoint. Cancer Cell. 2018;33:563–9. PubMed: 29634944.

120. Padron LJ, Maurer DM, O'Hara MH, et al. Sotigalimab and/or nivolumab with chemotherapy in first-line metastatic pancreatic cancer: clinical and immunologic analyses from the randomized phase 2 PRINCE trial. Nat Med. 2022;28:1167–77. https://doi.org/10.1038/s41591-022-01829-9.

121. Barlesi F, Lolkema M, Rohrberg KS, et al. 291 Phase Ib study of selicrelumab (CD40 agonist) in combination with atezolizumab (anti-PD-L1) in patients with advanced solid tumors. J ImmunoTher Cancer. 2020;8:291. https://doi.org/10.1136/jitc-2020-SITC2020.0291.

122. Byrne KT, Betts CB, Mick R, Sivagnanam S, Bajor DL, Laheru DA, Chiorean EG, O'Hara MH, Liudahl SM, Newcomb C, Alanio C, Ferreira AP, Park BS, Ohtani T, Huffman AP, Väyrynen SA, Dias Costa A, Kaiser JC, Lacroix AM, Redlinger C, Stern M, Nowak JA, Wherry EJ, Cheever MA, Wolpin BM, Furth EE, Jaffee EM, Coussens LM, Vonderheide RH. Neoadjuvant selicrelumab, an agonist CD40 antibody, induces changes in the tumor microenvironment in patients with resectable pancreatic cancer. Clin Cancer Res. 2021;27(16):4574–86. https://doi.org/10.1158/1078-0432.CCR-21-1047. Epub 2021 Jun 10. PMID: 34112709; PMCID: PMC8667686.

123. Jin D, Fan J, Wang L, Thompson LF, Liu A, Daniel BJ, et al. CD73 on tumor cells impairs antitumor T-cell responses: a novel mechanism of tumor-induced immune suppression. Cancer Res. 2010;70(6):2245–55.

124. Overman M, LoRusso P, Strickler J, et al. Safety, efficacy and pharmacodynamics (PD) of MEDI9447 (oleclumab) alone or in combination with durvalumab in advanced colorectal cancer (CRC) or pancreatic cancer (panc). J Clin Oncol. 2018;36(Suppl):abstr 4123.

125. Manji GA, et al. J Clin Oncol. 2021;39(3_suppl):404. https://doi.org/10.1200/JCO.2021.39.3_suppl.404.

126. Provenzano PPCC, Chang AE, et al. Enzymatic targeting of the stroma ablates physical barriers to treatment of pancreatic ductal adenocarcinoma. Cancer Cell. 2012;21:418–29.

127. Wong KMHK, Coveler AL, et al. Targeting the tumor stroma: the biology and clinical development of pegylated recombinant human hyaluronidase (PEGPH20). Curr Oncol Rep. 2017;19(47):1–9.

128. Ramanathan RKMS, Philip PA, et al. Phase Ib/II randomized study of FOLFIRINOX plus pegylated recombinant human hyaluronidase versus FOLFIRINOX alone in patients with metastatic pancreatic adenocarcinoma: SWOG S1313. J Clin Oncol. 2019;37(13):1062–9.

129. Van Cutsem E, Tempero MA, Sigal D, Oh DY, Fazio N, Macarulla T, et al. Randomized phase III trial of pegvorhyaluronidase alfa with nab-paclitaxel plus gemcitabine for patients with hyaluronan-high metastatic pancreatic adenocarcinoma. J Clin Oncol. 2020;38(27):3185–94. PubMed: 32706635.

130. Sherman MH, Yu RT, Engle DD, Ding N, Atkins AR, Tiriac H, et al. Vitamin D receptor-mediated stromal reprogramming suppresses pancreatitis and enhances pancreatic cancer therapy. Cell. 2014;159(1):80–93. PubMed: 25259922.

131. Pitarresi JRLX, Avendano A, et al. Disruption of stromal hedgehog signaling initiates RNF5-mediated proteasomal degradation of PTEN and accelerates pancreatic tumor growth. Life Sci Allian. 2018;1(5):1–12.

132. Olive KP, Jacobetz MA, Davidson CJ, Gopinathan A, McIntyre D, Honess D, et al. Inhibition of Hedgehog signaling enhances delivery of chemotherapy in a mouse model of pancreatic cancer. Science. 2009;324(5933):1457–61. PubMed: 19460966.

133. De Jesus-Acosta A, Sugar EA, O'Dwyer PJ, Ramanathan RK, Von Hoff DD, Rasheed Z, et al. Phase 2 study of vismodegib, a hedgehog inhibitor, combined with gemcitabine and

nab-paclitaxel in patients with untreated metastatic pancreatic adenocarcinoma. Br J Cancer. 2020;122(4):498–505. PubMed: 31857726.

134. Jiang H, Hegde S, Knolhoff BL, Zhu Y, Herndon JM, Meyer MA, et al. Targeting focal adhesion kinase renders pancreatic cancers responsive to checkpoint immunotherapy. Nat Med. 2016;22(8):851–60. PubMed: 27376576.

135. Piccozi VJ, et al. J Clin Oncol. 2018;36(15_suppl):4016. https://doi.org/10.1200/JCO.2018.36.15_suppl.4016.

136. Hassan R, Blumenschein GR Jr, Moore KN, Santin AD, Kindler HL, Nemunaitis JJ, Seward SM, Thomas A, Kim SK, Rajagopalan P, Walter AO, Laurent D, Childs BH, Sarapa N, Elbi C, Bendell JC. First-in-human, multicenter, phase I dose-escalation and expansion study of anti-mesothelin antibody-drug conjugate anetumab ravtansine in advanced or metastatic solid tumors. J Clin Oncol. 2020;38(16):1824–35. https://doi.org/10.1200/JCO.19.02085. Epub 2020 Mar 26. PMID: 32213105; PMCID: PMC7255978.

137. Park W. J Clin Oncol. 2020;38(15_suppl):TPS4667. https://doi.org/10.1200/JCO.2020.38.15_suppl.TPS4667.

138. Shi Y, Gao W, Lytle NK, et al. Targeting LIF-mediated paracrine interaction for pancreatic cancer therapy and monitoring. Nature. 2019;569:131–5. https://doi.org/10.1038/s41586-019-1130-6.

139. Laheru D, Lutz E, Burke J, Biedrzycki B, Solt S, Onners B, Tartakovsky I, Nemunaitis J, Le D, Sugar E, et al. Allogeneic granulocyte macrophage colony-stimulating factor–secreting tumor immunotherapy alone or in sequence with cyclophosphamide for metastatic pancreatic cancer: a pilot study of safety, feasibility, and immune activation. Clin Cancer Res. 2008;14:1455–63.

140. Le DT, Wang-Gillam A, Picozzi V, Greten TF, Crocenzi T, Springett G, Morse M, Zeh H, Cohen D, Fine RL, et al. Safety and survival with GVAX pancreas prime and listeria monocytogenes–expressing mesothelin (CRS-207) boost vaccines for metastatic pancreatic cancer. JCO. 2015;33:1325–33.

141. Chen S-H, Hung W-C, Wang P, Paul C, Konstantopoulos K. Mesothelin binding to CA125/MUC16 promotes pancreatic cancer cell motility and invasion via MMP-7 activation. Sci Rep. 2013;3:srep01870.

142. Soares KC, Rucki AA, Wu AA, Olino K, Xiao Q, Chai Y, et al. PD-1/PD-L1 blockade together with vaccine therapy facilitates effector T-cell infiltration into pancreatic tumors. J Immunother. 2015;38(1):1–11. PubMed: 25415283.

143. Tsujikawa T, Crocenzi T, Durham JN, Sugar EA, Wu AA, Onners B, et al. Evaluation of cyclophosphamide/GVAX pancreas followed by listeria-mesothelin (CRS-207) with or without nivolumab in patients with pancreatic cancer. Clin Cancer Res. 2020;26(14):3578–88. PubMed: 32273276.

144. Le DT, Lutz E, Uram JN, Sugar EA, Onners B, Solt S, Zheng L, Diaz L, Donehower RC, Jaffee E, et al. Evaluation of ipilimumab in combination with allogeneic pancreatic tumor cells transfected with a GM-CSF gene in previously treated pancreatic cancer. J Immunother. 2013;36:382–9. https://doi.org/10.1097/CJI.0b013e31829fb7a2.

145. Wu AA, Bever KM, Ho WJ, Fertig EJ, Niu N, Zheng L, Parkinson RM, Durham JN, Onners BL, Ferguson AK, et al. A phase II study of allogeneic GM-CSF–transfected pancreatic tumor vaccine (GVAX) with ipilimumab as maintenance treatment for metastatic pancreatic cancer. Clin Cancer Res. 2020;26:5129.

146. Oji Y, Nakamori S, Fujikawa M, Nakatsuka S-I, Yokota A, Tatsumi N, Abeno S, Ikeba A, Takashima S, Tsujie M, et al. Overexpression of the Wilms' tumor gene WT1 in pancreatic ductal adenocarcinoma. Cancer Sci. 2004;95:583–7.

147. Kaida M, Morita-Hoshi Y, Soeda A, Wakeda T, Yamaki Y, Kojima Y, Ueno H, Kondo S, Morizane C, Ikeda M, et al. Phase 1 trial of Wilms tumor 1 (WT1) peptide vaccine and gemcitabine combination therapy in patients with advanced pancreatic or biliary tract cancer. J Immunother. 2011;34:92–9.

148. Nishida S, Koido S, Takeda Y, Homma S, Komita H, Takahara A, Morita S, Ito T, Morimoto S, Hara K, et al. Wilms tumor gene (WT1) peptide–based cancer vaccine combined with gemcitabine for patients with advanced pancreatic cancer. J Immunother. 2014;37:105–14.

149. Koido S, Homma S, Okamoto M, Takakura K, Mori M, Yoshizaki S, Tsukinaga S, Odahara S, Koyama S, Imazu H, et al. Treatment with chemotherapy and dendritic cells pulsed with multiple Wilms' tumor 1 (WT1)–specific MHC class I/II–restricted epitopes for pancreatic cancer. Clin Cancer Res. 2014;20:4228–39.

150. Tsukinaga S, Kajihara M, Takakura K, Ito Z, Kanai T, Saito K, Takami S, Kobayashi H, Matsumoto Y, Odahara S, et al. Prognostic significance of plasma interleukin-6/-8 in pancreatic cancer patients receiving chemoimmunotherapy. World J Gastroenterol. 2015; 21:11168–78.

151. Mayanagi S, Kitago M, Sakurai T, Matsuda T, Fujita T, Higuchi H, Taguchi J, Takeuchi H, Itano O, Aiura K, et al. Phase I pilot study of Wilms tumor gene 1 peptide-pulsed dendritic cell vaccination combined with gemcitabine in pancreatic cancer. Cancer Sci. 2015;106:397–406.

152. Yanagisawa R, Koizumi T, Koya T, Sano K, Koido S, Nagai K, Kobayashi M, Okamoto M, Sugiyama H, Shimodaira S. WT1-pulsed dendritic cell vaccine combined with chemotherapy for resected pancreatic cancer in a phase I study. Anticancer Res. 2018;38(4):2217–25. https://doi.org/10.21873/anticanres.12464. PMID: 29599342.

153. Nishida S, Ishikawa T, Egawa S, Koido S, Yanagimoto H, Ishii J, Kanno Y, Kokura S, Yasuda H, Oba MS, et al. Combination gemcitabine and WT1 peptide vaccination improves progression-free survival in advanced pancreatic ductal adenocarcinoma: a phase II randomized study. Cancer Immunol Res. 2018;6:320–31.

154. Hanada S, Tsuruta T, Haraguchi K, Okamoto M, Sugiyama H, Koido S. Long-term survival of pancreatic cancer patients treated with multimodal therapy combined with WT1-targeted dendritic cell vaccines. Hum Vacc Immunother. 2018;15:397–406.

155. Nagai K, Adachi T, Harada H, Eguchi S, Sugiyama H, Miyazaki Y. Dendritic cell-based immunotherapy pulsed with Wilms tumor 1 peptide and mucin 1 as an adjuvant therapy for pancreatic ductal adenocarcinoma after curative resection: a phase I/IIa clinical trial. Anticancer Res. 2020;40:5765–76.

156. Suh H, Pillai K, Morris DL. Mucins in pancreatic cancer: biological role, implications in carcinogenesis and applications in diagnosis and therapy. Am J Cancer Res. 2017;7:1372–83.

157. Rong Y, Qin X, Jin D, Lou W, Wu L, Wang D, Wu W, Ni X, Mao Z, Kuang T, Zang YQ, Qin X. A phase I pilot trial of MUC1-peptide-pulsed dendritic cells in the treatment of advanced pancreatic cancer. Clin Exp Med. 2012;12(3):173–80. https://doi.org/10.1007/s10238-011-0159-0. Epub 2011 Sep 20. PMID: 21932124.

158. Taniuchi K, Nakagawa H, Nakamura T, Eguchi H, Ohigashi H, Ishikawa O, Katagiri T, Nakamura Y. Down-regulation of RAB6KIFL/KIF20A, a kinesin involved with membrane trafficking of discs large homologue 5, can attenuate growth of pancreatic cancer cell. Cancer Res. 2005;65:105–12.

159. Imai K, Hirata S, Irie A, Senju S, Ikuta Y, Yokomine K, Harao M, Inoue M, Tomita Y, Tsunoda T, et al. Identification of HLA-A2-restricted CTL epitopes of a novel tumour-associated antigen, KIF20A, overexpressed in pancreatic cancer. Br J Cancer. 2010;104:300–7.

160. Asahara S, Takeda K, Yamao K, Maguchi H, Yamaue H. Phase I/II clinical trial using HLA-A24-restricted peptide vaccine derived from KIF20A for patients with advanced pancreatic cancer. J Transl Med. 2013;11:291.

161. Miyazawa M, Katsuda M, Maguchi H, Katanuma A, Ishii H, Ozaka M, Yamao K, Imaoka H, Kawai M, Hirono S, et al. Phase II clinical trial using novel peptide cocktail vaccine as a postoperative adjuvant treatment for surgically resected pancreatic cancer patients. Int J Cancer. 2016;140:973–82.

162. Yamaue H, Tsunoda T, Tani M, Miyazawa M, Yamao K, Mizuno N, Okusaka T, Ueno H, Boku N, Fukutomi A, et al. Randomized phase II/III clinical trial of elpamotide for patients with advanced pancreatic cancer: PEGASUS—PC study. Cancer Sci. 2015;106:883–90.

163. Dong H, Qian N, Wang Y, Meng L, Chen D, Ji X, Feng W. Survivin expression and serum levels in pancreatic cancer. World J Surg Oncol. 2015;13:189.

164. Brown M, Zhang W, Yan D, Kenath R, Le LTT, Wang H, Delitto D, Ostrov D, Robertson K, Liu C, et al. The role of survivin in the progression of pancreatic ductal adenocarcinoma (PDAC) and a novel survivin-targeted therapeutic for PDAC. PLoS One. 2020;15:e0226917.

165. Shima H, Tsurita G, Wada S, Hirohashi Y, Yasui H, Hayashi H, Miyakoshi T, Watanabe K, Murai A, Asanuma H, Tokita S, Kubo T, Nakatsugawa M, Kanaseki T, Tsukahara T, Nakae Y, Sugita O, Ito YM, Ota Y, Kimura Y, Kutomi G, Hirata K, Mizuguchi T, Imai K, Takemasa I, Sato N, Torigoe T. Randomized phase II trial of survivin 2B peptide vaccination for patients with HLA-A24-positive pancreatic adenocarcinoma. Cancer Sci. 2019;110(8):2378–85. https:// doi.org/10.1111/cas.14106. Epub 2019 Jul 23. PMID: 31218770; PMCID: PMC6676125.

166. Jafri MA, Ansari SA, Alqahtani MH, Shay JW. Roles of telomeres and telomerase in cancer, and advances in telomerase targeted therapies. Genome Med. 2016;8:1–18.

167. Middleton G, Silcocks P, Cox T, Valle J, Wadsley J, Propper D, Coxon F, Ross P, Madhusudan S, Roques T, et al. Gemcitabine and capecitabine with or without telomerase peptide vaccine GV1001 in patients with locally advanced or metastatic pancreatic cancer (TeloVac): an open-label, randomised, phase 3 trial. Lancet Oncol. 2014;15:829–40.

168. Kim J, Reber HA, Dry SM, Elashoff D, Chen SL, Umetani N, Kitago M, Hines OJ, Kazanjian KK, Hiramatsu S, et al. Unfavourable prognosis associated with K-ras gene mutation in pancreatic cancer surgical margins. Gut. 2006;55:1598–605.

169. Kubuschok B, Pfreundschuh M, Breit R, Hartmann F, Sester M, Gärtner B, König J, Murawski N, Held G, Zwick C, et al. Mutated ras-transfected, EBV-transformed lymphoblastoid cell lines as a model tumor vaccine for boosting T-cell responses against pancreatic cancer: a pilot trial. Hum Gene Ther. 2012;23:1224–36.

170. Wedén S, Klemp M, Gladhaug IP, Møller M, Eriksen JA, Gaudernack G, Buanes T. Long-term follow-up of patients with resected pancreatic cancer following vaccination against mutant K-ras. Int J Cancer. 2010;128:1120–8.

171. Palmer DH, Valle JW, Ma YT, Faluyi O, Neoptolemos JP, Gjertsen TJ, Iversen B, Eriksen JA, Møller A-S, Aksnes A-K, et al. TG01/GM-CSF and adjuvant gemcitabine in patients with resected RAS-mutant adenocarcinoma of the pancreas (CT TG01-01): a single-arm, phase 1/2 trial. Br J Cancer. 2020;122:971–7.

172. Oettle H, Neuhaus P, Hochhaus A, Hartmann JT, Gellert K, Ridwelski K, Niedergethmann M, Zülke C, Fahlke J, Arning MB, et al. Adjuvant chemotherapy with gemcitabine and long-term outcomes among patients with resected pancreatic cancer. JAMA. 2013;310:1473–81.

173. Kinkead HL, Hopkins A, Lutz E, Wu AA, Yarchoan M, Cruz K, Woolman S, Vithayathil T, Glickman LH, Ndubaku CO, et al. Combining STING-based neoantigen-targeted vaccine with checkpoint modulators enhances antitumor immunity in murine pancreatic cancer. JCI Insight. 2018;3:e122857.

174. Foote JB, Kok M, Leatherman JM, Armstrong TD, Marcinkowski B, Ojalvo LS, Kanne DB, Jaffee E, Dubensky TW, Emens LA. A STING agonist given with OX40 receptor and PD-L1 modulators primes immunity and reduces tumor growth in tolerized mice. Cancer Immunol Res. 2017;5:468–79.

175. Bassani-Sternberg M, Digklia A, Huber F, Wagner D, Sempoux C, Stevenson BJ, Thierry A-C, Michaux J, Pak H, Racle J, et al. A phase Ib study of the combination of personalized autologous dendritic cell vaccine, aspirin, and standard of care adjuvant chemotherapy followed by nivolumab for resected pancreatic adenocarcinoma—a proof of antigen discovery feasibility in three patients. Front Immunol. 1832;2019:10.

176. Yanagimoto H, Shiomi H, Satoi S, Mine T, Toyokawa H, Yamamoto T, Tani T, Yamada A, Kwon AH, Komatsu N, Itoh K, Noguchi M. A phase II study of personalized peptide vaccination combined with gemcitabine for non-resectable pancreatic cancer patients. Oncol Rep. 2010;24(3):795–801. https://doi.org/10.3892/or_00000923. PMID: 20664989.

177. Qiu Y, Yun MM, Xu MB, Wang YZ, Yun S. Pancreatic carcinoma-specific immunotherapy using synthesised alpha-galactosyl epitope-activated immune responders: findings from a pilot study. Int J Clin Oncol. 2013;18(4):657–65. https://doi.org/10.1007/s10147-012-0434-4. Epub 2012 Jul 31. PMID: 22847800.

178. Mehrotra S, Britten CD, Chin S, et al. Vaccination with poly(IC:LC) and peptide-pulsed autologous dendritic cells in patients with pancreatic cancer. J Hematol Oncol. 2017;10:82. https://doi.org/10.1186/s13045-017-0459-2.

179. Hewitt DB, Nissen N, Hatoum H, Musher B, Seng J, Coveler AL, Al-Rajabi R, Yeo CJ, Leiby B, Banks J, Balducci L, Vaccaro G, LoConte N, George TJ, Brenner W, Elquza E, Vahanian N, Rossi G, Kennedy E, Link C, Lavu H. A phase 3 randomized clinical trial of chemotherapy with or without algenpantucel-L (hyperacute-pancreas) immunotherapy in subjects with borderline resectable or locally advanced unresectable pancreatic cancer. Ann Surg. 2022;275(1):45–53. https://doi.org/10.1097/SLA.0000000000004669. PMID: 33630475.

180. Bailey P, et al. Genomic analyses identify molecular subtypes of pancreatic cancer. Nature. 2016;531:47–52. https://doi.org/10.1038/nature16965.

181. Melisi D, et al. LY2109761, a novel transforming growth factor-beta receptor type I and type II dual inhibitor, as a therapeutic approach to suppressing pancreatic cancer metastasis. Mol Cancer Ther. 2008;7:829–40. https://doi.org/10.1158/1535-7163.MCT-07-0337.

182. Melisi D, Garcia-Carbonero R, Macarulla T, Pezet D, Deplanque G, Fuchs M, Trojan J, Oettle H, Kozloff M, Cleverly A, Smith C, Estrem ST, Gueorguieva I, Lahn MMF, Blunt A, Benhadji KA, Tabernero J. Galunisertib plus gemcitabine vs. gemcitabine for first-line treatment of patients with unresectable pancreatic cancer. Br J Cancer. 2018;119(10):1208–14. https://doi.org/10.1038/s41416-018-0246-z. Epub 2018 Oct 15. PMID: 30318515; PMCID: PMC6251034.

183. Melisi D, Oh DY, Hollebecque A, Calvo E, Varghese A, Borazanci E, Macarulla T, Merz V, Zecchetto C, Zhao Y, Gueorguieva I, Man M, Gandhi L, Estrem ST, Benhadji KA, Lanasa MC, Avsar E, Guba SC, Garcia-Carbonero R. Safety and activity of the TGFβ receptor I kinase inhibitor galunisertib plus the anti-PD-L1 antibody durvalumab in metastatic pancreatic cancer. J Immunother Cancer. 2021;9(3):e002068. https://doi.org/10.1136/jitc-2020-002068. PMID: 33688022; PMCID: PMC7944986.

184. Wang-Gillam A, Plambeck-Suess S, Goedegebuure P, Simon PO, Mitchem J, Hornick JR, Sorscher S, Picus J, Suresh R, Lockhart AC, et al. A phase I study of IMP321 and gemcitabine as the front-line therapy in patients with advanced pancreatic adenocarcinoma. Investig New Drugs. 2012;31:707–13.

185. Lu X. OX40 and OX40L interaction in cancer. Curr Med Chem. 2020;28:1–13.

186. Ma Y, Li J, Wang H, Chiu Y, Kingsley CV, Fry D, Delaney SN, Wei SC, Zhang J, Maitra A, et al. Combination of PD-1 inhibitor and OX40 agonist induces tumor rejection and immune memory in mouse models of pancreatic cancer. Gastroenterology. 2020;159:306–19.

187. Soerensen MM, et al. J Clin Oncol. 2018;36(15_suppl):e15155. https://doi.org/10.1200/JCO.2018.36.15_suppl.e15155.

188. Circelli L, Tornesello ML, Buonaguro FM, Buonaguro L. Use of adjuvants for immunotherapy. Hum Vacc Immunother. 2017;13:1774–7.

189. Khong H, Overwijk WW. Adjuvants for peptide-based cancer vaccines. J Immunother Cancer. 2016;4:56.

190. Nierkens S, Brok MHD, Roelofsen T, Wagenaars JAL, Figdor CG, Ruers TJ, Adema GJ. Route of administration of the TLR9 agonist CpG critically determines the efficacy of cancer immunotherapy in mice. PLoS One. 2009;4:e8368.

191. Leppänen J, Helminen O, Huhta H, Kauppila JH, Isohookana J, Haapasaari K-M, Lehenkari P, Saarnio J, Karttunen TJ. High toll-like receptor (TLR) 9 expression is associated with better prognosis in surgically treated pancreatic cancer patients. Virchows Arch. 2017;470:401–10.

192. Lanki M, Seppänen H, Mustonen H, Hagström J, Haglund C. Toll-like receptor 1 predicts favorable prognosis in pancreatic cancer. PLoS One. 2019;14:e0219245.

193. Lanki AM, Seppänen EH, Mustonen HK, Böckelman C, Juuti AT, Hagström J, Haglund CH. Toll-like receptor 2 and Toll-like receptor 4 predict favorable prognosis in local pancreatic cancer. Tumor Biol. 2018;40:1010428318801188.

194. Zambirinis C, Levie E, Nguy S, Avanzi A, Barilla R, Xu Y, Seifert L, Daley D, Greco SH, Deutsch M, et al. TLR9 ligation in pancreatic stellate cells promotes tumorigenesis. J Exp Med. 2015;212:2077–94.

195. Sun Y, Wu C, Ma J, Yang Y, Man X, Wu H, Li S. Toll-like receptor 4 promotes angiogenesis in pancreatic cancer via PI3K/AKT signaling. Exp Cell Res. 2016;347:274–82.
196. Jacobs C, Duewell P, Heckelsmiller K, Wei J, Bauernfeind F, Ellermeier J, Kisser U, Bauer CA, Dauer M, Eigler A, et al. An ISCOM vaccine combined with a TLR9 agonist breaks immune evasion mediated by regulatory T cells in an orthotopic model of pancreatic carcinoma. Int J Cancer. 2010;128:897–907.
197. Michaelis KA, Norgard MA, Zhu X, Levasseur PR, Sivagnanam S, Liudahl SM, Burfeind KG, Olson B, Pelz KR, Ramos DMA, et al. The TLR7/8 agonist R848 remodels tumor and host responses to promote survival in pancreatic cancer. Nat Commun. 2019;10:1–15.
198. Zou B-B, Wang F, Li L, Cheng F-W, Jin R, Luo X, Zhu L-X, Geng X, Zhang S-Q. Activation of Toll-like receptor 7 inhibits the proliferation and migration, and induces the apoptosis of pancreatic cancer cells. Mol Med Rep. 2015;12:6079–85.
199. Schölch S, Rauber C, Tietz A, Rahbari NN, Bork U, Schmidt T, Kahlert C, Haberkorn U, Tomai MA, Lipson K, et al. Radiotherapy combined with TLR7/8 activation induces strong immune responses against gastrointestinal tumors. Oncotarget. 2014;6:4663–76.
200. Narayanan JSS, Ray P, Hayashi T, Whisenant TC, Vicente D, Carson DA, Miller AM, Schoenberger SP, White RR. Irreversible electroporation combined with checkpoint blockade and TLR7 stimulation induces antitumor immunity in a murine pancreatic cancer model. Cancer Immunol Res. 2019;7:1714–26.
201. Dalgleish AG, Stebbing J, Adamson DJ, Arif SS, Bidoli P, Chang D, Cheeseman S, Diaz-Beveridge R, Fernandez-Martos C, Glynne-Jones R, et al. Randomised, open-label, phase II study of gemcitabine with and without IMM-101 for advanced pancreatic cancer. Br J Cancer. 2016;115:789–96.
202. Geboers B, Timmer F, Ruarus A, Pouw J, Schouten E, Bakker J, Puijk R, Nieuwenhuizen S, Dijkstra M, Tol MVD, et al. Irreversible electroporation and nivolumab combined with intratumoral administration of a toll-like receptor ligand, as a means of in vivo vaccination for metastatic pancreatic ductal adenocarcinoma (PANFIRE-III). A phase-I study protocol. Cancers. 2021;13:3902.
203. Jiang M, Chen P, Wang L, Li W, Chen B, Liu Y, Wang H, Zhao S, Ye L, He Y, et al. cGAS-STING, an important pathway in cancer immunotherapy. J Hematol Oncol. 2020;13:1–11.
204. Jing W, McAllister D, Vonderhaar EP, Palen K, Riese MJ, Gershan J, Johnson BD, Dwinell MB. STING agonist inflames the pancreatic cancer immune microenvironment and reduces tumor burden in mouse models. J Immunother Cancer. 2019;7:115.
205. Baird JR, Friedman D, Cottam B, Dubensky TW, Kanne DB, Bambina S, Bahjat KS, Crittenden MR, Gough MJ. Radiotherapy combined with novel STING-targeting oligonucleotides results in regression of established tumors. Cancer Res. 2015;76:50–61.
206. Hemminki O, Dos Santos JM, Hemminki A. Oncolytic viruses for cancer immunotherapy. J Hematol Oncol. 2020;13:1–15.
207. de Graaf J, de Vor L, Fouchier R, Hoogen BVD. Armed oncolytic viruses: a kick-start for antitumor immunity. Cytokine Growth Factor Rev. 2018;41:28–39.
208. Zhang L, Wang W, Wang R, Zhang N, Shang H, Bi Y, Chen D, Zhang C, Li L, Yin J, et al. Reshaping the immune microenvironment by oncolytic herpes simplex virus in murine pancreatic ductal adenocarcinoma. Mol Ther. 2020;29:744–61.
209. Watanabe K, Luo Y, Da T, Guedan S, Ruella M, Scholler J, Keith B, Young RM, Engels B, Sorsa S, et al. Pancreatic cancer therapy with combined mesothelin-redirected chimeric antigen receptor T cells and cytokine-armed oncolytic adenoviruses. JCI Insight. 2018;3:e99573.
210. Nakao A, Kasuya H, Sahin TT, Nomura N, Kanzaki A, Misawa M, Shirota T, Yamada S, Fujii T, Sugimoto H, et al. A phase I dose-escalation clinical trial of intraoperative direct intratumoral injection of HF10 oncolytic virus in non-resectable patients with advanced pancreatic cancer. Cancer Gene Ther. 2010;18:167–75.
211. Kasuya H, Kodera Y, Nakao A, Yamamura K, Gewen T, Zhiwen W, Hotta Y, Yamada S, Fujii T, Fukuda S, et al. Phase I dose-escalation clinical trial of HF10 oncolytic herpes virus in 17 Japanese patients with advanced cancer. Hepato-Gastroenterology. 2014;61:599–605.

212. Aguilar LK, Shirley L, Chung VM, Marsh C, Walker J, Coyle W, Marx H, Bekaii-Saab T, Lesinski GB, Swanson B, et al. Gene-mediated cytotoxic immunotherapy as adjuvant to surgery or chemoradiation for pancreatic adenocarcinoma. Cancer Immunol Immunother. 2015;64:727–36.

213. Noonan A, Farren M, Geyer SM, Huang Y, Tahiri S, Ahn D, Mikhail S, Ciombor KK, Pant S, Aparo S, et al. Randomized phase 2 trial of the oncolytic virus pelareorep (reolysin) in upfront treatment of metastatic pancreatic adenocarcinoma. Mol Ther. 2016;24:1150–8.

214. Mahalingam D, Wilkinson GA, Eng K, Fields P, Raber P, Moseley JL, Cheetham K, Coffey M, Nuovo G, Kalinski P, et al. Pembrolizumab in combination with the oncolytic virus pelareorep and chemotherapy in patients with advanced pancreatic adenocarcinoma: a phase Ib study. Clin Cancer Res. 2019;26:71–81.

215. Hirooka Y, Kasuya H, Ishikawa T, Kawashima H, Ohno E, Villalobos IB, Naoe Y, Ichinose T, Koyama N, Tanaka M, et al. A Phase I clinical trial of EUS-guided intratumoral injection of the oncolytic virus, HF10 for unresectable locally advanced pancreatic cancer. BMC Cancer. 2018;18:1–9.

216. Hajda J, Leuchs B, Angelova AL, Frehtman V, Rommelaere J, Mertens M, Pilz M, Kieser M, Krebs O, Dahm M, Huber B, Engeland CE, Mavratzas A, Hohmann N, Schreiber J, Jäger D, Halama N, Sedlaczek O, Gaida MM, Daniel V, Springfeld C, Ungerechts G. Phase 2 trial of oncolytic H-1 parvovirus therapy shows safety and signs of immune system activation in patients with metastatic pancreatic ductal adenocarcinoma. Clin Cancer Res. 2021;27(20):5546–56. https://doi.org/10.1158/1078-0432.CCR-21-1020. Epub 2021 Aug 23. PMID: 34426438.

217. Hashimoto Y, et al. J Clin Oncol. 2019;37(4_suppl):325. https://doi.org/10.1200/JCO.2019.37.4_suppl.325.

218. Musher BL, et al. J Clin Oncol. 2022;40(16_suppl):4138. https://doi.org/10.1200/JCO.2022.40.16_suppl.4138.

219. Garcia-Carbonero R, Bazan-Peregrino M, Gil-Martín M, Álvarez R, Macarulla T, Riesco-Martinez MC, Verdaguer H, Guillén-Ponce C, Farrera-Sal M, Moreno R, Mato-Berciano A, Maliandi MV, Torres-Manjon S, Costa M, Del Pozo N, Martínez de Villarreal J, Real FX, Vidal N, Capella G, Alemany R, Blasi E, Blasco C, Cascalló M, Salazar R. Phase I, multicenter, open-label study of intravenous VCN-01 oncolytic adenovirus with or without nab-paclitaxel plus gemcitabine in patients with advanced solid tumors. J Immunother Cancer. 2022;10(3):e003255. https://doi.org/10.1136/jitc-2021-003255. PMID: 35338084; PMCID: PMC8961117.

220. Haas AR, Tanyi JL, O'Hara MH, Gladney WL, Lacey SF, Torigian DA, Soulen MC, Tian L, McGarvey M, Nelson AM, et al. Phase I study of lentiviral-transduced chimeric antigen receptor-modified T cells recognizing mesothelin in advanced solid cancers. Mol Ther. 2019;27:1919–29. https://doi.org/10.1016/j.ymthe.2019.07.015.

221. Beatty GL, O'Hara M, Lacey SF, Torigian DA, Nazimuddin F, Chen F, Kulikovskaya IM, Soulen MC, McGarvey M, Nelson AM, et al. Activity of mesothelin-specific chimeric antigen receptor T cells against pancreatic carcinoma metastases in a phase 1 trial. Gastroenterology. 2018;155:29–32. https://doi.org/10.1053/j.gastro.2018.03.029.

222. Aoki T, Matsushita H, Hoshikawa M, Hasegawa K, Kokudo N, Kakimi K. Adjuvant combination therapy with gemcitabine and autologous $\gamma\delta$ T-cell transfer in patients with curatively resected pancreatic cancer. Cytotherapy. 2017;19:473–85. https://doi.org/10.1016/j.jcyt.2017.01.002.

223. Kumai T, Mizukoshi E, Hashiba T, Nakagawa H, Kitahara M, Miyashita T, Mochizuki T, Goto S, Kamigaki T, Takimoto R, et al. Effect of adoptive T-cell immunotherapy on immunological parameters and prognosis in patients with advanced pancreatic cancer. Cytotherapy. 2020;23:137–45. https://doi.org/10.1016/j.jcyt.2020.08.001.

224. Wang Y, Chen M, Wu Z, et al. CD133-directed CAR T cells for advanced metastasis malignancies: a phase I trial. Oncoimmunology. 2018;7(7):e1440169.

225. Liu Y, Guo Y, Wu Z, et al. Anti-EGFR chimeric antigen receptor-modified T cells in metastatic pancreatic carcinoma: a phase I clinical trial. Cytotherapy. 2020;22:573–80.

226. Feng K, Liu Y, Guo Y, Qiu J, Wu Z, Dai H, Yang Q, Wang Y, Han W. Phase I study of chimeric antigen receptor modified T cells in treating HER2-positive advanced biliary tract cancers and pancreatic cancers. Prot Cell. 2018;9:838–47.
227. Katz SC, Moody AE, Guha P, Hardaway JC, Prince E, LaPorte J, Stancu M, Slansky JE, Jordan KR, Schulick RD, Knight R, Saied A, Armenio V, Junghans RP. HITM-SURE: hepatic immunotherapy for metastases phase Ib anti-CEA CAR-T study utilizing pressure enabled drug delivery. J Immunother Cancer. 2020;8(2):e001097. https://doi.org/10.1136/jitc-2020-001097. PMID: 32843493; PMCID: PMC7449487.
228. Katz SC, Point GR, Cunetta M, Thorn M, Guha P, Espat NJ, Boutros C, Hanna N, Junghans RP. Regional CAR-T cell infusions for peritoneal carcinomatosis are superior to systemic delivery. Cancer Gene Ther. 2016;23:142–8.
229. Raj D, Yang MH, Rodgers D, Hampton EN, Begum J, Mustafa A, Lorizio D, Garces I, Propper D, Kench JG, et al. Switchable CAR-T cells mediate remission in metastatic pancreatic ductal adenocarcinoma. Gut. 2019;68:1052–64.
230. Cutmore LC, Brown NF, Raj D, Chauduri S, Wang P, Maher J, Wang Y, Lemoine NR, Marshall JF. Pancreatic cancer UK grand challenge: developments and challenges for effective CAR T cell therapy for pancreatic ductal adenocarcinoma. Pancreatology. 2020;20:394–408.
231. Raj D, Nikolaidi M, Garces I, Lorizio D, Castro NM, Caiafa SG, Moore K, Brown NF, Kocher HM, Duan XB, et al. CEACAM7 is an effective target for CAR T-cell therapy of pancreatic ductal adenocarcinoma. Clin Cancer Res. 2021;27:1538–52.
232. Anderson KG, Stromnes IM, Greenberg PD. Obstacles posed by the tumor microenvironment to T cell activity: a case for synergistic therapies. Cancer Cell. 2017;31(3):311–25. PubMed: 28292435.
233. Li S, Siriwon N, Zhang X, Yang S, Jin T, He F, Kim YJ, Mac J, Lu Z, Wang S, et al. Enhanced cancer immunotherapy by chimeric antigen receptor-modified T cells engineered to secrete checkpoint inhibitors. Clin Cancer Res. 2017;23:6982.
234. Yang C-Y, Fan MH, Miao CH, Liao YJ, Yuan R-H, Liu CL. Engineering chimeric antigen receptor T cells against immune checkpoint inhibitors PD-1/PD-L1 for treating pancreatic cancer. Mol Ther Oncolyt. 2020;17:571.
235. Lesch S, Blumenberg V, Stoiber S, Gottschlich A, Ogonek J, Cadilha BL, Dantes Z, Rataj F, Dorman K, Lutz J, et al. T cells armed with C-X-C chemokine receptor type 6 enhance adoptive cell therapy for pancreatic tumours Nat. Biomed Eng. 2021;21:1246–60.
236. Di Pilato M, Kfuri-Rubens R, Pruessmann JN, Ozga AJ, Messemaker M, Cadilha BL, Sivakumar R, Cianciaruso C, Warner RD, Marangoni F, et al. CXCR6 positions cytotoxic T cells to receive critical survival signals in the tumor microenvironment. Cell. 2021;184:4512–4530.e22.
237. Cadilha BL, Benmebarek MR, Dorman K, Oner A, Lorenzini T, Obeck H, Vanttinen M, Di Pilato M, Pruessmann JN, Stoiber S, et al. Combined tumor-directed recruitment and protection from immune suppression enable CAR T cell efficacy in solid tumors. Sci Adv. 2021;7:eabi5781.
238. Rezaei R, Ghaleh HEG, Farzanehpour M, Dorostkar R, Ranjbar R, Bolandian M, et al. Combination therapy with CAR T cells and oncolytic viruses: a new era in cancer immunotherapy. Cancer Gene Ther. 2021;29:647. https://doi.org/10.1038/s41417-021-00359-9.
239. Depil S, Duchateau P, Grupp SA, Mufti G, Poirot L. 'Off-the-shelf' allogeneic CAR T cells: development and challenges. Nat Rev Drug Discov. 2020;19:185–99.
240. Geller MA, Miller JS. Use of allogeneic NK cells for cancer immunotherapy. Immunotherapy. 2011;3:1445–59.
241. Froelich W. CAR NK cell therapy directed against pancreatic cancer. Oncol Times. 2021;43:46.
242. Li C, Yang N, Li H, Wang Z. Robo1-specific chimeric antigen receptor natural killer cell therapy for pancreatic ductal adenocarcinoma with liver metastasis. J Cancer Res Ther. 2020;16:393–6.

243. Boyd NR, Tiedemann M, Cartledge K, Cao M, Evtimov V, Shu R, Nguyen T, Nguyen N, Nisbet I, Boyd R, Trounson A. Off-the-shelf ipsc derived car-nk immunotherapy for solid tumors. Cytotherapy. 2020;22:S199.
244. Underwood J. Lymphoreticular infiltration in human tumours: prognostic and biological implications: a review. Br J Cancer. 1974;30:538.
245. Nguyen LT, Saibil SD, Sotov V, Le MX, Khoja L, Ghazarian D, Bonilla L, Majeed H, Hogg D, Joshua AM, et al. Phase II clinical trial of adoptive cell therapy for patients with metastatic melanoma with autologous tumor-infiltrating lymphocytes and low-dose interleukin-2. Cancer Immunol Immunother. 2019;68:773–85.
246. Klichinsky M, Ruella M, Shestova O, Lu XM, Best A, Zeeman M, Schmierer M, Gabrusiewicz K, Anderson NR, Petty NE, Cummins KD, Shen F, Shan X, Veliz K, Blouch K, Yashiro-Ohtani Y, Kenderian SS, Kim MY, O'Connor RS, Wallace SR, Kozlowski MS, Marchione DM, Shestov M, Garcia BA, June CH, Gill S. Human chimeric antigen receptor macrophages for cancer immunotherapy. Nat Biotechnol. 2020;38(8):947–53. https://doi.org/10.1038/s41587-020-0462-y. Epub 2020 Mar 23.
247. Leidner R, Sanjuan Silva N, Huang H, Sprott D, Zheng C, Shih YP, Leung A, Payne R, Sutcliffe K, Cramer J, Rosenberg SA, Fox BA, Urba WJ, Tran E. Neoantigen T-cell receptor gene therapy in pancreatic cancer. N Engl J Med. 2022;386(22):2112–9. https://doi.org/10.1056/NEJMoa2119662. PMID: 35648703.
248. Parikh AR, Szabolcs A, Allen JN, Clark JW, Wo JY, Raabe M, Thel H, Hoyos D, Mehta A, Arshad S, Lieb DJ, Drapek LC, Blaszkowsky LS, Giantonio BJ, Weekes CD, Zhu AX, Goyal L, Nipp RD, Dubois JS, Van Seventer EE, Foreman BE, Matlack LE, Ly L, Meurer JA, Hacohen N, Ryan DP, Yeap BY, Corcoran RB, Greenbaum BD, Ting DT, Hong TS. Radiation therapy enhances immunotherapy response in microsatellite stable colorectal and pancreatic adenocarcinoma in a phase II trial. Nat Can. 2021;2(11):1124–35. https://doi.org/10.1038/s43018-021-00269-7. Epub 2021 Nov 18. PMID: 35122060; PMCID: PMC8809884.
249. Scheffer HJ, Stam AG, Geboers B, Vroomen LG, Ruarus A, De Bruijn B, Tol MPVD, Kazemier G, Meijerink MR, De Gruijl TD. Irreversible electroporation of locally advanced pancreatic cancer transiently alleviates immune suppression and creates a window for antitumor T cell activation. Oncoimmunology. 2019;8:1652532.
250. Pandit H, Hong YK, Li Y, Rostas J, Pulliam Z, Li SP, Martin RCG. Evaluating the Regulatory Immunomodulation Effect of Irreversible Electroporation (IRE) in Pancreatic Adenocarcinoma. Ann Surg Oncol. 2019;26:800–6.
251. Geboers B, Scheffer HJ, Graybill PM, Ruarus AH, Nieuwenhuizen S, Puijk RS, Tol PMVD, Davalos RV, Rubinsky B, De Gruijl TD, et al. High-voltage electrical pulses in oncology: irreversible electroporation, electrochemotherapy, gene electrotransfer, electrofusion, and electroimmunotherapy. Radiology. 2020;295:254–72.
252. Yang J, Eresen A, Shangguan J, Ma Q, Yaghmai V, Zhang Z. Irreversible electroporation ablation overcomes tumor-associated immunosuppression to improve the efficacy of DC vaccination in a mice model of pancreatic cancer. OncoImmunology. 2021;10:1875638.
253. Zhao J, Wen X, Tian L, Li T, Xu C, Wen X, Melancon MP, Gupta S, Shen B, Peng W, et al. Irreversible electroporation reverses resistance to immune checkpoint blockade in pancreatic cancer. Nat Commun. 2019;10:1–14.
254. O'Neill C, Hayat T, Hamm J, Healey M, Zheng Q, Li Y, Martin RC. A phase 1b trial of concurrent immunotherapy and irreversible electroporation in the treatment of locally advanced pancreatic adenocarcinoma. Surgery. 2020;168:610–6.
255. Ruarus AH, Vroomen L, Geboers B, van Veldhuisen E, Puijk RS, Nieuwenhuizen S, et al. Percutaneous irreversible electroporation in locally advanced and recurrent pancreatic cancer (PANFIRE-2): a multicenter, prospective, single-arm, phase II study. Radiology. 2020;294(1):212–20. PubMed: 31687922.
256. Lin M, Liang S, Wang X, Liang Y, Zhang M, Chen J, Niu L, Xu K. Percutaneous irreversible electroporation combined with allogeneic natural killer cell immunotherapy for patients with unresectable (stage III/IV) pancreatic cancer: a promising treatment. J Cancer Res Clin Oncol. 2017;143:2607–18.

257. Lin M, Zhang X, Liang S, Luo H, Alnaggar M, Liu A, Yin Z, Chen J, Niu L, Jiang Y. Irreversible electroporation plus allogenic Vγ9Vδ2 T cells enhances antitumor effect for locally advanced pancreatic cancer patients. Signal Transduct Target Ther. 2020;5:1–9.

258. Mills BN, Connolly KA, Ye J, Murphy J, Uccello T, Han BJ, Zhao T, Drage MG, Murthy A, Qiu H, et al. Stereotactic body radiation and interleukin-12 combination therapy eradicates pancreatic tumors by repolarizing the immune microenvironment. Cell Rep. 2019;29:406–21.

259. Yasmin-Karim S, Bruck PT, Moreau M, Kunjachan S, Chen GZ, Kumar R, Grabow S, Dougan SK, Ngwa W. Radiation and local anti-CD40 generate an effective in situ vaccine in preclinical models of pancreatic cancer. Front Immunol. 2018;9:2030.

260. Xie C, Duffy AG, Brar G, Fioravanti S, Mabry-Hrones D, Walker M, Bonilla CM, Wood BJ, Citrin DE, Gil Ramirez EM, et al. Immune checkpoint blockade in combination with stereotactic body radiotherapy in patients with metastatic pancreatic ductal adenocarcinoma. Clin Cancer Res. 2020;26:2318–26.

261. Lin C, Verma V, Lazenby A, Ly QP, Berim LD, Schwarz JK, Madiyalakan M, Nicodemus CF, Hollingsworth MA, Meza JL, et al. Phase I/II trial of neoadjuvant oregovomab-based chemoimmunotherapy followed by stereotactic body radiotherapy and nelfinavir for locally advanced pancreatic adenocarcinoma. Am J Clin Oncol. 2019;42:755–60.

262. Pushalkar S, Hundeyin M, Daley D, Zambirinis CP, Kurz E, Mishra A, et al. The pancreatic cancer microbiome promotes oncogenesis by induction of innate and adaptive immune suppression. Cancer Discov. 2018;8:403.

263. Thomas RM, Jobin C. Microbiota in pancreatic health and disease: the next frontier in microbiome research. Nat Rev Gastroenterol Hepatol. 2020;17(1):53–64. PubMed: 31811279.

264. Sethi V, Kurtom S, Tarique M, Lavania S, Malchiodi Z, Hellmund L, et al. Gut microbiota promotes tumor growth in mice by modulating immune response. Gastroenterology. 2018;155:33.

265. Ren Z, Jiang J, Xie H, Li A, Lu H, Xu S, et al. Gut microbial profile analysis by MiSeq sequencing of pancreatic carcinoma patients in China. Oncotarget. 2017;8(56):95176–91. PubMed: 29221120.

266. Geller LT, Barzily-Rokni M, Danino T, Jonas OH, Shental N, Nejman D, et al. Potential role of intratumor bacteria in mediating tumor resistance to the chemotherapeutic drug gemcitabine. Science. 2017;357(6356):1156–60. PubMed: 28912244.

267. Riquelme E, Maitra A, McAllister F. Immunotherapy for pancreatic cancer: more than just a gut feeling. Cancer Discov. 2018;8(4):386–8. PubMed: 29610286.

268. Riquelme EZY, Zhang L, et al. Tumor microbiome diversity and composition influence pancreatic cancer outcomes. Cell. 2019;178:795–806. PubMed: 31398337.

269. Baruch EN, Youngster I, Ben-Betzalel G, Ortenberg R, Lahat A, Katz L, et al. Fecal microbiota transplant promotes response in immunotherapy-refractory melanoma patients. Science. 2021;371(6529):602–9. PubMed: 33303685.

270. Davar D, Dzutsev AK, McCulloch JA, Rodrigues RR, Chauvin JM, Morrison RM, et al. Fecal microbiota transplant overcomes resistance to anti-PD-1 therapy in melanoma patients. Science. 2021;371(6529):595–602. PubMed: 33542131.

271. Sokol ES, Pavlick D, Khiabanian H, et al. Pan-canceranalysisofBRCA1and BRCA2 genomic alterations and their association with genomic instability as measured by genome-wide loss of heterozygosity. JCO Precis Oncol. 2020;4:442–65. https://doi.org/10.1200/PO.19.00345.

272. Park W, Chen J, Chou JF, et al. Genomic methods identify homologous recombination deficiency in pancreas adenocarcinoma and optimize treatment selection. Clin Cancer Res. 2020;26:3239–47.

273. Momtaz P, O'Connor CA, Chou JF, et al. Pancreas cancer and BRCA: a critical subset of patients with improving therapeutic outcomes. Cancer. 2021;127:4393–402.

274. Golan T, Hammel P, Reni M, et al. Maintenance olaparib for germline BRCA-mutated metastatic pancreatic cancer. N Engl J Med. 2019;381(4):317–27. https://doi.org/10.1056/NEJMoa1903387.

275. Strickland KC, Howitt BE, Shukla SA, et al. Association and prognostic significance of BRCA1/2-mutation status with neoantigen load, number of tumor-infiltrating

lymphocytes and expression of PD-1/PD-L1 in high grade serous ovarian cancer. Oncotarget. 2016;7(12):13587–98. https://doi.org/10.18632/oncotarget.7277.

276. Seeber A. Proceedings ASCO. Alexandria, VA: ASCO; 2019.

277. Renouf DJ, et al. Predictive value of germline ATM mutations in the CCTG PA.7 trial: gemcitabine (GEM) and nab-paclitaxel (Nab-P) versus GEM, nab-P, durvalumab (D) and tremelimumab (T) as first-line therapy in metastatic pancreatic ductal adenocarcinoma (mPDAC). J Clin Oncol. 2021;39(15_suppl):4135. https://doi.org/10.1200/JCO.2021.39.15_suppl.4135.

278. Zhang Q, Green MD, Lang X, Lazarus J, Parsels JD, Wei S, et al. Inhibition of ATM increases interferon signaling and sensitizes pancreatic cancer to immune checkpoint blockade therapy. Cancer Res. 2019;79(15):3940–51. PubMed: 31101760.

279. Terrero G, Datta J, Dennison J, Sussman D, Lohse I, Merchant N, Hosein P. Ipilimumab/nivolumab therapy in patients with metastatic pancreatic or biliary cancer with homologous recombination deficiency pathogenic germline variants. JAMA Oncol. 2022;8:1. https://doi.org/10.1001/jamaoncol.2022.0611.

280. Lundy J, McKay O, Croagh D, et al. Exceptional response to olaparib and pembrolizumab for pancreatic adenocarcinoma with germline BRCA1 mutation and high tumor mutation burden: case report and literature review. JCO Precis Oncol. 2022;6:e2100437.

281. Reiss KA, Mick R, Teitelbaum U, O'Hara M, Schneider C, Massa R, Karasic T, Tondon R, Onyiah C, Gosselin MK, Donze A, Domchek SM, Vonderheide RH. Niraparib plus nivolumab or niraparib plus ipilimumab in patients with platinum-sensitive advanced pancreatic cancer: a randomised, phase 1b/2 trial. Lancet Oncol. 2022;23:1009. https://doi.org/10.1016/S1470-2045(22)00369-2. PMID: 35810751.

Liquid Biopsies for Pancreatic Cancer: Is It Ready for Prime Time?

7

Kathleen Monahan and Ben George

Introduction

The general concept of circulating tumor cells dates back almost 150 years when Australian physician Thomas Ashworth observed cells in the blood that were identical to the primary tumor of a man with metastatic cancer postmortem. This seminal discovery contributed to our understanding of the hematogenous spread of malignancy, and exploitation of this concept would later inspire the development of techniques used to isolate these cells. The term "liquid biopsy" has been used to describe various methods aimed at obtaining any tumor material—either whole tumor cells or a component of tumor cells—from body fluids such as blood, CSF, or pleural fluid. Liquid biopsies are less invasive than tissue biopsies and have demonstrated utility with regards to early detection, diagnosis, treatment selection, and monitoring treatment response in some cancers. Additionally, liquid biopsies have the potential to account for spatiotemporal heterogeneity and dynamic clonal evolution, circumventing the inherent challenges associated with tissue-based genomic profiling.

There is growing interest in the use of liquid biopsies for screening, surveillance, and therapeutic decision making along the treatment continuum of PDAC [1]. PDAC is the third leading cause of cancer related death in the USA with a 5-year

K. Monahan
Division of Hematology and Oncology, Medical College of Wisconsin, Milwaukee, WI, USA

B. George (✉)
Division of Hematology and Oncology, Medical College of Wisconsin, Milwaukee, WI, USA

Mary Ann and Charles LaBahn Pancreatic Cancer Program, Medical College of Wisconsin, Milwaukee, WI, USA
e-mail: bgeorge@mcw.edu

survival rate of 11% [2]. Early detection, and elimination of minimal residual disease (MRD) after curative intent multimodality therapy, as well as dynamic utilization of systemic therapies informed by clonal evolution of the somatic genome are pivotal to improving the overall outcome of PDAC patients. Thus, there is an urgent, unmet need to refine liquid biopsies and explore opportunities for its systematic use in the diagnosis and treatment of PDAC.

In this chapter we will review core concepts related to liquid biopsies and their use in PDAC with emphasis on utility in screening/early detection, MRD assessment, surveillance, and/or therapeutic decision making.

Liquid Biopsy Methods

While most often occurring with blood samples, liquid biopsies can be performed on any bodily fluid including cerebral spinal fluid, pleural effusion, and ascites [3]. In PDAC, liquid biopsy can even be performed on pancreatic juices as they tend to be rich in tumor derived products, but this involves invasive procedures [4]. Various techniques have been established to detect and isolate both circulating tumor cells (CTCs) as well as material from tumor cells in the form of circulating DNA and exosomes—an overview is provided below.

Circulating Tumor Cells (CTCs)

Tumor cells enter the vasculature both passively and actively. Leaky blood vessels in combination with pressure from tumor growth or invasive procedures can push cells beyond the primary tumor site [5]. Additionally, in some instances, epithelial-mesenchymal transition (EMT) impacts the metastatic potential of tumor cells, promoting a tumor cell's ability to detach from surrounding tissue, mobilize, gain access to systemic circulation, and subsequently grow in other tissue environments [6]. Once tumor cells gain access to the vasculature, only a small proportion remain in circulation to avoid the immune system and/or shearing stress destruction [7]. Mechanisms to avoid destruction include upregulation of protective cell surface markers including CD47 and utilization of platelets to serve as a shield [8]. In PDAC specifically, the complex microenvironment of tumor cells, stromal tissue, and extracellular matrix promote angiogenesis and immune suppression further instigating movement of CTCs into circulation [9]. Clusters of heterogenous cell clusters called circulating tumor micro-emboli (CTM) commonly occur in pancreatic cancer as well and are thought to be primed to colonize metastatic sites [10].

CTCs remain scarce, particularly in early stage disease, accounting for approximately 1 of every 1×10^8 circulating blood cells and so detection is challenging. Moreover, in PDAC large CTCs or clusters may become trapped within the portal venous system prior to entering systemic circulation. Currently, there is only one US Food and Drug Administration (FDA) approved method to isolate CTCs called CellSearch that utilizes antibodies targeting known cell surface markers CD45, EpCAM, and cytokeratin. Through the process of EMT and other genotypic/phenotypic transformation, some CTCs lose these cell surface markers; therefore, both cell surface marker dependent and independent strategies for CTC detection are being developed such size-based separation [11–13]. Though difficult to isolate, CTCs are being utilized for detection, prognostication , and monitoring treatment response.. Additionally, CTCs retain the whole genome of a tumor cell facilitating single-cell transcriptomic analysis [14].

Circulating Free DNA and Circulating Tumor DNA

The term cell-free DNA (cfDNA) refers to extracellular DNA isolated from blood or other bodily fluids. cfDNA arising from cancer cells is termed circulating tumor DNA (ctDNA) and contains cancer-specific genetic alterations. cfDNA and ctDNA are released from normal and malignant cells respectively either through cell death processes (apoptosis and necrosis) or through excretion [15]. Both can be isolated from plasma or serum, but plasma yields better sample quality due to decreased contamination from leukocyte DNA [16]. Compared to cfDNA (average length of 166 base pairs (bps)) ctDNA is generally more fragmented (average length of about 140 bps) [17]. The relative amount of cfDNA that is ctDNA is referred to as the variant allele frequency (VAF) and is highly variable. In early stage cancer, VAF of ctDNA is often less than 1%, compared to the metastatic setting where it is often much higher, with reports ranging from 5% to 80% depending on histology, tumor burden, and location of disease [18].

Targeted as well as untargeted deep sequencing of ctDNA can provide important tumor-related genomic information for individual patients, particularly when tumor tissue is unavailable either due to inaccessible location or paucity of tumor cells. Furthermore, ctDNA is more representative of the spatial heterogeneity of cancer cells [19]. Therefore, deep sequencing of multi-base gene regions utilizing ctDNA may better represent intra-tumoral heterogeneity.

Recent advances in ctDNA technology have improved the sensitivity of ctDNA based assays. Targeted deep sequencing and droplet digital PCR (ddPCR) have the capability to detect high-frequency mutations in PDAC with mutant allele-frequencies (MAF) ≥0.1%, thereby greatly improving sensitivity [20, 21]. While targeted sequencing and ddPCR can rapidly and economically detect known mutations in ctDNA, these techniques are limited by requiring predefined gene mutations of interest, which are then amplified using prespecified sets of primers. Comprehensive genomic profiling (CGP) platforms also known as next-generation sequencing (NGS) platforms have been able to surmount these challenges since they have the capability to screen for unknown mutations, as well as structural and copy-number variations, which cannot be detected by PCR-based methods [22]. NGS technologies permit high-throughput analysis, whole genome sequencing and detection of somatic gene mutations at similar VAFs as those detectable with ddPCR [23, 24]. Additionally, CGP/NGS platforms permit characterization of tumor mutational burden (TMB) and microsatellite instability (MSI) using ctDNA, thus serving as a predictive tool for immune checkpoint inhibitor therapies [25, 26].

While ddPCR, and CGP/NGS improve upon the limitations of conventional PCR, neither of these platforms characterize epigenetic changes. Recent advances in high-throughput quantitative methylation assays now offer rapid and accurate identification of tumor DNA methylation using peripheral blood samples [27]. DNA methylation profiling has also demonstrated reliability in predicting tumor of origin in patients with cancer of unknown primary [28]. Recently, epigenome and ATAC-sequencing have been leveraged to simultaneously profile gene expression and open chromatin regions, and genome-scale DNA methylation (using reduced representation bisulfite sequencing; RBBS) [29, 30]. Additionally, isolation of cell-free methylated-DNA using immunoprecipitation coupled with NGS and PCR-based sequencing techniques can be used to improve specificity and reduce background noise [31]. In PDAC specifically, differential hydroxy methylation of genes related to pancreas development or function and cancer pathogenesis have been shown to reliably detect PDAC using peripheral blood samples. As with DNA sequencing techniques, the sensitivity and specificity of this method improves with more advanced cancer which in turn correlates with higher ctDNA fraction [32].

One notable drawback of NGS is that it is more expensive than ddPCR; however, the cost is decreasing dramatically and NGS is increasingly being utilized in routine clinical practice. NGS-based RNA sequencing of both tumor and peripheral blood using whole transcriptome sequencing platforms have also become commercially available, allowing for the identification of differentially expressed genes as well as identification of fusions, variant transcripts, and point mutations. Several commercial CGP/NGS liquid biopsy platforms are now being used to guide clinical decisions for individuals with PDAC and other solid tumors.

Exosomes

Exosomes are very small extracellular vesicles derived from various cells, including tumor cells, which contain proteins and genetic material that can be isolated and analyzed. Exosome release into circulation is not dependent on tumor cell destruction or CTCs moving into the vasculature [33]. Since the material is contained in vesicles, the genetic material also has a longer circulating half-life than ctDNA [34]. These factors present interesting potential for screening and early detection, but active research in PDAC is ongoing [35].

Additional Targets

Other potential liquid biopsy targets being explored in pancreatic cancer include RNA, platelets, and immune cells. Both mRNA and non-coding RNA are being investigated as targets; they have the advantage that they are released both actively and with apoptosis, so cell death is not required for their detection. Both immune cells and platelets are utilized by PDAC cells to evade destruction by the host immune system; changes in normal characteristics of these host cells can be targeted for cancer detection and monitoring.

Screening and Diagnosis

Screening and Early Detection

The US Preventative Task Force currently has no recommendations to routinely screening for PADC outside of high-risk populations. Individuals carrying high risk for developing pancreatic cancer in their lifetime include those with certain genetic predisposition syndromes or those with more than 1 first degree relative with PADC [36]. The inherited cancer syndromes with the highest risk of developing PDAC include Peutz-jeghers (STK11 gene), Familial Atypical Multiple Mole Melanoma syndrome (CDKN2A gene), and Hereditary pancreatitis (PRSS1, SPINK1 genes) [36, 37]. Other well-known genetic mutations such as BRCA2, BRCA1, and DNA mismatch repair genes are also associated with increased risk [37]. Current screening modalities include either yearly EUS or MRCP with variable age of onset of testing [38].

The use of ctDNA as a form of screening for PDAC in both average and high-risk populations is being actively investigated. A meta-analysis of seven protocols utilizing ctDNA as a screening test demonstrated a pooled sensitivity of on 0.64 [39]. Even though ctDNA can be released in the absence of cell destruction, it is thought that more advanced disease with tissue necrosis may be needed to reach adequate concentrations for detection [39]. Screening sensitivity seems to improve when ctDNA detection is combined with detection of other biomarkers such as CEA and CA-19-9, with early detection rates being 69% or better in difficult to detect cancers such as PDAC [40]. In addition to protein-based biomarkers, exosomes, nucleosomes, RNA, epigenetic evaluation, and autoantibodies are being evaluated to enhance ctDNA analysis.

A major barrier to utilizing ctDNA as a screening test remains the cost-prohibitive nature of sequencing all coding regions of DNA (as opposed to utilizing hotspot/panel based testing) [41]. The GRAIL Galleri test is an example of screening test currently being evaluated by a large clinical trial in the UK that does not utilize mutation detection but rather patterns of DNA methylation. With the ability to screen for over 50 different malignancies with one testing application, this could potentially circumvent major financial barriers overall. Another complicating factor is clonal hematopoiesis of indeterminate potential (CHIP), a process that becomes more prevalent with age with an occurrence of over 10% in individuals over seventy. Individuals with CHIP have a 0.5–1% probability of developing hematologic malignancy and interesting carry high mortality and have high incidence of solid tumor malignancy [42, 43]. These clonal hematopoietic cells create interference with ctDNA assays as they can release DNA fragments containing mutations associated with other malignancies [44]. There is currently no way to appropriately differentiate the source of ctDNA, which may lead to false positive results [44].

Diagnosis and Treatment

Liquid biopsy may be a useful, non-invasive, adjunct to diagnosis of PDAC when a solid pancreatic mass is noted on imaging. Current standard for diagnosis of localized PDAC includes cross-sectional imaging in combination with tissue biopsy—often via endoscopic ultrasound guided fine needle aspiration (EUS-FNA.) In a small study directly comparing CA 19-9, CTCs, and ctDNA to EUS-FNA in the setting of known pancreatic mass, ctDNA was comparable to standard biomarker CA 19-9 but failed to prove superior [45]. The sensitivity and specificity for PADC diagnosis were 73% and 88% for EUS-FNA, 67% and 80% for CTC, 65% and 75% for ctDNA, and 79% and 93% for CA19.9, respectively [45]. The low sensitivity associated with ctDNA is likely due to its lower concentration in patients with localized disease compared to metastatic PDAC.

Liquid biopsies utilizing ctDNA show even greater potential in diagnosis of actionable mutations, particularly in the metastatic setting. Tumors often display a high degree of spatiotemporal heterogeneity, and a tissue sample only allows for analysis of a limited population of cells [46]. Sampling ctDNA provides ability to address the spatiotemporal heterogeneity associated with tumors in a non-invasive fashion [47–49]. In a small study comparing tissue biopsy versus liquid biopsy for the detection of genomic alterations in head and neck squamous cell carcinoma, colorectal cancer, and melanoma, 79% of the mutations detected were unique to liquid biopsy and not seen in the tissue biopsy [50]. If mutations are missed with tissue-based genomic profiling— due to spatial heterogeneity—this could translate to missed opportunities for targeted therapies [46]. While there are limited targeted therapies approved for the treatment of PDAC, this will change in the coming years with improvements in precision medicine assays and therapeutics.

Liquid biopsies present a dynamic, non-invasive opportunity to assess for clonal evolution in response to therapeutic selection pressure [51]. There is scarcity of data in this sphere for pancreatic cancer; nonetheless, as assays and therapies evolve, liquid biopsies will likely capture clonal evolution and treatment resistance ahead of cross-sectional imaging. More importantly, such data may dictate precision therapeutics aimed to address evolving cancer clonality. Liquid biopsies offer the additional advantage that germline alterations can be picked up in addition to alterations in the somatic genome. Detection of some pathogenic germline alterations have treatment implications in addition to the transmissible heritable risk mandating screening of relevant family members.

Risk Stratification

Preoperative Setting

Multimodality therapy (chemotherapy, radiotherapy, and surgery) form the cornerstone of curative intent therapy for patients with localized PDAC. Despite aggressive multimodality therapy, systemic recurrence rates after surgery remain high [52, 53]. Since systemic failure due to presence of radiographically occult micro-metastatic disease at the time of surgery is high, risk stratification and optimal patient selection for a curative intent surgery—with potential for morbidity—is crucial.

Currently, CA 19-9—which is elevated in 70–80% of patients with localized PDAC—serves as a biomarker to predict resectability with elevated levels at diagnosis being associated higher likelihood of recurrence and development of metastatic disease [54]. Circulating tumor DNA has also been studied to predict prognosis in resectable PDAC prior to surgery. In one study, the detection of ctDNA prior to surgery by targeting mutations in *KRAS* predicted both decreased median recurrence free survival (RFS) (6 vs. 16 months; $p < 0.001$) and decreased overall survival (OS) (14 vs. 28 months; $p < 0.0001$) [55]. In another study, presence of ctDNA at time of diagnosis correlated with a relapse rate of 83% [56]. This rate of relapse appeared to be mitigated by the use of neoadjuvant chemotherapy if ctDNA was eliminated prior to surgery [56]. Number of ctDNA alterations and variant allelic fraction of ctDNA detected at diagnosis also seem to correlate with resectability [47].

Additionally, pathologic complete response (pCR) can sometimes be obtained with neoadjuvant chemotherapy or chemoradiation alone; however, a small study demonstrated that half of these patients with pCR after neoadjuvant therapy still had detectable ctDNA and CTCs [57].

Postoperative Setting

The ability to detect minimal residual disease (MRD) after curative intent therapy can provide useful information regarding the risk of relapse and possibly guide additional adjuvant therapy. Studies have looked at use of both CTCs and ctDNA to assess for MRD after curative intent multimodality therapy. It is intuitive that CTCs would decrease with systemic chemotherapy, but a decrease in CTCs is noted with surgery as well. Persistence of CTCs after curative intent therapy indicates a higher risk of relapse [58, 59]. Some CTCs undergo EMT and it has been reported that CTCs carrying mesenchymal markers indicate decreased survival [59].

The presence of ctDNA after surgery carries poor prognosis in PDAC and indicates the risk of relapse as high as 100% [56]. Detection of ctDNA or MRD after completion of curative intent therapy assumes even greater relevance if additional adjuvant therapy can result in cure. Such data are currently not available in PDAC, but more established in colorectal cancer (CRC) [60]. As liquid biopsy capabilities in PDAC become more refined, prospective trials to establish the role of perioperative systemic therapy guided by MRD status will be pivotal.

Surveillance

The use of various liquid biopsy techniques to enhance surveillance after completion of curative intent therapy is an area of active exploration. Currently, cross-sectional imaging remains the gold standard for surveillance after curative intent treatment, but small studies suggest that ctDNA can be detected in the blood several months prior to radiographic evidence of recurrence. In a surveillance study of patients with CRC, MRD was noted 16.5 months prior to radiologic evidence [60]. There is intuitive appeal to the idea that earlier pursuit of treatment in PDAC- based on MRD status when disease burden is arguably microscopic—may result in better long-term survival, but definitive data are not available in this realm.

Future Directions

Comprehensive genomic profiling based on tissue biopsies ushered in a new era of targeted therapies in oncology. Our recognition of the concepts of clonal evolution, spatiotemporal heterogeneity, and MRD mandate scalable, non-invasive techniques that can facilitate longitudinal monitoring of treatment response. Additionally, early detection and surveillance is a crucial component of our efforts to reduce cancer burden globally. Liquid biopsies—while still imperfect and in need of significant refinement—have all the requisite hallmarks to transform early detection, surveillance, and treatment of cancer. The next decade promises transformative changes in cancer care, leveraging enhanced liquid biopsy techniques, burgeoning bioinformatic/computational capabilities, and precision cancer therapeutics.

References

1. Vincent A, et al. Pancreatic cancer. Lancet. 2011;378(9791):607–20.
2. Siegel RL, Miller KD, Wagle NS, Jemal A. Cancer statistics, 2023. CA Cancer J Clin. 2023;73(1):17–48.
3. Villatoro S, et al. Prospective detection of mutations in cerebrospinal fluid, pleural effusion, and ascites of advanced cancer patients to guide treatment decisions. Mol Oncol. 2019;13(12):2633–45.

4. Yamaguchi Y, et al. Detection of mutations of p53 tumor suppressor gene in pancreatic juice and its application to diagnosis of patients with pancreatic cancer: comparison with K-ras mutation. Clin Cancer Res. 1999;5(5):1147–53.

5. McDonald DM, Baluk P. Significance of blood vessel leakiness in cancer. Cancer Res. 2002;62(18):5381–5.

6. Książkiewicz M, Markiewicz A, Zaczek AJ. Epithelial-mesenchymal transition: a hallmark in metastasis formation linking circulating tumor cells and cancer stem cells. Pathobiology. 2012;79(4):195–208.

7. Steinert G, et al. Immune escape and survival mechanisms in circulating tumor cells of colorectal cancer. Cancer Res. 2014;74(6):1694–704.

8. Cooke NM, et al. Aspirin and P2Y12 inhibition attenuate platelet-induced ovarian cancer cell invasion. BMC Cancer. 2015;15:627.

9. Samandari M, et al. Liquid biopsies for management of pancreatic cancer. Transl Res. 2018;201:98–127.

10. Hong Y, Fang F, Zhang Q. Circulating tumor cell clusters: what we know and what we expect (Review). Int J Oncol. 2016;49(6):2206–16.

11. Yu M, et al. Circulating breast tumor cells exhibit dynamic changes in epithelial and mesenchymal composition. Science. 2013;339(6119):580–4.

12. Kallergi G, et al. Evaluation of isolation methods for circulating tumor cells (CTCs). Cell Physiol Biochem. 2016;40(3-4):411–9.

13. Ozkumur E, et al. Inertial focusing for tumor antigen-dependent and -independent sorting of rare circulating tumor cells. Sci Transl Med. 2013;5(179):179ra47.

14. Yu J, et al. Pancreatic circulating tumor cell detection by targeted single-cell next-generation sequencing. Cancer Lett. 2020;493:245–53.

15. Lee JS, et al. Liquid biopsy in pancreatic ductal adenocarcinoma: current status of circulating tumor cells and circulating tumor DNA. Mol Oncol. 2019;13(8):1623–50.

16. Parpart-Li S, et al. The effect of preservative and temperature on the analysis of circulating tumor DNA. Clin Cancer Res. 2017;23(10):2471–7.

17. Underhill HR, et al. Fragment length of circulating tumor DNA. PLoS Genet. 2016;12(7):e1006162.

18. Diaz LA Jr, Bardelli A. Liquid biopsies: genotyping circulating tumor DNA. J Clin Oncol. 2014;32(6):579–86.

19. Parikh AR, et al. Liquid versus tissue biopsy for detecting acquired resistance and tumor heterogeneity in gastrointestinal cancers. Nat Med. 2019;25(9):1415–21.

20. Park G, et al. Utility of targeted deep sequencing for detecting circulating tumor DNA in pancreatic cancer patients. Sci Rep. 2018;8(1):11631.

21. Sugimori M, et al. Quantitative monitoring of circulating tumor DNA in patients with advanced pancreatic cancer undergoing chemotherapy. Cancer Sci. 2020;111(1):266–78.

22. Zill OA, et al. Cell-free DNA next-generation sequencing in pancreatobiliary carcinomas. Cancer Discov. 2015;5(10):1040–8.

23. Newman AM, et al. An ultrasensitive method for quantitating circulating tumor DNA with broad patient coverage. Nat Med. 2014;20(5):548–54.

24. Pécuchet N, et al. Analysis of base-position error rate of next-generation sequencing to detect tumor mutations in circulating DNA. Clin Chem. 2016;62(11):1492–503.

25. Dong J, et al. Advances in targeted therapy and immunotherapy for non-small cell lung cancer based on accurate molecular typing. Front Pharmacol. 2019;10:230.

26. Wang Z, et al. Assessment of blood tumor mutational burden as a potential biomarker for immunotherapy in patients with non-small cell lung cancer with use of a next-generation sequencing cancer gene panel. JAMA Oncol. 2019;5(5):696–702.

27. Eads CA, et al. MethyLight: a high-throughput assay to measure DNA methylation. Nucleic Acids Res. 2000;28(8):E32.

28. Moran S, et al. Epigenetic profiling to classify cancer of unknown primary: a multicentre, retrospective analysis. Lancet Oncol. 2016;17(10):1386–95.

29. Swanson E, et al. Simultaneous trimodal single-cell measurement of transcripts, epitopes, and chromatin accessibility using TEA-seq. Elife. 2021;10:e63632.
30. Xu W, et al. A plate-based single-cell ATAC-seq workflow for fast and robust profiling of chromatin accessibility. Nat Protoc. 2021;16(8):4084–107.
31. Shen SY, et al. Sensitive tumour detection and classification using plasma cell-free DNA methylomes. Nature. 2018;563(7732):579–83.
32. Guler GD, et al. Detection of early stage pancreatic cancer using 5-hydroxymethylcytosine signatures in circulating cell free DNA. Nat Commun. 2020;11(1):5270.
33. San Lucas FA, et al. Minimally invasive genomic and transcriptomic profiling of visceral cancers by next-generation sequencing of circulating exosomes. Ann Oncol. 2016;27(4):635–41.
34. Marrugo-Ramírez J, Mir M, Samitier J. Blood-based cancer biomarkers in liquid biopsy: a promising non-invasive alternative to tissue biopsy. Int J Mol Sci. 2018;19(10):2877.
35. Erb U, Zöller M. Progress and potential of exosome analysis for early pancreatic cancer detection. Expert Rev Mol Diagn. 2016;16(7):757–67.
36. Klein AP. Pancreatic cancer epidemiology: understanding the role of lifestyle and inherited risk factors. Nat Rev Gastroenterol Hepatol. 2021;18(7):493–502.
37. Goggins M, et al. Management of patients with increased risk for familial pancreatic cancer: updated recommendations from the International Cancer of the Pancreas Screening (CAPS) Consortium. Gut. 2020;69(1):7–17.
38. Canto MI, et al. Frequent detection of pancreatic lesions in asymptomatic high-risk individuals. Gastroenterology. 2012;142(4):796–804; quiz e14–5.
39. Zhu Y, et al. Diagnostic value of various liquid biopsy methods for pancreatic cancer: a systematic review and meta-analysis. Medicine (Baltimore). 2020;99(3):e18581.
40. Cohen JD, et al. Combined circulating tumor DNA and protein biomarker-based liquid biopsy for the earlier detection of pancreatic cancers. Proc Natl Acad Sci U S A. 2017;114(38):10202–7.
41. Campos-Carrillo A, et al. Circulating tumor DNA as an early cancer detection tool. Pharmacol Ther. 2020;207:107458.
42. Genovese G, et al. Clonal hematopoiesis and blood-cancer risk inferred from blood DNA sequence. N Engl J Med. 2014;371(26):2477–87.
43. Jaiswal S, et al. Age-related clonal hematopoiesis associated with adverse outcomes. N Engl J Med. 2014;371(26):2488–98.
44. Hu Y, et al. False-positive plasma genotyping due to clonal hematopoiesis. Clin Cancer Res. 2018;24(18):4437–43.
45. Sefrioui D, et al. Diagnostic value of CA19.9, circulating tumour DNA and circulating tumour cells in patients with solid pancreatic tumours. Br J Cancer. 2017;117(7):1017–25.
46. Gerlinger M, et al. Intratumor heterogeneity and branched evolution revealed by multiregion sequencing. N Engl J Med. 2012;366(10):883–92.
47. Patel H, et al. Clinical correlates of blood-derived circulating tumor DNA in pancreatic cancer. J Hematol Oncol. 2019;12(1):130.
48. Vietsch EE, van Eijck CH, Wellstein A. Circulating DNA and Micro-RNA in patients with pancreatic cancer. Pancreat Disord Ther. 2015;5(2):156.
49. Pishvaian MJ, et al. A pilot study evaluating concordance between blood-based and patient-matched tumor molecular testing within pancreatic cancer patients participating in the Know Your Tumor (KYT) initiative. Oncotarget. 2017;8(48):83446–56.
50. Liebs S, et al. Applicability of liquid biopsies to represent the mutational profile of tumor tissue from different cancer entities. Oncogene. 2021;40(33):5204–12.
51. Fisher R, Pusztai L, Swanton C. Cancer heterogeneity: implications for targeted therapeutics. Br J Cancer. 2013;108(3):479–85.
52. Dunne RF, Hezel AF. Genetics and biology of pancreatic ductal adenocarcinoma. Hematol Oncol Clin North Am. 2015;29(4):595–608.
53. Katz MH, et al. Long-term survival after multidisciplinary management of resected pancreatic adenocarcinoma. Ann Surg Oncol. 2009;16(4):836–47.

54. Ballehaninna UK, Chamberlain RS. The clinical utility of serum CA 19-9 in the diagnosis, prognosis and management of pancreatic adenocarcinoma: an evidence based appraisal. J Gastrointest Oncol. 2012;3(2):105–19.
55. Hadano N, et al. Prognostic value of circulating tumour DNA in patients undergoing curative resection for pancreatic cancer. Br J Cancer. 2016;115(1):59–65.
56. Lee B, et al. Circulating tumor DNA as a potential marker of adjuvant chemotherapy benefit following surgery for localized pancreatic cancer. Ann Oncol. 2019;30(9):1472–8.
57. Yin L, et al. Improved assessment of response status in patients with pancreatic cancer treated with neoadjuvant therapy using somatic mutations and liquid biopsy analysis. Clin Cancer Res. 2021;27(3):740–8.
58. Gemenetzis G, et al. Circulating tumor cells dynamics in pancreatic adenocarcinoma correlate with disease status: results of the prospective CLUSTER study. Ann Surg. 2018;268(3):408–20.
59. Poruk KE, et al. Circulating tumor cell phenotype predicts recurrence and survival in pancreatic adenocarcinoma. Ann Surg. 2016;264(6):1073–81.
60. Tie J, et al. Circulating tumor DNA analysis detects minimal residual disease and predicts recurrence in patients with stage II colon cancer. Sci Transl Med. 2016;8(346):346ra92.

Supportive Care Challenges and Management in Pancreatic Cancer

8

Jacqueline Tschanz, Ernai Hernadez Sanchez, and Shalini Dalal

Pancreatic cancer frequently presents at later stages, contributing to its poor prognosis. Patients often present with pain and/or jaundice once the tumor has progressed enough to obstruct or damage surrounding structures. Patients may also present with weight loss or gastrointestinal symptoms such as nausea, vomiting, or diarrhea. Symptom burden among these patients can lead to poor quality of life or functionality. Understanding and treating these symptoms can lead to improved quality of life and improved ability to tolerate cancer treatment.

Pain

Pain is an intricate symptom in pancreatic cancer patients, and its multifactorial characteristics make management challenging. In this chapter, we discuss the prevalence, pathophysiology, and different approaches to pain management in pancreatic cancer patients, including specific pharmacotherapy and non-invasive therapies.

Pain is highly prevalent in cancer patients. In health and symptom surveys from the Pancreatic Cancer Action Network, 93% of respondents cited pain as a symptom, and 83% rated the pain as moderate or severe [1]. Approximately 90% of patients cited having discussions with their doctors about their pain, yet half ended up in the emergency room with uncontrolled pain and about one-third were hospitalized for pain management [1]. Poorly managed pain has significant effects on other aspects of life. Pain has been associated with poor sleep, decreased caloric intake, and social or work-related functionality loss. Better pain control has shown to not only improvement these deficits but also shown to improve survivability [2]. Poor functionality or heavy symptom burden can preclude someone from various chemotherapy options and the potential to decrease the disease burden.

J. Tschanz · E. H. Sanchez · S. Dalal (✉)
Department of Palliative Care, MD Anderson Cancer Center, Houston, TX, USA
e-mail: sdalal@mdanderson.org

© The Author(s), under exclusive license to Springer Nature Switzerland AG 2023
S. Pant (ed.), *Pancreatic Cancer*, https://doi.org/10.1007/978-3-031-38623-7_8

Pathophysiology of Pain in Pancreatic Cancer

Pain in pancreatic cancer is multifactorial and complicated. There are two main mechanisms of pain in pancreatic cancer: pancreatic neuropathy and pancreatic duct obstruction [3]. Both these etiologies lead to further inflammation and worsened pain severity.

Neuropathic Pain

Nerve pain in pancreatic cancer can come from direct invasion from the cancer cells, mass effect, or cancer-driven nerve growth. Direct invasion and infiltration of the cancer cells can lead to inflammation [4], and 70% of all pancreatic tumors have been found to have malignant involvement of the sheaths around the axons [5]. Involvement can include intrapancreatic nerves or extrapancreatic nerve plexuses, i.e., celiac plexus. Mass effect or this perineural invasion can lead to an increase in inflammation and release of neurotransmitters, such as substance P and glutamate, which are possible sources of pain in this patient population [6]. Neuropathy in pancreatic cancer is associated with hypertrophy of the nerves as well [7]. Higher levels of nerve growth factor (NGF), which support the maintenance, growth, and proliferation of neurons, have been associated with increased pain intensity in pancreatic cancer [8].

Obstruction

Pancreatic cancer mass obstructs the main pancreatic duct, leading to its blockage and pain from upstream intraductal and interstitial pressures [9]. The obstruction affects the exocrine pancreas function, decreasing the secretion of the exocrine pancreatic enzymes, and thereby, furthering abdominal pain, particularly postprandial pain, and malabsorption can occur [10]. Relief of pain has been demonstrated in studies with pancreatic ductal stenting which lowers the interstitial pressure [11, 12]. In addition, the replacement of enzymes in pancreatic insufficiency and malabsorption from other conditions have also demonstrated improvements in abdominal pain [13–15].

Pain Management

Pain management in pancreatic cancer can be broadly divided into conventional and non-conventional approaches (Table 8.1). Conventional options include pharmacological therapies such as non-opioid and opioid medications and non-pharmacological therapies such as radiation-focused and non-radiation-focused therapies. Non-conventional approaches refer to integrative therapies.

Table 8.1 Pain management approaches in pancreatic cancer

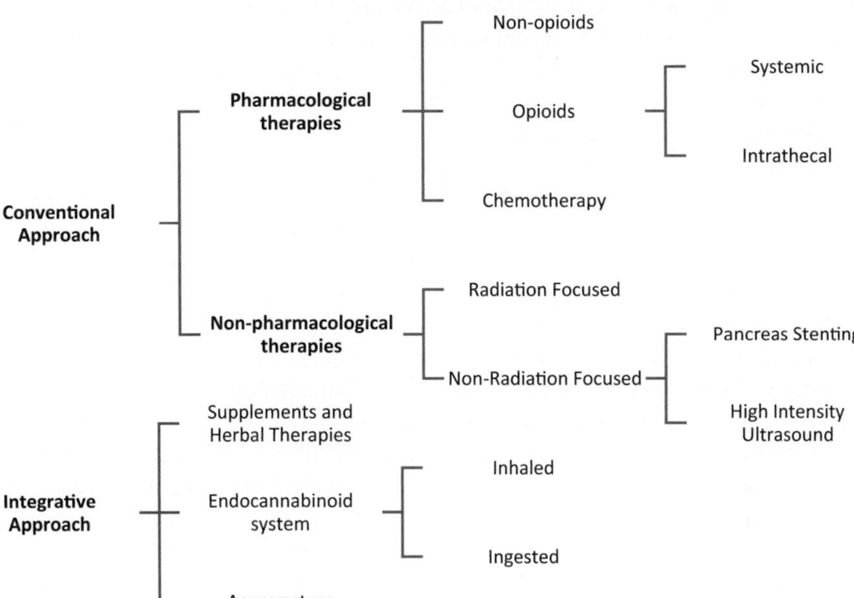

Pharmacological Therapies

Non-opioids

Nonsteroidal Anti-Inflammatory Medications and Acetaminophen

The vast majority of patients will attempt to treat pain with over-the-counter medications such as nonsteroidal anti-inflammatory medications (NSAIDs) or acetaminophen. There are more than 20 different NSAIDs produced worldwide. They work by decreasing inflammation by blocking cyclooxygenase and thereby decreasing prostaglandins, prostacyclins, and thromboxane [16]. Acetaminophen (also known as N-acetyl-p-aminophenol, APAP, or paracetamol) has an unknown mechanism of action. It may work within the central nervous system to activate serotonergic inhibitory pathways [17]. Both treat mild to moderate pain and have concerning toxicities with long-term or high dose use. There is a concern for liver damage in using high doses of acetaminophen. Its metabolites deplete glutathione and damage liver mitochondria leading to cell death. NSAIDs are associated with damage to the gastric mucosa, ulcer formation, and kidney damage.

Opioids

Opioids remain the mainstay of care for treating pain in pancreatic cancer. This class of analgesics works on the mu-receptors in central and peripheral nervous systems. Most opioids are pure mu-receptor agonists; however, some act on other receptors. Methadone and levorphanol also exhibit N-methyl-D-aspartate receptor antagonism, and tramadol, tapentadol, methadone, and levorphanol have been shown to inhibit monoamine reuptake as well [18]. Buprenorphine is a partial mu-receptor agonist and needs further research in cancer pain [19].

The goal of opioid therapy is to maximize the functionality of patients while minimizing medication side effects. A general approach to initiating treatment is to start with an immediate release (IR) opioid on an as needed basis for moderate to severe pain. If patients require frequent dosing, they will benefit from the addition of extended-release (ER) opioids to provide more consistent plasma levels of the drug [20]. Patients are continued on their IR opioid for breakthrough pain at a dose of 10–20% of their ER medication [20].

Opioid side effects include constipation, sedation, pruritus, opioid-induced neurotoxicity (OIN), and respiratory depression. Constipation occurs secondary to increase gastric tone and decreased peristalsis and secretion. This side effect should be managed prophylactically to avoid progressive severity of symptoms such as worsening abdominal pain, nausea, and anorexia, which may already be present in patients due to their pancreatic cancer. OIN symptoms include delirium, hallucinations, sedation, cognitive impairment, myoclonus, and hyperalgesia. If present, opioids may need to be decreased or rotated to another [21]. In general, use of concomitant sedating medications such as benzodiazepines, gabapentin, or anticholinergics should be avoided to decrease the potential of OIN with opioids.

Non-medical opioid use (NMOU) is the use of prescribed opioids in ways that were not directed, such as using opioids outside of personal prescription or use of opioids for indications other than pain. Opioids are potentially abusable drugs. Recent literature suggests that approximately 20% of cancer patients exhibit some level of NMOU [22]. Universal screening for NMOU risk is recommended for all patients initiated on opioids, with periodic monitoring during the course of opioid therapy [23]. Patients need to be screened for risk factors, including personal or family history of substance abuse or mental health disorders [24, 25]. Continued monitoring for aberrant behaviors such as early refill requests, doctor shopping, urine drug screening, and inconsistent prescription drug monitoring programs data are essential [22, 23]. Patients who are at high risk for NMOU may require more frequent monitoring with shorter follow-up intervals, periodic urine drug testing, and review of prescription drug monitoring programs, and we recommend referral to pain management specialists [23]. Naloxone nasal sprays or injectables should be prescribed to patients. Their families and caregivers should be educated on signs of overdose such as excessive sedation and decreased respiratory drive and how to appropriately deliver the medication.

Intrathecal Drug Delivery

Intrathecal drug delivery systems (IDDSs) consist of a pump placed under the skin with a tunneled catheter directly into the intrathecal space by the spinal cord. The medication used is generally an opioid analgesic, and patients can immediately note improvement in the pain. The advantage of this delivery is the reduction in pain using opioid doses that are substantially lower than what is needed with peripheral or oral administration and thus fewer side effects. Patients can have other medications added for further benefits, such as muscle relaxants or anesthetics agents. Patients can achieve significant and prolonged control of the pain. Complications are generally mild with post-procedure headaches, but patients can also get an implant infection or dehiscence of procedure wounds [26, 27].

An observational study designed to evaluate the 11-year results (2006–2017) of IDDSs for refractory pancreas cancer pain [28] demonstrated 50–75% reductions in mean pain levels [26]. In a 2002 randomized controlled trial of IDDS versus comprehensive medical management (CMM) in 146 evaluable cancer patients with refractory pain at 4 weeks, pain control was shown to be superior in the IDDS arm with fewer opioid-induced side effects [29].

Chemotherapy

Improvement of pain is a frequently studied outcome of systemic chemotherapy, and the management of pancreatic cancer can also improve both pain and patients' quality of life. Significant pain improvement has been found in studies of both first-line and second-line chemotherapy [30–32].

Non-pharmacological Therapies

Radiation Focused

Radiation therapy is a non-invasive intervention to treat tumors and has been found to reduce pain significantly. This likely improves pain by either alleviating the obstruction of the pancreatic ducts, decreasing the perineural invasion, or decreasing the tumor mass. Patients are generally treated with 6–30 Gy in 1–10 fractions. Response rates vary by fractions and study but have improved pain in 60–100% of patients [33, 34]. A strategy called stereotactic body radiation therapy can be used to limit the amount of radiation the surrounding organs receive. Due to the unique position of the pancreas in relation to other organs, the beam of radiation will meet the body at different angles to continue to treat the tumor with decreased time penetrating elsewhere and thus less damage to the other vital organs [35]. A recent systematic review has shown that between 16.5 Gy and 45 Gy in one to six fractions resulted in pain response rates of over 80%, with 54% of patients reporting complete pain resolution [36]. The study also showed a significant reduction in nausea, fatigue, weight loss, and anorexia.

Non-radiation Focused

Stenting of Pancreas

The obstruction of the ducts can also be mechanically unobstructed. Stenting of the ducts has been found to decrease pain since it will decrease both the upstream and interstitial pressures [12, 37].

High-Intensity Ultrasound

Ultrasound can be used as part of another noninvasive way to ablate and disrupt targeted tissue [38]. This procedure is being used for various solid tumors, pancreatic cancer included [39]. The heat can cause a rapid temperature increase in a small volume in tumors to induce necrosis and cavitation of the tumor. This necrosis can further damage outward to a larger volume due to mechanical damage from the cavitation pressures and gas formation. Aside from treating cancer at the tumor site, the procedure has been shown to decrease pain as well [40], likely from a decrease in mass tumor effect or possibly acting directly on nerve fibers in the tumor and celiac plexus.

Neurolytic Procedures

Patients can also have improved pain from neurolytic procedures that involve application of chemical agents to result in a permanent or temporary degeneration of targeted nerve fibers to interrupt neuronal transmission. Celiac plexus neurolysis (CPN) and thoracoscopic splanchnicectomy (TS) are invasive neurolytic procedures that may improve pain and/or decrease the need for opioids in managing pain related to an upper abdominal malignancy, such as pancreatic cancer. Recent studies support the use and efficacy of neurolytic procedures early in the management of pain, such as after one or two trials of opioid therapy have been inadequate for pain control. The neurolytic injectate is usually 50–100% ethyl alcohol. For CPN, several techniques may be used to approach the celiac plexus, such as percutaneous (aided by fluoroscopy or computed tomographic imaging), surgical placement, or endoscopic ultrasound. Several CPN studies have demonstrated significant improvements in pain at 2, 4, or 8 weeks [41, 42], and in some studies, this was associated with lower opioid usage [43]. The 2011 Cochrane review (six RCTs, published 1993–2008) [44] demonstrated significantly lower pain scores at 4 weeks (-0.43; 95% confidence interval [CI], -0.73, -0.14; $p = 0.004$], with a trend toward lower pain at 8 weeks (-0.44; 95% CI, -0.89, -0.23; $p = 0.06$]. In subsequent reviews by Nagels et al. (2013, five RCTs) and Zhong et al. (2014, eight RCTs), statistical improvements in pain scores with CPN were found at 4 but not at 8 weeks [45, 46]. Thus, current evidence suggests that percutaneous CPN improves pain scores at 4 weeks, which may not be sustained over time. However, all three meta-analyses demonstrated significant reductions in opioid consumption at 4 and 8 weeks or last report.

Integrative Therapies

A substantial number of patients with pancreatic cancer do not achieve satisfactory relief with first-line pharmacotherapy and noninvasive second-line therapies. This common scenario may be addressed in many ways with the following non-conventional therapies.

Supplementation and Herbal Therapies

Patients commonly supplement their prescribed medical therapies with over-the-counter herbal remedies [47]. Many of these herbal medicines or nutraceuticals lack evidence-based support for significant improvement of pain or other symptoms. Some have been shown to cause organ damage or interact with medications or chemotherapy by increasing toxicities or decreasing efficacy [48, 49]. The safest recommendation for patients is thus to discontinue use while receiving treatment.

Cannabinoids

Cannabinoids act on central and peripheral nervous systems. Receptors have been found to act on the gastrointestinal tract, immune system, and more directly nerves and the brain [50, 51]. Endocannabinoids, endogenous cannabinoids, affect metabolism through these receptors. The drug has historically been inhaled or orally ingested.

Medical marijuana has been becoming increasingly available to patients. As of 2022, 37 states allow the legal use of medical marijuana. Cannabis has been touted as treating diverse problems, including pain, nausea, loss of appetite, inflammation, poor mood, and even seizures [52]. There are synthetic forms of THC that have been approved to treat nausea and vomiting, but limited data support its use in analgesia.

Acupuncture

Acupuncture is a nonpharmacologic intervention consisting of small, thin needles placed in specific areas known as "meridian points" that are thought to more specifically affect neurotransmitter release [53]. Data has been mixed; studies that show significant pain relief have shown the onset of analgesia after about a day and can last for days [54]. Patients interested in this intervention should be referred to the appropriate specialist.

References

1. Westermann MLA, Rahib L. The need for improvement in the management of fatigue, depression and pain in pancreatic cancer. J Clin Oncol. 2019;37(suppl 4):429.
2. Hameed M, Hameed H, Erdek M. Pain management in pancreatic cancer. Cancers (Basel). 2010;3:43–60.

3. Coveler AL, Mizrahi J, Eastman B, Apisarnthanarax SJ, Dalal S, McNearney T, Pant S, Precision Promise C. Pancreas cancer-associated pain management. Oncologist. 2021;26:e971–82.

4. Demir IE, Schorn S, Schremmer-Danninger E, Wang K, Kehl T, Giese NA, Algul H, Friess H, Ceyhan GO. Perineural mast cells are specifically enriched in pancreatic neuritis and neuropathic pain in pancreatic cancer and chronic pancreatitis. PLoS One. 2013;8:e60529.

5. Yi SQ, Miwa K, Ohta T, Kayahara M, Kitagawa H, Tanaka A, Shimokawa T, Akita K, Tanaka S. Innervation of the pancreas from the perspective of perineural invasion of pancreatic cancer. Pancreas. 2003;27:225–9.

6. Barreto SG, Saccone GT. Pancreatic nociception—revisiting the physiology and pathophysiology. Pancreatology. 2012;12:104–12.

7. Ceyhan GO, Bergmann F, Kadihasanoglu M, Altintas B, Demir IE, Hinz U, Muller MW, Giese T, Buchler MW, Giese NA, Friess H. Pancreatic neuropathy and neuropathic pain—a comprehensive pathomorphological study of 546 cases. Gastroenterology. 2009;136:177–186 e1.

8. Zhu Z, Kleeff J, Kayed H, Wang L, Korc M, Buchler MW, Friess H. Nerve growth factor and enhancement of proliferation, invasion, and tumorigenicity of pancreatic cancer cells. Mol Carcinog. 2002;35:138–47.

9. Koulouris AI, Banim P, Hart AR. Pain in patients with pancreatic cancer: prevalence, mechanisms, management and future developments. Dig Dis Sci. 2017;62:861–70.

10. Warshaw AL, Banks PA, Fernandez-Del Castillo C. AGA technical review: treatment of pain in chronic pancreatitis. Gastroenterology. 1998;115:765–76.

11. Costamagna G, Alevras P, Palladino F, Rainoldi F, Mutignani M, Morganti A. Endoscopic pancreatic stenting in pancreatic cancer. Can J Gastroenterol. 1999;13:481–7.

12. Wehrmann T, Riphaus A, Frenz MB, Martchenko K, Stergiou N. Endoscopic pancreatic duct stenting for relief of pancreatic cancer pain. Eur J Gastroenterol Hepatol. 2005;17:1395–400.

13. Whitcomb DC, Lehman GA, Vasileva G, Malecka-Panas E, Gubergrits N, Shen Y, Sander-Struckmeier S, Caras S. Pancrelipase delayed-release capsules (CREON) for exocrine pancreatic insufficiency due to chronic pancreatitis or pancreatic surgery: a double-blind randomized trial. Am J Gastroenterol. 2010;105:2276–86.

14. Trapnell BC, Maguiness K, Graff GR, Boyd D, Beckmann K, Caras S. Efficacy and safety of Creon 24,000 in subjects with exocrine pancreatic insufficiency due to cystic fibrosis. J Cyst Fibros. 2009;8:370–7.

15. Gubergrits N, Malecka-Panas E, Lehman GA, Vasileva G, Shen Y, Sander-Struckmeier S, Caras S, Whitcomb DC. A 6-month, open-label clinical trial of pancrelipase delayed-release capsules (Creon) in patients with exocrine pancreatic insufficiency due to chronic pancreatitis or pancreatic surgery. Aliment Pharmacol Ther. 2011;33:1152–61.

16. Vane JR. Inhibition of prostaglandin synthesis as a mechanism of action for aspirin-like drugs. Nat New Biol. 1971;231:232–5.

17. Smith HS. Potential analgesic mechanisms of acetaminophen. Pain Physician. 2009;12:269–80.

18. Morrone LA, Scuteri D, Rombola L, Mizoguchi H, Bagetta G. Opioids resistance in chronic pain management. Curr Neuropharmacol. 2017;15:444–56.

19. Schmidt-Hansen M, Bromham N, Taubert M, Arnold S, Hilgart JS. Buprenorphine for treating cancer pain. Cochrane Database Syst Rev. 2015;2018:CD009596.

20. Perez-Hernandez C, Blasco A, Gandara A, Manas A, Rodriguez-Lopez MJ, Martinez V, Fernandez-Nistal A, Montoto C. Prevalence and characterization of breakthrough pain in patients with cancer in Spain: the CARPE-DIO study. Sci Rep. 2019;9:17701.

21. Nersesyan H, Slavin KV. Current aproach to cancer pain management: availability and implications of different treatment options. Ther Clin Risk Manag. 2007;3:381–400.

22. Carmichael AN, Morgan L, Del Fabbro E. Identifying and assessing the risk of opioid abuse in patients with cancer: an integrative review. Subst Abus Rehabil. 2016;7:71–9.

23. Dalal S, Bruera E. Pain management for patients with advanced cancer in the opioid epidemic era. Am Soc Clin Oncol Educ Book. 2019;39:24–35.

24. Turk DC, Swanson KS, Gatchel RJ. Predicting opioid misuse by chronic pain patients: a systematic review and literature synthesis. Clin J Pain. 2008;24:497–508.

25. Edlund MJ, Martin BC, Fan MY, Devries A, Braden JB, Sullivan MD. Risks for opioid abuse and dependence among recipients of chronic opioid therapy: results from the TROUP study. Drug Alcohol Depend. 2010;112:90–8.
26. Carvajal G, Dupoiron D, Seegers V, Lebrec N, Bore F, Dubois PY, Leblanc D, Delorme T, Jubier-Hamon S. Intrathecal drug delivery systems for refractory pancreatic cancer pain: observational follow-up study over an 11-year period in a comprehensive cancer center. Anesth Analg. 2018;126:2038–46.
27. Dupoiron D. Intrathecal therapy for pain in cancer patients. Curr Opin Support Palliat Care. 2019;13:75–80.
28. Dupoiron D, Leblanc D, Demelliez-Merceron S, Bore F, Seegers V, Dubois PY, Pechard M, Robard S, Delorme T, Jubier-Hamon S, Carvajal G, Lebrec N. Optimizing initial intrathecal drug ratio for refractory cancer-related pain for early pain relief. A retrospective monocentric study. Pain Med. 2019;20:2033–42.
29. Smith TJ, Staats PS, Deer T, Stearns LJ, Rauck RL, Boortz-Marx RL, Buchser E, Catala E, Bryce DA, Coyne PJ, Pool GE, et al. Implantable drug delivery systems study, randomized clinical trial of an implantable drug delivery system compared with comprehensive medical management for refractory cancer pain: impact on pain, drug-related toxicity, and survival. J Clin Oncol. 2002;20:4040–9.
30. Wang-Gillam A, Li CP, Bodoky G, Dean A, Shan YS, Jameson G, Macarulla T, Lee KH, Cunningham D, Blanc JF, Hubner RA, Chiu CF, Schwartsmann G, Siveke JT, Braiteh F, Moyo V, Belanger B, Dhindsa N, Bayever E, Von Hoff DD, Chen LT, N.-S. Group. Nanoliposomal irinotecan with fluorouracil and folinic acid in metastatic pancreatic cancer after previous gemcitabine-based therapy (NAPOLI-1): a global, randomised, open-label, phase 3 trial. Lancet. 2016;387:545–57.
31. Gourgou-Bourgade S, Bascoul-Mollevi C, Desseigne F, Ychou M, Bouche O, Guimbaud R, Becouarn Y, Adenis A, Raoul JL, Boige V, Berille J, Conroy T. Impact of FOLFIRINOX compared with gemcitabine on quality of life in patients with metastatic pancreatic cancer: results from the PRODIGE 4/ACCORD 11 randomized trial. J Clin Oncol. 2013;31:23–9.
32. Burris HA 3rd, Moore MJ, Andersen J, Green MR, Rothenberg ML, Modiano MR, Cripps MC, Portenoy RK, Storniolo AM, Tarassoff P, Nelson R, Dorr FA, Stephens CD, Von Hoff DD. Improvements in survival and clinical benefit with gemcitabine as first-line therapy for patients with advanced pancreas cancer: a randomized trial. J Clin Oncol. 1997;15:2403–13.
33. Morganti AG, Trodella L, Valentini V, Barbi S, Macchia G, Mantini G, Turriziani A, Cellini N. Pain relief with short-term irradiation in locally advanced carcinoma of the pancreas. J Palliat Care. 2003;19:258–62.
34. Ebrahimi G, Rasch CRN, van Tienhoven G. Pain relief after a short course of palliative radiotherapy in pancreatic cancer, the Academic Medical Center (AMC) experience. Acta Oncol. 2018;57:697–700.
35. Ryan JF, Rosati LM, Groot VP, Le DT, Zheng L, Laheru DA, Shin EJ, Jackson J, Moore J, Narang AK, Herman JM. Stereotactic body radiation therapy for palliative management of pancreatic adenocarcinoma in elderly and medically inoperable patients. Oncotarget. 2018;9:16427–36.
36. Buwenge M, Macchia G, Arcelli A, Frakulli R, Fuccio L, Guerri S, Grassi E, Cammelli S, Cellini F, Morganti AG. Stereotactic radiotherapy of pancreatic cancer: a systematic review on pain relief. J Pain Res. 2018;11:2169–78.
37. Costamagna G, Pandolfi M. Endoscopic stenting for biliary and pancreatic malignancies. J Clin Gastroenterol. 2004;38:59–67.
38. Maloney E, Hwang JH. Emerging HIFU applications in cancer therapy. Int J Hyperth. 2015;31:302–9.
39. Zhou Y. High-intensity focused ultrasound treatment for advanced pancreatic cancer. Gastroenterol Res Pract. 2014;2014:205325.
40. Xiong LL, Hwang JH, Huang XB, Yao SS, He CJ, Ge XH, Ge HY, Wang XF. Early clinical experience using high intensity focused ultrasound for palliation of inoperable pancreatic cancer. JOP. 2009;10:123–9.

41. Zhang CL, Zhang TJ, Guo YN, Yang LQ, He MW, Shi JZ, Ni JX. Effect of neurolytic celiac plexus block guided by computerized tomography on pancreatic cancer pain. Dig Dis Sci. 2008;53:856–60.
42. Wong GY, Schroeder DR, Carns PE, Wilson JL, Martin DP, Kinney MO, Mantilla CB, Warner DO. Effect of neurolytic celiac plexus block on pain relief, quality of life, and survival in patients with unresectable pancreatic cancer: a randomized controlled trial. JAMA. 2004;291:1092–9.
43. Mercadante S. Celiac plexus block versus analgesics in pancreatic cancer pain. Pain. 1993;52:187–92.
44. Arcidiacono PG, Calori G, Carrara S, McNicol ED, Testoni PA. Celiac plexus block for pancreatic cancer pain in adults. Cochrane Database Syst Rev. 2011;2019:CD007519.
45. Nagels W, Pease N, Bekkering G, Cools F, Dobbels P. Celiac plexus neurolysis for abdominal cancer pain: a systematic review. Pain Med. 2013;14:1140–63.
46. Zhong W, Yu Z, Zeng JX, Lin Y, Yu T, Min XH, Yuan YH, Chen QK. Celiac plexus block for treatment of pain associated with pancreatic cancer: a meta-analysis. Pain Pract. 2014;14:43–51.
47. Cornman-Homonoff J, Holzwanger DJ, Lee KS, Madoff DC, Li D. Celiac plexus block and neurolysis in the management of chronic upper abdominal pain. Semin Intervent Radiol. 2017;34:376–86.
48. Zhou X, Li CG, Chang D, Bensoussan A. Current status and major challenges to the safety and efficacy presented by Chinese herbal medicine. Medicines (Basel). 2019;6:14.
49. Jermini M, Dubois J, Rodondi PY, Zaman K, Buclin T, Csajka C, Orcurto A, et al. Complementary medicine use during cancer treatment and potential herb-drug interactions from a cross-sectional study in an academic Centre. Sci Rep. 2019;9:5078.
50. Guindon J, Hohmann AG. The endocannabinoid system and pain. CNS Neurol Disord Drug Targets. 2009;8:403–21.
51. Starowicz FDK. Cannabinoids and pain: sites and mechanisms of action. New York: Elsevier; 2017.
52. Abrams DI. Integrating cannabis into clinical cancer care. Curr Oncol. 2016;23:S8–S14.
53. Lau CHY, Wu X, Chung VCH, Liu X, Hui EP, Cramer H, Lauche R, Wong SYS, Lau AYL, Sit RWS, Ziea ETC, Ng BFL, Wu JCY. Acupuncture and related therapies for symptom management in palliative cancer care: systematic review and meta-analysis. Medicine (Baltimore). 2016;95:e2901.
54. Lee IS, Cheon S, Park JY. Central and peripheral mechanism of acupuncture analgesia on visceral pain: a systematic review. Evid Based Complement Alternat Med. 2019;2019:1304152.

Physical Activity and Nutrition Optimization in Pancreatic Cancer

9

Maria Q. B. Petzel, Chelsea S. Ebrus, Jessica Tse Cheng, Nathan Parker, and An Ngo-Huang

Chapter Introduction

Physical activity and nutritional optimization have largely become incorporated into the clinical management of patients with pancreatic cancer (PC). Patients with PC are at risk of malnutrition, weight loss, muscle loss in cachexia or sarcopenia, and declines in physical function. Historically, oncology clinicians advised patients with cancer to avoid exercise; however, this approach has changed. Exercise is deemed safe and well-tolerated during and after cancer treatment. Exercise has been found to improve physical fitness, physical functioning, quality of life, and fatigue.

M. Q. B. Petzel
Department of Surgical Oncology, The University of Texas MD Anderson Cancer Center, Houston, TX, USA

Department of Clinical Nutrition, The University of Texas MD Anderson Cancer Center, Houston, TX, USA
e-mail: mpetzel@mdanderson.org

C. S. Ebrus
Department of Clinical Nutrition, The University of Texas MD Anderson Cancer Center, Houston, TX, USA
e-mail: csebrus@mdanderson.org

J. T. Cheng
Department of Supportive Care Medicine, City of Hope Orange County Lennar Foundation Cancer Center, Irvine, CA, USA
e-mail: jescheng@coh.org

N. Parker
Department of Health Outcomes and Behavior, Moffitt Cancer Center, Tampa, FL, USA
e-mail: nathan.parker@moffitt.org

A. Ngo-Huang (⊠)
Department of Palliative, Rehabilitation, and Integrative Medicine, The University of Texas MD Anderson Cancer Center, Houston, TX, USA
e-mail: ango2@mdanderson.org

Furthermore, individualized nutrition intervention improves multiple domains including improved weight, muscle mass, quality of life, and fatigue.

Physical Activity Trends and Outcomes

Physical activity includes all bodily movement by the musculoskeletal system that requires energy expenditure and ranges between leisure activity to moderate to vigorous physical activity. A targeted exercise program comprising of aerobic exercise and resistance (strengthening) exercise is recommended for cancer patients. By 2018, randomized controlled exercise trials in cancer survivors burgeoned with multiple national efforts calling for further incorporation of exercise into clinical cancer care [1–3]. The American College of Sports Medicine (ACSM) convened at the International Multidisciplinary Roundtable to update the Exercise Guidelines for Cancer Survivors [4]. The exercise recommendation is for moderate-intensity aerobic exercise for 30 min at least three times per week for 8–12 weeks and resistance exercises twice a week using at least two sets of 8–15 repetitions at 60% or more of one repetition maximum. Further included were exercise programming considerations for specific cancer survivors such as those with bone loss/bone metastases, older adults, ostomy, peripheral neuropathy, and symptom clusters. Additional patient benefits identified with exercise included reduced anxiety and fewer depressive symptoms [4]. A systematic review in 2021 evaluating home-based and supervised aerobic and resistance exercise trials including early-stage and advanced pancreatic cancer showed exercise interventions were associated with improvements in cancer-related fatigue, physical function, and psychological distress [5].

Preoperative exercise, a part of prehabilitation, is an increasingly adopted strategy to optimize physical function and treatment tolerance in anticipation of surgery. There is increasing interest in the benefits of multimodal prehabilitation programs for cancer patients. A recent systematic review and meta-analysis by Daniels et al. comprehensively evaluated prehabilitation interventions in elective abdominal cancer surgery in older patients including 33 studies with 3962 patients total, a minority of which had pancreatic cancer [6]. The interventions included exercise, nutrition, psychological input, comprehensive geriatric assessment and optimization, smoking cessation, and multimodal interventions. All multimodal studies included exercise and at least one other intervention. A meta-analysis of 10 studies showed that multimodal intervention programs had significant benefit with a risk difference of −0.1 (95% CI -0.18 to −0.02; $P = 0.01$, $I^2 = 18\%$) for overall complications. Authors found that exercise interventions can improve the cardiopulmonary exercise test and 6-min walk test (6MWT) preoperatively. Adherence for the majority of the studies was high. Overall, evidence shows that multimodal prehabilitation is likely more beneficial than a single intervention [6].

Exercise prehabilitation for PC patients, who are often elderly, frail, and sarcopenic, can improve physical function. Ngo-Huang et al. conducted a prospective single-arm trial with 50 participants (mean age 66 years) with resectable pancreatic adenocarcinoma (PDAC) receiving preoperative chemotherapy or chemoradiation [7]. To establish feasibility of exercise, patients were advised to participate in at least

60 min per week of moderate intensity aerobic exercise (e.g., brisk walking, elliptical, stationary bicycles) and 60 min per week of full body strengthening exercise divided into two separate sessions. Study staff demonstrated all strengthening exercise in person and called participants at least once every 2 weeks to encourage adherence and to monitor for adverse events. Participants completed daily exercise logs and wore accelerometers to track their physical activity. Moreover, individualized dietary counseling emphasizing high protein intake was provided to all participants. Patients, on average, met the ACSM guidelines for aerobic exercise with mean accelerometer-measured physical activity of 158.7 ± 146.7 min per week of moderate-to-vigorous physical activity. They had significant improvement in the 6MWT and 5 times sit-to-stand (5xSTS) during the preoperative period, and this was associated with improved quality of life. This result is especially remarkable because the improvement in physical function was clinically meaningful during a period where decline in physical function is common [8]. The 6MWT has been associated with intraoperative and postoperative complications [9–11], length of stay [12], and functional recovery [13]. The 5xSTS has been associated with activities of daily living and disability and is a predictor of falls [14]. Concordant with guidelines to avoid inactivity, increased light physical activity on accelerometry was associated with improved health-related quality of life, while sedentary activity was associated with decreased quality of life [7]. Physical activity motivators included interpersonal and environmental factors, particularly social support from friends and neighborhood aesthetics. Additional motivators included desire to complete and recover from treatment and support and accountability from healthcare providers [15].

Pre-clinical animal studies have demonstrated some of the positive effects of exercise in delaying PC growth; however, the underlying mechanisms of these effects are unclear [16]. For instance, there is evidence that exercise for PC patients directly impacts tumor biology by modifying tumor vascularity. Schadler et al. used mouse models to show that moderate aerobic exercise-induced shear stress led to a tumor vessel remodeling, normalizing effect that allowed for improved chemotherapy delivery [17]. When exercise was used in addition to chemotherapy, there was a significant decrease in tumor growth. The same group of researchers then compared tumor biology of historical control patients who did not receive an exercise intervention to a group of patients who participated in the prehabilitation exercise trial [7]. The exercise prehabilitation group showed differences in tumor vasculature including significantly higher microvessel density and more elongated blood vessels [18].

Exercise rehabilitation postoperatively, during adjuvant therapy, and in survivorship for PC patients can be similarly beneficial. Postoperatively, even progressive mobilization on the same day of surgery compared to the day after surgery showed benefit in oxygenation [19]. A randomized-controlled study of postoperative home-based resistance training for 3 months improved sleep and fatigue in patients with PC [20]. A systematic review of exercise for patients with PC found that during adjuvant treatment, exercise is safe and effective in mitigating impaired physical function, quality of life, and fatigue [21]. In survivorship, although 70% of PC survivors are willing to participate in diet and exercise interventions [22], less than 25% of patients after resection for PC met exercise guidelines [23], highlighting a wide gap in physical activity, with patients potentially missing the beneficial effects.

Physical Activity and Body Composition

The negative impacts of cancer and cancer therapies extend to body composition—patients who receive multimodal cancer treatments tend to lose muscle. Skeletal muscle loss, particularly in the context of excess adiposity, is associated with worse treatment and survivorship outcomes across the spectrum of cancer diagnoses. Patients diagnosed with PC tend to be older, and they frequently present with muscle loss attributable to older age, physical inactivity, or a combination of these factors, defined as sarcopenia. A recent review found rates of sarcopenia ranging from 21% to 65% in patients with PC [24]. Additionally, these patients may have cachexia, which is defined as loss of muscle concurrently with adipose tissue depletion as part of general weight loss and tissue wasting. Cachexia is particularly common among individuals diagnosed with PC, with prevalence extending across PC stages and treatment regimens. Cachexia occurs from a variety of factors: reduced food intake, elevated energy expenditure from tumor metabolism, excess catabolism, and overall inflammation [25]. An estimated 80% of patients with PC are cachectic, and 30% of PC deaths are due to cachexia alone [26].

To date, several studies have enumerated changes in body composition that occur throughout the PC treatment continuum. In a recent study among patients with borderline resectable and locally advanced tumors who underwent neoadjuvant chemotherapy and/or chemoradiation therapy prior to surgical exploration, there was significant fat loss and a significant minimal increase in skeletal muscle mass in ones who were underwent surgical resection versus ones who did not have surgery [27]. Even for patients receiving curative treatment, body weight, body fat, and skeletal muscle mass are significantly lower 3 months after surgical resection, as patients cope with nutritional challenges along with reduction in physical activity [28]. Moreover, this muscle loss tends to persist long-term [29]. Patients who present with advanced disease (stages III–IV) and who receive palliative chemotherapy tend to lose skeletal muscle mass rapidly, and the radiodensity (i.e., quality) of their muscle also deteriorates [30]. Muscle loss has been associated with delays, reductions, or premature cessation of treatment and shorter survival among patients with PC [31]. Maintaining or increasing skeletal muscle mass during and following PC treatment presents an important target for exercise oncology interventions in order to improve treatment outcomes, survivorship, physical functioning, and quality of life.

To date, few studies have examined changes in body composition as outcomes of exercise interventions. In a comparison of patients with PC enrolled in a preoperative exercise program (prehabilitation) to historical controls who did not receive exercise training, investigators found better maintenance of skeletal muscle mass in the exercise group [32]. In a randomized trial comparing 3 months of supervised resistance training to usual care for cachectic PC patients, exercisers demonstrated significant increases in upper and lower limb skeletal muscle mass compared to controls [33]. Preliminary evidence is favorable, but there is a clear need for more research on the potential benefits of exercise to improve body composition outcomes for patients during and following treatment for PC. Future studies should aim to increase the rigor and intensity of exercise programming (particularly resistance training) to determine whether guideline-concordance training can move the needle on body composition and associated clinical and quality of life outcomes [34].

Nutrition in Pancreatic Cancer

Individuals with PC are at high risk for nutrition problems due to tumor anatomical location and its potential effects on digestion and absorption. Nutrition status may be affected by the cancer itself and/or treatment. It can vary with stage of disease [35] and change through the continuum of care [36]. Malnutrition occurs in 50–90% of patients with PC [35, 37, 38]. Malnutrition (including comorbid diagnoses of cachexia and sarcopenia) is associated with decreased survival, treatment tolerance and response, quality of life, and performance status as well as increased postoperative length of stay, hospital admission/readmission, and post-surgical infection [25, 37–42]. Nutrition status can be improved through medical nutrition therapy, though cachexia is unlikely to be reversed by conventional nutrition support measures alone. Multimodal interventions including nutrition and exercise components for treatment of cachexia show promise.

Nutrition Screening and Referral to the Registered Dietitian

Routine use of nutrition screening tools can identify patients with malnutrition, cachexia, or risk thereof. Assessment by a registered dietitian (RD) can identify early stages of cachexia and potentially modifiable factors—food intake, catabolic drive, muscle mass, and physical function [38, 42–44]. Nutrition counseling should focus on recommendations for increased energy intake including energy-dense foods, a protein-rich diet (with specific calorie and protein goals), potentially increased meal frequency, and oral supplementation of nutrients [42, 43].

In a study of patients with unresectable PC not receiving anti-cancer therapy, nutrition intervention, including a weekly RD visit, demonstrated significantly greater median survival (8.6 versus 5.5 months) in weight-stable vs. weight-losing subjects. The RD visit comprised of a weekly phone call to discuss pain, nausea, pancreatic enzyme replacement optimization, and nutrient dense meals [45].

Nutrition Intervention

Energy dense, high-fat foods, and oral nutrition supplement (ONS) drinks are often recommended to increase intake in patients with cancer. General nutrition recommendations for PC patients are outlined in Table 9.1. Studies have demonstrated improved total energy and protein intake in patients adherent to ONS recommendations resulting in improved weight, muscle mass, quality of life, and fatigue [46].

Table 9.1 General nutrition recommendations for pancreatic cancer patients

- Schedule oral intake, plan meals/snacks the day before
- Eat small frequent meals (6–8/day)
- Get plenty of fluids
- Limit use/portions of fat (as needed)
- Choose nutrient dense foods
- Be active
- Take pancreatic enzyme replacement therapy (if prescribed)
- Consider regular use of oral nutrition supplement drinks

However, adherence to recommendations varies in these studies from approximately 50–70% [46, 47]. The European Society for Clinical Nutrition and Metabolism practice guidelines, among others, recommend a food-first approach, incorporating ONS when diet modification is inadequate to meet goals [43].

In cachectic PC patients, caloric supplementation resulted in decreased loss of muscle tissue and increased survival time, regardless of nutritional product used [38]. Though preliminary studies of supplementation with L-carnitine, branched chain amino acids, and/or lactoferrins have shown promise, practice recommendations are still limited [38, 43, 48]. Stronger evidence has shown benefit with use of omega-3 fatty acids (supplemental or in ONS) [43, 49]; however, results are dependent on adequate intake. A randomized controlled trial in 2019 found patients adherent with use of omega-3-enriched ONS had greater skeletal muscle mass ratio (post- vs pre-intervention); however, only 45% of patients consumed >50% of the study dose of ONS [49]. Clinicians should guide patients in selecting appropriate ONS products and encouraging adherence.

Macronutrient Needs

Calorie Needs

It is commonly assumed that patients with PC are hypermetabolic; however, studies show a range of metabolic needs [50–52]. Therefore, initial prediction of calorie needs should align with recommendations for cancer patients in general—25–30 kilocalories per kilogram (kcal/kg) body weight per day (if obese, use ideal body weight) [43]. Needs should be periodically reassessed and adjusted based on the clinical effects on body weight and muscle mass (assessed through physical exam, anthropometric measures, or validated body composition measures such as dual-energy absorptiometry or bioelectrical impedance) [43, 53].

Protein Needs

Similarly, there is no protein recommendation specific to patients with PC; therefore, estimates for cancer patients in general should be used—1–1.5 grams per kilogram (g/kg) of body weight per day [43]. This is similar to the recommendations for older adults (>65 years old)—1–1.2 g/kg per day for maintenance and up to 1.6 g/kg per day to build lean body mass [48]. Additionally, it is important that individuals distribute protein through the day (25–30 grams per meal) to optimize muscle protein synthesis and maintenance [48, 54].

Common Nutrition Symptoms in PC

Nutrition impact symptoms may be present at the time of diagnosis or lead to a diagnosis of PC. Moreover, these symptoms may present as side effects of treatment or manifest as progression of disease [55, 56]. Table 9.2 outlines many of these common symptoms in PC and the medical and nutritional management strategies. The more complex symptoms of diarrhea and pancreatic exocrine insufficiency are discussed in more detail below.

Diarrhea

Diarrhea is common in patients with PC and may be a result of multiple sources including pancreatic exocrine insufficiency, side effects of chemotherapy or radiation therapy, surgery, or advanced disease. Regardless of etiology, interventions for diarrhea include diet modification (Table 9.3), medications (Table 9.4), and absorptive fiber.

Absorptive Fiber

Patients with diarrhea and/or rapid intestinal transit may benefit from the use of absorptive fiber taken following meals (and at bedtime if indicated). A dose of absorptive fiber is 3.4 g psyllium powder or 1-teaspoon methylcellulose powder blended with 2 ounces water. (may substitute fiber wafers/crisps in place of psyllium powder.) Fiber should be taken after a meal, and individuals should avoid drinking fluid for 1 h after. Patients start with once a day dosing and gradually increase as needed up to four times per day (three times a day after meals and at bedtime) [80–82].

Table 9.2 Common nutrition impact symptoms and management for pancreatic cancer patients

Nutrition issue	Symptoms	Medical management	Nutrition intervention
Diabetes mellitus and hyperglycemia [57, 58]	Prolonged hyperglycemia, hypoglycemic episodes	Antidiabetic drugs, insulin	• Minimize refined carbohydrates • Minimize sugar-sweetened beverages and fruit juice • Avoid skipping meals • Balance meals with protein, carbs, and fat
Delayed gastric emptying [59–62]	Bloating, fullness, nausea, vomiting, decreased appetite	Prokinetic medications such as metoclopramide and erythromycin.	• Diet low in fat and fiber • Small, frequent meals • Chew foods well • Nutrient-dense liquids/supplements • Nutrition support if condition persists >/=1 week
Gastric outlet obstruction/small bowel obstruction [63–72]	Abdominal pain, distention, nausea, vomiting, early satiety, decreased appetite, weight loss, dehydration	Gastrojejunostomy bypass	• Diet low in fat and fiber during healing phase • Regular diet as tolerated long-term
		Duodenal stent	• Soft diet low in fiber
		Decompression gastrostomy tube	• Soft diet low in fiber • Potential for jejunostomy tube for enteral feedings
Malabsorption [57, 73]	Steatorrhea, ongoing diarrhea, weight loss, nutrition deficiencies	Pancreatic enzyme replacement therapy (PERT) (see PERT section)	• Medium chain triglyceride (MCT) oil substituted for other fats • Mild restriction of fat intake (<75 g fat daily) in patients with severe steatorrhea
Ascites [59, 74–76]	Bloating, early satiety, decreased appetite	Diuretics, paracentesis	• Diet low in fat and fiber • Small, frequent meals • Nutrient-dense liquids/supplements • Avoid fluids at mealtimes • Consider a no added salt diet (~2 g sodium)

Table 9.3 Diet and behavior modification for management of diarrhea [77]

Foods to increase
High soluble fiber foods
– Banana
– Peeled apple, apple sauce (unsweetened)
– Oats
– Barley
Sodium foods
– Salted pretzels or crackers
– Broth (room temperature)
Potassium foods
– Potato (without skin)
– Banana
– Coconut water
Foods to minimize
High insoluble fiber foods
– Beans, peas, legumes
– Whole grains
– Fruits and vegetables with thick skins/peels
High sugar foods
Foods that contain sugar alcohol
High-fat and fried foods
Milk products unless low-lactose or lactose-free
Behavior modifications
Maintain adequate hydration
– Favor electrolyte containing fluids and oral rehydration solutions
– Minimize fluid intake at meals, push fluids between meals
– Limit caffeine, alcohol, and carbonated beverages
– Avoid hot liquids
Eat smaller meals, more frequently

Table 9.4 Medications for diarrhea [78, 79]

Medication	Common dosing	Maximum dose
Loperamide (Imodium® AD)[a]	4 mg by mouth once then 2 mg after each bowel movement	16 mg per day
	2–4 mg four times a day (every 6 h)	
Diphenoxylate/atropine (Lomotil®)[a]	1–2 tablets by mouth 3–4 times a day	8 tablets per day
Deodorized tincture of opium	0.3–1 mL by mouth 4 times a day	6 mL per day
Codeine[b]	15–30 mg by mouth three or four times a day	

[a]May be used together, each taken every 6 h, alternating use resulting in individual taking one or the other every 3 h

[b]Used less commonly due to sedation and nausea

Table 9.5 Clinical symptoms of pancreatic exocrine insufficiency [78, 86, 92–94]

- Abdominal bloating
- Cramping or abdominal pain after meals
- Excessive gas (burping, flatulence)
- Indigestion
- Foul-smelling gas or stools
- Unexplained weight loss
- Stool changes:
  - Fatty or oily (frothy, foamy)
  - Frequent
  - Floating
  - Light-colored or yellow
  - Loose

Other Considerations

- Metformin, commonly used for diabetes mellitus management, may contribute to gastrointestinal (GI) side effects including diarrhea. Gradual dose escalation is advised and/or consideration of extended-release preparation if appropriate [83].
- Diarrhea may be a transient side effect following a celiac plexus block [78]. Diet strategies (Table 9.3) may be helpful during the acute recovery following neurolysis.
- For those suspected to have bile acid related diarrhea, a bile acid sequestrant (cholestyramine, colestipol) may be prescribed [82].

Pancreatic Exocrine Insufficiency

Pancreatic exocrine insufficiency (PEI) in PC may be due to loss of pancreatic parenchyma, obstructed duct, changes in GI tract synchrony, and/or reduced pancreatic secretions [84, 85]. Consequences of PEI (untreated) include malnutrition, sarcopenia, vitamin and mineral deficiencies, reduced quality of life, and reduced survival [44, 86, 87]. PEI is reported in 50–100% of PC patients [84, 88, 89]. Patients who present without PEI may develop it over time [90]. It may be a consequence of or worsen due to surgery (pancreaticoduodenectomy more often than distal pancreatectomy) [35, 36, 87, 91] or radiation therapy [90] .

In clinical practice, diagnosis may be based on presence of symptoms (Table 9.5) and/or diagnostic test results (Table 9.6). Use of diagnostic tests in the clinical setting varies due to limited availability, level of invasiveness, varied sensitivity and specificity, and/or the cumbersome nature of stool collection [44]. Diagnosis based only on clinical symptoms may lead to false negatives as patients may have significant reduction in exocrine secretion without manifestation of symptoms [87]. Currently, there is no universally accepted guideline for assessment of PEI in PC patients [87]. Diagnosis based on clinical symptoms is appropriate, but in the absence of symptoms, fecal elastase should be evaluated in unresected patients and those without surgical alteration of the stomach or intestine [44]. Fecal fat studies or empiric prescription of PERT should be considered in asymptomatic patients with a

Table 9.6 Diagnostic tests for pancreatic exocrine insufficiency [86, 92, 94]

- Coefficient of fat absorption
- Fecal chymotrypsin level
- Fecal elastase (fecal elastase 1)
- Fecal fat excretion
- 13C-labeled mixed triglyceride breath test

history of pancreaticoduodenectomy [44, 85]. Patients presenting without PEI should be regularly reassessed throughout the course of treatment and disease [44].

Management of PEI with Pancreatic Enzyme Replacement Therapy

When PEI is present, pancreatic enzymes (pancrelipase) should be prescribed. Pancreatic enzyme replacement therapy (PERT) is demonstrated to have a positive effect on body weight, stool frequency, total calorie, and total protein intake even in the absence of symptomatic improvement [95]. It is associated with improved nutrition status, quality of life, and survival in patients with unresectable as well as resected disease [36, 96–99]. Dominguez-Munoz et al. found, in a retrospective analysis of patients with unresectable PC, a median 3-month survival benefit for patients on PERT vs not [96]. Similarly, Roberts et al. found a survival benefit of over 4 months in patients on PERT vs not [97].

Despite these benefits, PERT may not be prescribed to the majority of patients who need it due to undiagnosed PEI and suboptimal communication between patient and clinician [97, 100].

Pancreatic enzymes may be dosed based on an assumed general intake of food at meals and snacks (meal-based dosing), the patient's body weight, or the fat content of the diet. The most common practice in PC is meal-based dosing. Recommended starting doses range from 20,000 to 80,000 lipase units per meal and approximately half the dose per snack [36, 39, 57, 84, 85, 87, 88, 91, 96, 101–103]. This wide range of initial dosing reflects the wide range of diet variation—some patients present already self-restricting the fat content of the diet or meal sizes (or meal sizes may be restricted due to surgery) and thus require lower doses of PERT, while patients who consume regular-sized meals or large amounts of fat may need higher doses [104]. To best mimic the normal physiologic response to eating, the enzyme dose should be divided and administered at the start, throughout the meal, and at the end [57, 101, 105].

Based on characteristics of stools, clinical symptoms, and nutrition intake, enzymes may be titrated up every several days to identify the optimal dose to minimize or avoid PEI symptoms [86, 87, 101, 106]. Supplemental pancreatic enzyme dosages should not exceed 10,000 lipase units per kilogram of body weight per day or 2500 lipase units per kilogram per meal up to 4 times a day [101]. Figure 9.1 is a guide through the process of starting PERT, titrating dose, and troubleshooting concerns. It is important to continue to reassess compliance with PERT when making changes. Close monitoring by an RD can help patients achieve optimal management of PEI [44, 107].

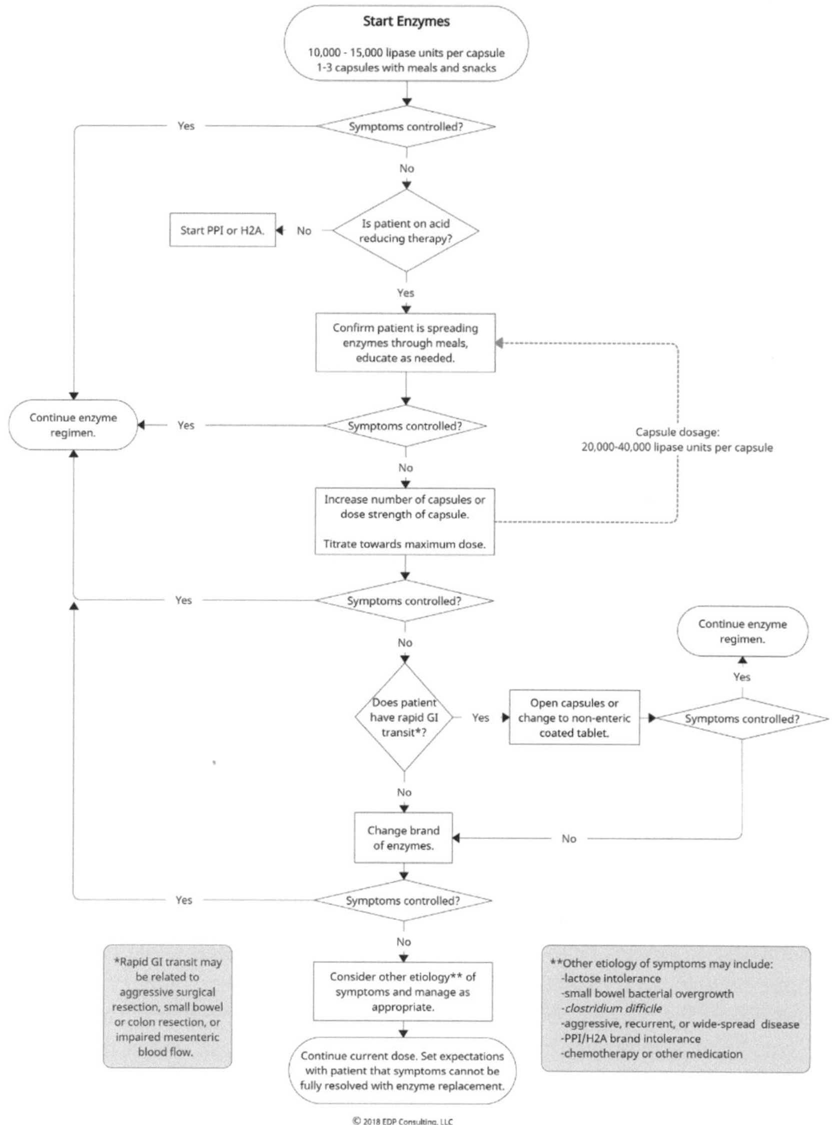

Fig. 9.1 Pancreatic enzyme replacement therapy initiation and optimization

Of note, the cost of enzymes can preclude use, and patients may seek to use an over-the-counter (OTC) preparation or may ration their supply of pancrelipase. OTC enzyme preparations may include bromelain, papain, trypsin, and chymotrypsin, or may be a combination product [108]. There is a lack of strong data to support use of these supplements, and as with all OTC supplements, individuals should be counseled regarding concerns with the non-regulated industry and directed toward patient financial assistance programs.

Special Populations: Perioperative Nutrition, Nutrition at End of Life, and Long-Term Survivors

Perioperative Nutrition

Preoperative nutrition and prehabilitation has prevented declines in nutrition in patients who suffered skeletal muscle loss [109]. Preoperative nutrition intervention is important to reduce the risk of surgical complications. Oral or enteral use of immunonutrition (IM) (formulas containing arginine, omega-3 fatty acids, and nucleotides) is recommended for patients undergoing major abdominal surgery [43]. Use is associated with reduced infectious complications, surgical complications, and hospital length of stay in surgical GI cancer patients [110–118]. IM has been found beneficial in both well-nourished and malnourished individuals [35, 110]. The strongest body of evidence supports the use for 5–7 days before surgery in patients with PC [118–120], with potential additional benefit after surgery [118]. Higher rates of surgical site infection, hospital-acquired infection, or pancreatic fistula have been reported in patients undernourished before pancreatic resection [121]. Preoperative nutrition support is indicated for patients with severe nutrition risk, to improve postoperative outcomes [35, 121–123].

Nutrition Support

Nutrition support, in the form of either enteral nutrition (EN) or parenteral nutrition (PN), can be essential for patients' nutrition status. EN is preferred over PN due its beneficial effects on the digestive system and reduced risk for infection as compared to PN. PN should only be utilized when a patient cannot be fed via their digestive tract, such as cases of ileus, GI obstruction, severe shock, intestinal ischemia, and high output fistulas [122, 124].

Special consideration should be given to EN formulas for PC patients with PEI. For those patients, it is ideal to use a semi-elemental, high medium chain triglyceride formula to limit the need for supplemental PERT during tube feeding [125, 126]. For patients with severe PEI or where semi-elemental formula produces a financial burden to the patient, administration of PERT with EN may still be necessary.

End of Life

Once a patient enters a refractory cachexia stage, the focus of interventions should shift to palliation and symptom control [42, 127]. In this stage, risks and encumbrance of artificial nutrition support tend to outweigh potential value, as these efforts have not been shown to reverse cachexia [42, 127]. PN should not be routinely prescribed near the end of life though guidelines recommend consideration of PN if

Table 9.7 Potential micronutrient deficiency in long-term pancreatic cancer survivors [93, 104]

Vitamin A
Vitamins B6 and B12
Vitamin D
Vitamin E
Copper
Iron
Selenium
Zinc

the GI tract is not functional and only in the absence of heavy metastatic disease burden and if vital prognosis is conditioned by nutritional status rather than disease [35].

Long-Term Survivors

Because of the limited long-term survival of PC, studies of long-term survivors are limited. Nutrition recommendations are based on small populations and case studies of patients with nutritional deficiencies. These patients are at increased risk for vitamin and mineral deficiencies (Table 9.7) as well as bone density loss due to inadequate food intake, loss of absorptive site, and alterations in physiology, synchrony, and chemistry of the GI tract [87, 104]. Evaluation for micronutrient deficiency is recommended about 1 year after surgical resection or sooner if patient has signs or symptoms of malabsorption or deficiency. For those with normal serum levels, annual reevaluation is recommended. For deficiency, repletion should be attempted and serum levels should be rechecked about 3 months later [104].

The existing literature suggests it is important to monitor bone density in long-term PC survivors. Recommendations for bone health are the same as those for the general population (re: calcium intake, vitamin D, and weight-bearing activity) but should advise use of calcium citrate supplements for better absorption versus calcium carbonate.

Summary

Regardless of the stage of PC, nutrition therapy can improve treatment outcomes and empower patients and families. For those patients who survive long term, the nutrition implications of the disease and treatments are likely to endure for the rest of their lives, and continued nutrition intervention may be necessary. It is important to help patients cope with nutrition issues throughout the course of treatment and disease.

Conclusions

Given the risk of muscle loss, weakness, deconditioning, nutritional deficits, and weight loss due to PC and its treatments, supportive care interventions to optimize nutrition and physical activity are essential. These interventions should start early, ideally at the time of diagnosis and initiation of treatment. Recommendations for physical activity should align with those of American College of Sports Medicine guidelines for cancer survivors, including moderate-intensity aerobic exercise for at least 30 min at least three times per week and resistance exercises at least twice a week [4]. These recommendations should be formulated based on patients' physical status and activity tolerance with opportunity for advancement of physical activity recommendations. The nutritional implications from disease and treatments for pancreatic cancer require frequent monitoring and adjustment of nutritional support, PERT, supplements, and strategies to mitigate gastrointestinal and nutritional challenges. Thus, support by a clinical dietitian is essential throughout the pancreatic cancer continuum of care.

References

1. National Comprehensive Cancer Network. NCCN clinical practice guidelines in oncology—survivorship. 2018;Version 2.2018. 9.
2. Cormie P, Atkinson M, Bucci L, Cust A, Eakin E, Hayes S, et al. Clinical oncology Society of Australia position statement on exercise in cancer care. Med J Aust. 2018;209(4):184–7.
3. Segal R, Zwaal C, Green E, Tomasone JR, Loblaw A, Petrella T. Exercise for people with cancer: a clinical practice guideline. Curr Oncol. 2017;24(1):40–6.
4. Campbell KL, Winters-Stone KM, Wiskemann J, May AM, Schwartz AL, Courneya KS, et al. Exercise guidelines for cancer survivors: consensus statement from international multidisciplinary roundtable. Med Sci Sports Exerc. 2019;51(11):2375–90.
5. Luo H, Galvao DA, Newton RU, Lopez P, Tang C, Fairman CM, et al. Exercise medicine in the management of pancreatic cancer: a systematic review. Pancreas. 2021;50(3):280–92.
6. Daniels SL, Lee MJ, George J, Kerr K, Moug S, Wilson TR, et al. Prehabilitation in elective abdominal cancer surgery in older patients: systematic review and meta-analysis. BJS Open. 2020;4(6):1022–41.
7. Ngo-Huang A, Parker NH, Bruera E, Lee RE, Simpson R, O'Connor DP, et al. Home-based exercise Prehabilitation during preoperative treatment for pancreatic cancer is associated with improvement in physical function and quality of life. Integr Cancer Ther. 2019;18:1534735419894061.
8. Cloyd JM, Hyman S, Huwig T, Monsour C, Santry H, Wills C, et al. Patient experience and quality of life during neoadjuvant therapy for pancreatic cancer: a systematic review and study protocol. Support Care Cancer. 2021;29(6):3009–16.
9. Moriello C, Mayo NE, Feldman L, Carli F. Validating the six-minute walk test as a measure of recovery after elective colon resection surgery. Arch Phys Med Rehabil. 2008;89(6):1083–9.
10. Hayashi K, Yokoyama Y, Nakajima H, Nagino M, Inoue T, Nagaya M, et al. Preoperative 6-minute walk distance accurately predicts postoperative complications after operations for hepato-pancreato-biliary cancer. Surgery. 2017;161(2):525–32.

11. Keeratichananont W, Thanadetsuntorn C, Keeratichananont S. Value of preoperative 6-minute walk test for predicting postoperative pulmonary complications. Ther Adv Respir Dis. 2016;10(1):18–25.

12. Lai Y, Su J, Qiu P, Wang M, Zhou K, Tang Y, et al. Systematic short-term pulmonary rehabilitation before lung cancer lobectomy: a randomized trial. Interact Cardiovasc Thorac Surg. 2017;25(3):476–83.

13. Gillis C, Li C, Lee L, Awasthi R, Augustin B, Gamsa A, et al. Prehabilitation versus rehabilitation: a randomized control trial in patients undergoing colorectal resection for cancer. Anesthesiology. 2014;121(5):937–47.

14. Zhang F, Ferrucci L, Culham E, Metter EJ, Guralnik J, Deshpande N. Performance on five times sit-to-stand task as a predictor of subsequent falls and disability in older persons. J Aging Health. 2013;25(3):478–92.

15. Parker NH, Lee RE, O'Connor DP, Ngo-Huang A, Petzel MQB, Schadler K, et al. Supports and barriers to home-based physical activity during preoperative treatment of pancreatic cancer: a mixed-methods study. J Phys Act Health. 2019;16(12):1113–22.

16. Hsueh HY, Pita-Grisanti V, Gumpper-Fedus K, Lahooti A, Chavez-Tomar M, Schadler K, et al. A review of physical activity in pancreatic ductal adenocarcinoma: epidemiology, intervention, animal models, and clinical trials. Pancreatology. 2022;22(1):98–111.

17. Schadler KL, Thomas NJ, Galie PA, Bhang DH, Roby KC, Addai P, et al. Tumor vessel normalization after aerobic exercise enhances chemotherapeutic efficacy. Oncotarget. 2016;7(40):65429–40.

18. Florez Bedoya CA, Cardoso ACF, Parker N, Ngo-Huang A, Petzel MQ, Kim MP, et al. Exercise during preoperative therapy increases tumor vascularity in pancreatic tumor patients. Sci Rep. 2019;9(1):13966.

19. Fagevik Olsén M, Becovic S, Dean E. Short-term effects of mobilization on oxygenation in patients after open surgery for pancreatic cancer: a randomized controlled trial. BMC Surg. 2021;21(1):185.

20. Steindorf K, Clauss D, Tjaden C, Hackert T, Herbolsheimer F, Bruckner T, et al. Quality of life, fatigue, and sleep problems in pancreatic cancer patients—a randomized trial on the effects of exercise. Dtsch Arztebl Int. 2019;116(27–28):471–8.

21. O'Connor D, Brown M, Eatock M, Turkington RC, Prue G. Exercise efficacy and prescription during treatment for pancreatic ductal adenocarcinoma: a systematic review. BMC Cancer. 2021;21(1):43.

22. Arthur AE, Delk A, Demark-Wahnefried W, Christein JD, Contreras C, Posey JA 3rd, et al. Pancreatic cancer survivors' preferences, barriers, and facilitators related to physical activity and diet interventions. J Cancer Surviv. 2016;10(6):981–9.

23. Parker NH, Basen-Engquist K, Rubin ML, Li Y, Prakash L, Ngo-Huang A, et al. Factors influencing exercise following pancreatic tumor resection. Ann Surg Oncol. 2021;28(4):2299–309.

24. Mintziras I, Miligkos M, Wachter S, Manoharan J, Maurer E, Bartsch DK. Sarcopenia and sarcopenic obesity are significantly associated with poorer overall survival in patients with pancreatic cancer: systematic review and meta-analysis. Int J Surg. 2018;59:19–26.

25. Poulia KA, Sarantis P, Antoniadou D, Koustas E, Papadimitropoulou A, Papavassiliou AG, et al. Pancreatic cancer and cachexia-metabolic mechanisms and novel insights. Nutrients. 2020;12(6):1543.

26. Michaelis KA, Zhu X, Burfeind KG, Krasnow SM, Levasseur PR, Morgan TK, et al. Establishment and characterization of a novel murine model of pancreatic cancer cachexia. J Cachexia Sarcopenia Muscle. 2017;8(5):824–38.

27. Sandini M, Patino M, Ferrone CR, Alvarez-Perez CA, Honselmann KC, Paiella S, et al. Association between changes in body composition and neoadjuvant treatment for pancreatic cancer. JAMA Surg. 2018;153(9):809–15.

28. Kurokawa H, Akezaki Y, Tominaga R, Okamoto M, Kikuuchi M, Hamada M, et al. Changes in physical function and effects on QOL in patients after pancreatic cancer surgery. Healthcare (Basel). 2021;9(7):882.

29. Cloyd JM, Nogueras-Gonzalez GM, Prakash LR, Petzel MQB, Parker NH, Ngo-Huang AT, et al. Anthropometric changes in patients with pancreatic cancer undergoing preoperative therapy and Pancreatoduodenectomy. J Gastrointest Surg. 2018;22(4):703–12.
30. Babic A, Rosenthal MH, Bamlet WR, Takahashi N, Sugimoto M, Danai LV, et al. Postdiagnosis loss of skeletal muscle, but not adipose tissue, is associated with shorter survival of patients with advanced pancreatic cancer. Cancer Epidemiol Biomark Prev. 2019;28(12):2062–9.
31. Basile D, Corvaja C, Caccialanza R, Aprile G. Sarcopenia: looking to muscle mass to better manage pancreatic cancer patients. Curr Opin Support Palliat Care. 2019;13(4):279–85.
32. Parker NH, Gorzelitz J, Ngo-Huang A, Caan BJ, Prakash L, Garg N, et al. The role of home-based exercise in maintaining skeletal muscle during preoperative pancreatic cancer treatment. Integr Cancer Ther. 2021;20:1534735420986615.
33. Kamel FH, Basha MA, Alsharidah AS, Salama AB. Resistance training impact on mobility, muscle strength and lean mass in pancreatic cancer cachexia: a randomized controlled trial. Clin Rehabil. 2020;34(11):1391–9.
34. Clifford B, Koizumi S, Wewege MA, Leake HB, Ha L, Macdonald E, et al. The effect of resistance training on body composition during and after cancer treatment: a systematic review and meta-analysis. Sports Med. 2021;51(12):2527–46.
35. Vedie AL, Neuzillet C. Pancreatic cancer: best supportive care. Presse Med. 2019;48(3 Pt 2):e175–e85.
36. Kim E, Kang JS, Han Y, Kim H, Kwon W, Kim JR, et al. Influence of preoperative nutritional status on clinical outcomes after pancreatoduodenectomy. HPB (Oxford). 2018;20(11):1051–61.
37. Vashi P, Popiel B, Lammersfeld C, Gupta D. Outcomes of systematic nutritional assessment and medical nutrition therapy in pancreatic cancer. Pancreas. 2015;44(5):750–5.
38. Mueller TC, Burmeister MA, Bachmann J, Martignoni ME. Cachexia and pancreatic cancer: are there treatment options? World J Gastroenterol. 2014;20(28):9361–73.
39. Ottery F. Supportive nutritional management of the patient with pancreatic cancer. Oncology (Williston Park). 1996;10(9 Suppl):26–32.
40. Bruera E. ABC of palliative care. Anorexia, cachexia, and nutrition. BMJ. 1997;315(7117):1219–22.
41. Dev R. Measuring cachexia-diagnostic criteria. Ann Palliat Med. 2019;8(1):24–32.
42. Fearon K, Strasser F, Anker SD, Bosaeus I, Bruera E, Fainsinger RL, et al. Definition and classification of cancer cachexia: an international consensus. Lancet Oncol. 2011;12(5):489–95.
43. Muscaritoli M, Arends J, Bachmann P, Baracos V, Barthelemy N, Bertz H, et al. ESPEN practical guideline: clinical nutrition in cancer. Clin Nutr. 2021;40(5):2898–913.
44. Hendifar AE, Petzel MQB, Zimmers TA, Denlinger CS, Matrisian LM, Picozzi VJ, et al. Pancreas cancer-associated weight loss. Oncologist. 2018;24:691.
45. Davidson W, Ash S, Capra S, Bauer J. Weight stabilisation is associated with improved survival duration and quality of life in unresectable pancreatic cancer. Clin Nutr. 2004;23(2):239–47.
46. Kim SH, Lee SM, Jeung HC, Lee IJ, Park JS, Song M, et al. The effect of nutrition intervention with oral nutritional supplements on pancreatic and bile duct cancer patients undergoing chemotherapy. Nutrients. 2019;11(5):1145.
47. Solheim TS, Laird BJA, Balstad TR, Stene GB, Bye A, Johns N, et al. A randomized phase II feasibility trial of a multimodal intervention for the management of cachexia in lung and pancreatic cancer. J Cachexia Sarcopenia Muscle. 2017;8(5):778–88.
48. Deutz NE, Bauer JM, Barazzoni R, Biolo G, Boirie Y, Bosy-Westphal A, et al. Protein intake and exercise for optimal muscle function with aging: recommendations from the ESPEN expert group. Clin Nutr. 2014;33(6):929–36.
49. Akita H, Takahashi H, Asukai K, Tomokuni A, Wada H, Marukawa S, et al. The utility of nutritional supportive care with an eicosapentaenoic acid (EPA)-enriched nutrition agent during pre-operative chemoradiotherapy for pancreatic cancer: prospective randomized control study. Clin Nutr. 2019;33:148–53.

50. Cao DX, Wu GH, Zhang B, Quan YJ, Wei J, Jin H, et al. Resting energy expenditure and body composition in patients with newly detected cancer. Clin Nutr. 2010;29(1):72–7.

51. Falconer JS, Fearon KC, Plester CE, Ross JA, Carter DC. Cytokines, the acute-phase response, and resting energy expenditure in cachectic patients with pancreatic cancer. Ann Surg. 1994;219(4):325–31.

52. Sasaki M, Okamoto H, Johtatsu T, Kurihara M, Iwakawa H, Tanaka T, et al. Resting energy expenditure in patients undergoing pylorus preserving pancreatoduodenectomies for bile duct cancer or pancreatic tumors. J Clin Biochem Nutr. 2011;48(3):183–6.

53. Cederholm T, Jensen GL, Correia M, Gonzalez MC, Fukushima R, Higashiguchi T, et al. GLIM criteria for the diagnosis of malnutrition—a consensus report from the global clinical nutrition community. J Cachexia Sarcopenia Muscle. 2019;10(1):207–17.

54. Paddon-Jones D, Rasmussen BB. Dietary protein recommendations and the prevention of sarcopenia. Curr Opin Clin Nutr Metab Care. 2009;12(1):86–90.

55. DiMagno EP, Reber HA, Tempero MA. AGA technical review on the epidemiology, diagnosis, and treatment of pancreatic ductal adenocarcinoma. American Gastroenterological Association Gastroenterology. 1999;117(6):1464–84.

56. National Cancer Institute. Pancreatic Cancer Treatment (PDQ(R))-Health Professional Version 2020 [updated 5/15/2020]. https://www.cancer.gov/types/pancreatic/hp/pancreatic-treatment-pdq.

57. Sarner M. Treatment of pancreatic exocrine deficiency. World J Surg. 2003;27(11):1192–5.

58. Poulson J. The management of diabetes in patients with advanced cancer. J Pain Symptom Manag. 1997;13(6):339–46.

59. Academy of Nutrition and Dietetics. Gastroparesis. Nutrition Care Manual 2020; https://www.nutritioncaremanual.org/client_ed.cfm?ncm_client_ed_id=168. Accessed 18 May 2020.

60. Beane JD, House MG, Miller A, et al. Optimal management of delayed gastric emptying after pancreatectomy: an analysis of 1,089 patients. Surgery. 2014;156(4):939–46.

61. Camilleri M, Parkman HP, Shafi MA, Abell TL, Gerson L. American College of G. clinical guideline: management of gastroparesis. Am J Gastroenterol. 2013;108(1):18–37; quiz 38.

62. August DA, Huhmann MB, American Society for P, Enteral Nutrition Board of D.A.S.P.E.N. Clinical guidelines: nutrition support therapy during adult anticancer treatment and in hematopoietic cell transplantation. JPEN J Parenter Enteral Nutr. 2009;33(5):472–500.

63. Koop AH, Palmer WC, Stancampiano FF. Gastric outlet obstruction: a red flag, potentially manageable. Cleve Clin J Med. 2019;86(5):345–53.

64. Oh SY, Edwards A, Mandelson M, et al. Survival and clinical outcome after endoscopic duodenal stent placement for malignant gastric outlet obstruction: comparison of pancreatic cancer and nonpancreatic cancer. Gastrointest Endosc. 2015;82(3):460–468 e462.

65. Orr J, Lockwood R, Gamboa A, Slaughter JC, Obstein KL, Yachimski P. Enteral stents for malignant gastric outlet obstruction: low reintervention rates for obstruction due to pancreatic adenocarcinoma versus other etiologies. J Gastrointest Surg. 2020;25:720.

66. Manuel-Vazquez A, Latorre-Fragua R, Ramiro-Perez C, Lopez-Marcano A, la Plaza-Llamas R, Ramia JM. Laparoscopic gastrojejunostomy for gastric outlet obstruction in patients with unresectable hepatopancreatobiliary cancers: a personal series and systematic review of the literature. World J Gastroenterol. 2018;24(18):1978–88.

67. Yoshida Y, Fukutomi A, Tanaka M, et al. Gastrojejunostomy versus duodenal stent placement for gastric outlet obstruction in patients with unresectable pancreatic cancer. Pancreatology. 2017;17(6):983–9.

68. Perone JA, Riall TS, Olino K. Palliative care for pancreatic and periampullary cancer. Surg Clin North Am. 2016;96(6):1415–30.

69. National Comprehensive Cancer Network. NCCN Clinical Practice Guidelines in Oncology Pancreatic Adenocarcinoma Version 1.2020. 2019; https://www.nccn.org/professionals/physician_gls/pdf/pancreatic.pdf. Accessed 18 May 2020.

70. Adler DG, Baron TH. Endoscopic palliation of malignant gastric outlet obstruction using self-expanding metal stents: experience in 36 patients. Am J Gastroenterol. 2002;97(1):72–8.

71. Dormann A, Meisner S, Verin N, Wenk LA. Self-expanding metal stents for gastroduodenal malignancies: systematic review of their clinical effectiveness. Endoscopy. 2004;36(6):543–50.
72. Pothuri B, Montemarano M, Gerardi M, et al. Percutaneous endoscopic gastrostomy tube placement in patients with malignant bowel obstruction due to ovarian carcinoma. Gynecol Oncol. 2005;96(2):330–4.
73. Babayan VK. Medium chain triglycerides and structured lipids. Lipids. 1987;22(6):417–20.
74. White A. Outpatient interventions for hepatology patients with fluid retention: a review and synthesis of the literature. Gastroenterol Nurs. 2014;37(3):236–44.
75. Moore KP, Aithal GP. Guidelines on the management of ascites in cirrhosis. Gut. 2006;55(Suppl 6):vi1-12.
76. Yu AS, Hu KQ. Management of ascites. Clin Liver Dis. 2001;5(2):541–68. viii
77. National Cancer Institute. Nutrition in cancer care (PDQ(R))- Health professionals. Nutrition in cancer care (PDQ(R))- Health professionals. 2020; https://www.cancer.gov/about-cancer/treatment/side-effects/appetite-loss/nutrition-hp-pdq#_74. Accessed 1 May 2020.
78. Rabow MW, Petzel MQB, Adkins SH. Symptom management and palliative Care in Pancreatic Cancer. Cancer J. 2017;23(6):362–73.
79. Bisanz A, Tucker AM, Amin DM, et al. Summary of the causative and treatment factors of diarrhea and the use of a diarrhea assessment and treatment tool to improve patient outcomes. Gastroenterol Nurs. 2010;33(4):268–81; quiz 282–263.
80. Murphy J, Stacey D, Crook J, Thompson B, Panetta D. Testing control of radiation-induced diarrhea with a psyllium bulking agent: a pilot study. Can Oncol Nurs J. 2000;10(3):96–100.
81. Singh B. Psyllium as therapeutic and drug delivery agent. Int J Pharm. 2007;334(1–2):1–14.
82. Bisanz A, Tucker AM, Amin DM, Patel D, Calderon BB, Joseph MM, et al. Summary of the causative and treatment factors of diarrhea and the use of a diarrhea assessment and treatment tool to improve patient outcomes. Gastroenterol Nurs. 2010;33(4):268–81; quiz 82–3.
83. Cui Y, Andersen DK. Pancreatogenic diabetes: special considerations for management. Pancreatology. 2011;11(3):279–94.
84. Phillips ME. Pancreatic exocrine insufficiency following pancreatic resection. Pancreatology. 2015;15(5):449–55.
85. Sabater L, Ausania F, Bakker OJ, Boadas J, Dominguez-Munoz JE, Falconi M, et al. Evidence-based guidelines for the management of exocrine pancreatic insufficiency after pancreatic surgery. Ann Surg. 2016;264(6):949–58.
86. Dominguez-Munoz JE. Diagnosis and treatment of pancreatic exocrine insufficiency. Curr Opin Gastroenterol. 2018;34(5):349–54.
87. Nikfarjam M, Wilson JS, Smith RC. Australasian pancreatic club pancreatic enzyme replacement therapy guidelines working G. diagnosis and management of pancreatic exocrine insufficiency. Med J Aust. 2017;207(4):161–5.
88. Bartel MJ, Asbun H, Stauffer J, Raimondo M. Pancreatic exocrine insufficiency in pancreatic cancer: a review of the literature. Dig Liver Dis. 2015;47(12):1013–20.
89. Imrie CW, Connett G, Hall RI, Charnley RM. Review article: enzyme supplementation in cystic fibrosis, chronic pancreatitis, pancreatic and periampullary cancer. Aliment Pharmacol Ther. 2010;32(Suppl 1):1–25.
90. Horst E, Seidel M, Micke O, Rube C, Glashorster M, Schafer U, et al. Accelerated radiochemotherapy in pancreatic cancer is not necessarily related to a pathologic pancreatic function decline in the early period. Int J Radiat Oncol Biol Phys. 2002;52(2):304–9.
91. Capurso G, Traini M, Piciucchi M, Signoretti M, Arcidiacono PG. Exocrine pancreatic insufficiency: prevalence, diagnosis, and management. Clin Exp Gastroenterol. 2019;12:129–39.
92. Powell-Brett S, de Liguori CN, Roberts K. Understanding pancreatic exocrine insufficiency and replacement therapy in pancreatic cancer. Eur J Surg Oncol. 2021;47(3 Pt A):539–44.
93. Petzel MQB. Medical nutrition therapy for pancreatic cancer. In: Voss AC, Williams V, editors. Oncology nutrition for clinical practice. 2nd ed. Chicago IL: Academy of Nutrition and Dietetics; 2021. p. 434–71.

94. Sabater L, Ausania F, Bakker OJ, et al. Evidence-based guidelines for the management of exocrine pancreatic insufficiency after pancreatic surgery. Ann Surg. 2016;264(6):949–58.
95. Bruno MJ, Haverkort EB, Tijssen GP, Tytgat GN, van Leeuwen DJ. Placebo controlled trial of enteric coated pancreatin microsphere treatment in patients with unresectable cancer of the pancreatic head region. Gut. 1998;42(1):92–6.
96. Dominguez-Munoz JE, Nieto-Garcia L, Lopez-Diaz J, Larino-Noia J, Abdulkader I, Iglesias-Garcia J. Impact of the treatment of pancreatic exocrine insufficiency on survival of patients with unresectable pancreatic cancer: a retrospective analysis. BMC Cancer. 2018;18(1):534.
97. Roberts KJ, Bannister CA, Schrem H. Enzyme replacement improves survival among patients with pancreatic cancer: results of a population based study. Pancreatology. 2019;19(1):114–21.
98. Roberts KJ, Schrem H, Hodson J, Angelico R, Dasari BVM, Coldham CA, et al. Pancreas exocrine replacement therapy is associated with increased survival following pancreatoduodenectomy for periampullary malignancy. HPB (Oxford). 2017;19(10):859–67.
99. Gooden HM, White KJ. Pancreatic cancer and supportive care—pancreatic exocrine insufficiency negatively impacts on quality of life. Support Care Cancer. 2013;21(7):1835–41.
100. Landers A, Muircroft W, Brown H. Pancreatic enzyme replacement therapy (PERT) for malabsorption in patients with metastatic pancreatic cancer. BMJ Support Palliat Care. 2016;6(1):75–9.
101. Fieker A, Philpott J, Armand M. Enzyme replacement therapy for pancreatic insufficiency: present and future. Clin Exp Gastroenterol. 2011;4:55–73.
102. Layer P, Keller J, Lankisch PG. Pancreatic enzyme replacement therapy. Curr Gastroenterol Rep. 2001;3(2):101–8.
103. Ellison NM, Chevlen E, Still CD, Dubagunta S. Supportive care for patients with pancreatic adenocarcinoma: symptom control and nutrition. Hematol Oncol Clin North Am. 2002;16(1):105–21.
104. Petzel MQB, Hoffman L. Nutrition implications for long-term survivors of pancreatic cancer surgery [formula: see text]. Nutr Clin Pract. 2017;32(5):588–98.
105. Struyvenberg MR, Martin CR, Freedman SD. Practical guide to exocrine pancreatic insufficiency—breaking the myths. BMC Med. 2017;15(1):29.
106. Creon R. Package insert. North Chicago, IL: AbbVie Inc.; 2015.
107. Toouli J, Biankin AV, Oliver MR, Pearce CB, Wilson JS, Wray NH, et al. Management of pancreatic exocrine insufficiency: Australasian pancreatic Club recommendations. Med J Aust. 2010;193(8):461–7.
108. Edakkanambeth Varayil J, Bauer BA, Hurt RT. Over-the-counter enzyme supplements: what a clinician needs to know. Mayo Clin Proc. 2014;89(9):1307–12.
109. Tsukagoshi M, Harimoto N, Araki K, Kubo N, Watanabe A, Igarashi T, et al. Impact of preoperative nutritional support and rehabilitation therapy in patients undergoing pancreaticoduodenectomy. Int J Clin Oncol. 2021;26(9):1698–706.
110. Burden S, Todd C, Hill J, Lal S. Pre-operative nutrition support in patients undergoing gastrointestinal surgery. Cochrane Database Syst Rev. 2012;11:CD008879.
111. Martin RC 2nd, Agle S, Schlegel M, Hayat T, Scoggins CR, McMasters KM, et al. Efficacy of preoperative immunonutrition in locally advanced pancreatic cancer undergoing irreversible electroporation (IRE). Eur J Surg Oncol. 2017;43(4):772–9.
112. Silvestri S, Franchello A, Deiro G, Galletti R, Cassine D, Campra D, et al. Preoperative oral immunonutrition versus standard preoperative oral diet in well nourished patients undergoing pancreaticoduodenectomy. Int J Surg. 2016;31:93–9.
113. Gade J, Levring T, Hillingso J, Hansen CP, Andersen JR. The effect of preoperative oral immunonutrition on complications and length of hospital stay after elective surgery for pancreatic cancer—a randomized controlled trial. Nutr Cancer. 2016;68(2):225–33.
114. Shirakawa H, Kinoshita T, Gotohda N, Takahashi S, Nakagohri T, Konishi M. Compliance with and effects of preoperative immunonutrition in patients undergoing pancreaticoduodenectomy. J Hepatobiliary Pancreat Sci. 2012;19(3):249–58.

115. Suzuki D, Furukawa K, Kimura F, Shimizu H, Yoshidome H, Ohtsuka M, et al. Effects of perioperative immunonutrition on cell-mediated immunity, T helper type 1 (Th1)/Th2 differentiation, and Th17 response after pancreaticoduodenectomy. Surgery. 2010;148(3):573–81.
116. Gilliland TM, Villafane-Ferriol N, Shah KP, Shah RM, Tran Cao HS, Massarweh NN, et al. Nutritional and metabolic derangements in pancreatic cancer and pancreatic resection. Nutrients. 2017;9(3):243.
117. Adiamah A, Skorepa P, Weimann A, Lobo DN. The impact of preoperative immune modulating nutrition on outcomes in patients undergoing surgery for gastrointestinal cancer: a systematic review and meta-analysis. Ann Surg. 2019;270(2):247–56.
118. Miyauchi Y, Furukawa K, Suzuki D, Yoshitomi H, Takayashiki T, Kuboki S, et al. Additional effect of perioperative, compared with preoperative, immunonutrition after pancreaticoduodenectomy: a randomized, controlled trial. Int J Surg. 2019;61:69–75.
119. Yang FA, Chen YC, Tiong C. Immunonutrition in patients with pancreatic cancer undergoing surgical intervention: a systematic review and meta-analysis of randomized controlled trials. Nutrients. 2020;12(9):2798.
120. Takagi K, Umeda Y, Yoshida R, Yagi T, Fujiwara T. Systematic review on immunonutrition in partial pancreatoduodenectomy. Langenbeck's Arch Surg. 2020;405(5):585–93.
121. Jeune F, Coriat R, Prat F, Dousset B, Vaillant JC, Gaujoux S. Pancreatic cancer surgical management. Presse Med. 2019;48(3 Pt 2):e147–e58.
122. Weimann A, Braga M, Carli F, Higashiguchi T, Hubner M, Klek S, et al. ESPEN guideline: clinical nutrition in surgery. Clin Nutr. 2017;36(3):623–50.
123. Gianotti L, Besselink MG, Sandini M, Hackert T, Conlon K, Gerritsen A, et al. Nutritional support and therapy in pancreatic surgery: a position paper of the international study group on pancreatic surgery (ISGPS). Surgery. 2018;164(5):1035–48.
124. Jankowski M, Las-Jankowska M, Sousak M, Zegarski W. Contemporary enteral and parenteral nutrition before surgery for gastrointestinal cancers: a literature review. World J Surg Oncol. 2018;16(1):94.
125. Alexander DD, Bylsma LC, Elkayam L, Nguyen DL. Nutritional and health benefits of semi-elemental diets: a comprehensive summary of the literature. World J Gastrointest Pharmacol Ther. 2016;7(2):306–19.
126. Ferrie S, Graham C, Hoyle M. Pancreatic enzyme supplementation for patients receiving enteral feeds. Nutr Clin Pract. 2011;26(3):349–51.
127. Sadeghi M, Keshavarz-Fathi M, Baracos V, Arends J, Mahmoudi M, Rezaei N. Cancer cachexia: diagnosis, assessment, and treatment. Crit Rev Oncol Hematol. 2018;127:91–104.

Index

S. Pant (ed.), *Pancreatic Cancer*, https://doi.org/10.1007/978-3-031-38623-7